Environmental Triggers for Rheumatic Diseases

Editor

BRYANT R. ENGLAND

RHEUMATIC DISEASE CLINICS OF NORTH AMERICA

www.rheumatic.theclinics.com

Consulting Editor
MICHAEL H. WEISMAN

November 2022 • Volume 48 • Number 4

ELSEVIER

1600 John F. Kennedy Boulevard ● Suite 1800 ● Philadelphia, Pennsylvania, 19103-2899
http://www.theclinics.com

RHEUMATIC DISEASE CLINICS OF NORTH AMERICA Volume 48, Number 4

November 2022 ISSN 0889-857X, ISBN 13: 978-0-323-98667-0

Editor: Joanna Collett
Developmental Editor: Karen Solomon

Rheumatic Disease Clinics of North America (ISSN 0889-857X) is published quarterly by Elsevier Inc., 360 Park Avenue South, New York, NY 10010-1710. Months of issue are February, May, August, and November. Business and editorial offices: 1600 John F. Kennedy Boulevard, Suite 1800, Philadelphia, PA 19103-2899. Periodicals postage paid at New York, NY and additional mailing offices. Subscription prices are USD 366.00 per year for US individuals, USD 1020.00 per year for US institutions, USD 100.00 per year for US students and residents, USD 431.00 per year for Canadian individuals, USD 1040.00 per year for Canadian institutions, USD 100.00 per year for Canadian students/residents, USD 470.00 per year for international individuals, USD 1040.00 per year for international institutions, and USD 230.00 per year for foreign students/residents. To receive student/ resident rate, orders must be accompanied by name of affiliated institution, date of term, and the *signature* of program/residency coordinator on institution letterhead. Orders will be billed at individual rate until proof of status received. Foreign air speed delivery is included in all *Clinics* subscription prices. All prices are subject to change without notice. **POSTMASTER:** Send address changes to *Rheumatic Disease Clinics of North America*, Elsevier Health Sciences Division, Subscription Customer Service, 3251 Riverport Lane, Maryland Heights, MO 63043. **Customer Service: 1-800-654-2452 (US and Canada). From outside of the US and Canada: 314-447- 8871. Fax: 314-447-8029. For print support, e-mail: JournalsCustomerService-usa@elsevier.com. For online support, e-mail: JournalsOnlineSupport-usa@elsevier.com.**

Reprints. For copies of 100 or more of articles in this publication, please contact the Commercial Reprints Department, Elsevier Inc., 360 Park Avenue South, New York, New York, 10010-1710; Tel.: +1-212-633- 3874, Fax: +1-212-633-3820, and E-mail: reprints@elsevier.com.

Rheumatic Disease Clinics of North America is covered in *MEDLINE/PubMed (Index Medicus), Current Contents/Clinical Medicine, Science Citation Index, ISI/BIOMED,* and *EMBASE/Excerpta Medica.*

Contributors

CONSULTING EDITOR

MICHAEL H. WEISMAN, MD
Adjunct Professor of Medicine, Stanford University, Distinguished Professor of Medicine Emeritus, David Geffen School of Medicine at UCLA, Professor of Medicine Emeritus, Cedars-Sinai Medical Center, Los Angeles, California, USA

EDITOR

BRYANT R. ENGLAND, MD, PhD
Assistant Professor of Medicine, Division of Rheumatology and Immunology, Department of Internal Medicine, VA Nebraska-Western Iowa Health Care System, University of Nebraska Medical Center, Omaha, Nebraska, USA

AUTHORS

ZAREEN AHMAD, MD, FRCPC
Assistant Professor of Medicine, University of Toronto, Toronto Scleroderma Program, Mount Sinai Hospital, Toronto, Ontario, Canada

HANA ALAHMARI, MBBS
Scleroderma Clinical Research Fellow, Toronto Scleroderma Program, Mount Sinai Hospital, Toronto, Ontario, Canada

JOSHUA F. BAKER, MD, MSCE
Division of Rheumatology, Department of Epidemiology and Biostatistics, University of Pennsylvania, Philadelphia VA Medical Center, Philadelphia, Pennsylvania, USA

SASHA BERNATSKY, MD
Centre for Outcomes Research and Evaluation, Research Institute of the McGill University Health Centre, Montreal, Quebec, Canada

WENG IAN CHE, MMSc
Department of Medicine, Solna, Eugeniahemmet, T2, Karolinska Universitetssjukhuset, Solna, Clinical Epidemiology Division, Department of Medicine, Solna, Karolinska Institutet, Stockholm, Sweden

KAREN H. COSTENBADER, MD
Division of Rheumatology, Inflammation and Immunity, Brigham and Women's Hospital, Harvard Medical School, Boston, Massachusetts, USA

CYNTHIA S. CROWSON, PhD
Professor of Medicine and Biostatistics, Division of Rheumatology, Department of Quantitative Health Sciences, Mayo Clinic, Rochester, Minnesota, USA

JOHN M. DAVIS III, MD, MS
Professor of Medicine, Division of Rheumatology, Mayo Clinic, Rochester, Minnesota, USA

KEVIN D. DEANE, MD, PhD
Professor of Medicine, Division of Rheumatology, University of Colorado Denver Anschutz Medical Campus, Aurora, Colorado, USA

NANCY DESAI, MD
Division of Rheumatology, University of Pennsylvania, Philadelphia, Pennsylvania, USA

BRYANT R. ENGLAND, MD, PhD
Assistant Professor of Medicine, Division of Rheumatology and Immunology, Department of Internal Medicine, VA Nebraska-Western Iowa Health Care System, University of Nebraska Medical Center, Omaha, Nebraska, USA

YVETTE FARRAN, MD
Rheumatology Fellow, Division of Rheumatology, Department of Internal Medicine, John P. and Kathrine G. McGovern School of Medicine, The University of Texas Health Science Center at Houston, Houston, Texas, USA

LYDIA FEDERICO, BA
Division of Rheumatology, University of Pennsylvania, Philadelphia, Pennsylvania, USA

YVONNE M. GOLIGHTLY, PT, PhD
Department of Epidemiology, Division of Physical Therapy, Thurston Arthritis Research Center, Injury Prevention Research Center, The University of North Carolina at Chapel Hill, Chapel Hill, North Carolina, USA

LINDSAY N. HELGET, MD
VA Nebraska-Western Iowa Health Care System, Assistant Professor of Medicine, Department of Internal Medicine, University of Nebraska Medical Center, Omaha, Nebraska, USA

MARIE HOLMQVIST, MD, PhD
Department of Medicine, Solna, Eugeniahemmet, T2, Karolinska Universitetssjukhuset, Solna, Clinical Epidemiology Division, Department of Medicine, Solna, Karolinska Institutet, Division of Rheumatology, Department of Medicine, Solna, Karolinska Institutet, Stockholm, Sweden

MARK HWANG, MD, MS
Assistant Professor of Medicine, Division of Rheumatology, Department of Internal Medicine, John P. and Kathrine G. McGovern School of Medicine, The University of Texas Health Science Center at Houston, Houston, Texas, USA

SØREN JACOBSEN, MD
Copenhagen Lupus and Vasculitis Clinic, Rigshospitalet, Copenhagen University Hospital, Denmark

SINDHU R. JOHNSON, MD, PhD, FRCPC
Associate Professor of Medicine, Director, Toronto Scleroderma Program, Division of Rheumatology, Department of Medicine, Toronto Western Hospital, Mount Sinai Hospital, Institute of Health Policy, Management and Evaluation, University of Toronto, Toronto, Ontario, Canada

GUY KATZ, MD
Rheumatology Unit, Division of Rheumatology, Allergy, and Immunology, Massachusetts General Hospital, Boston, Massachusetts, USA

VANESSA L. KRONZER, MD, MSCI
Assistant Professor of Medicine, Division of Rheumatology, Mayo Clinic, Rochester, Minnesota, USA

JIA LI LIU, MD
McGill University, Montreal, Quebec, Canada

BRENT A. LUEDDERS, MD
Fellow, Division of Rheumatology and Immunology, University of Nebraska Medical Center, VA Nebraska-Western Iowa Health Care System, Omaha, Nebraska, USA

INGRID E. LUNDBERG, MD, PhD
Rheumatology, Karolinska University Hospital, Division of Rheumatology, Department of Medicine, Solna, Karolinska Institutet, ME Gastro, Derm and Rheuma, Theme Inflammation and Aging, Karolinska University Hospital, Stockholm, Sweden

TED R. MIKULS, MD, MSPH
Veterans Affairs Nebraska-Western Iowa Health Care System, Stokes-Shackelford Professor of Rheumatology, Department of Internal Medicine, University of Nebraska Medical Center, Omaha, Nebraska, USA

CHRISTINE G. PARKS, PhD
Epidemiology Branch, Department of Health and Human Services, National Institutes of Environmental Health Sciences, National Institutes of Health, Research Triangle Park, North Carolina, USA

JILL A. POOLE, MD
Professor, Division of Allergy and Immunology, University of Nebraska Medical Center, Omaha, Nebraska, USA

AUSTIN POST, BS
Division of Physical Therapy Education, College of Medicine, University of Nebraska Medical Center, Omaha, Nebraska, USA

JOHN REVEILLE, MD
Professor of Medicine, Division of Rheumatology, Department of Internal Medicine, John P. and Kathrine G. McGovern School of Medicine, The University of Texas Health Science Center at Houston, Houston, Texas, USA

MATTHEW TAO, MD
Division of Physical Therapy Education, Department of Orthopedic Surgery and Rehabilitation, University of Nebraska Medical Center, Omaha, Nebraska, USA

GEOFFREY M. THIELE, PhD
Umbach Professor of Rheumatology, Division of Rheumatology and Immunology, University of Nebraska Medical Center, VA Nebraska-Western Iowa Health Care System, Omaha, Nebraska, USA

ZACHARY S. WALLACE, MD, MSc
Clinical Epidemiology Program, Rheumatology Unit, Division of Rheumatology, Allergy, and Immunology, Mongan Institute, Massachusetts General Hospital, Harvard Medical School, Boston, Massachusetts, USA

ELIZABETH WELLSANDT, PT, DPT, PhD, OCS
Doctorate of Physical Therapy, Board Certified in Orthopedic Physical Therapy, Division of Physical Therapy Education, Department of Orthopedic Surgery and Rehabilitation, University of Nebraska Medical Center, Omaha, Nebraska, USA

DAVID M. WERNER, PT, DPT, OCS, CSCS
Doctorate of Physical Therapy, Board Certified in Orthopedic Physical Therapy, Certified Strength and Conditioning Specialist, Division of Physical Therapy Education, Medical Sciences Interdepartmental Area Program, University of Nebraska Medical Center, Omaha, Nebraska, USA

JENNIFER M.P. WOO, PhD
Epidemiology Branch, Department of Health and Human Services, National Institutes of Environmental Health Sciences, National Institutes of Health, Research Triangle Park, North Carolina, USA

Contents

Most rheumatic diseases have a stronger environmental than hereditary etiology. This article summarizes the key environmental risk factors for rheumatic diseases, the data sources that generated these findings, and the key pitfalls with existing research that every rheumatology clinician should know. Emerging research opportunities hold promise to revolutionize this field, and soon.

Rheumatoid arthritis (RA) occurs as the result of a complex interplay of environmental factors in a genetically susceptible individual. There is considerable evidence that the lungs may serve as an initial site of tolerance loss in the generation of RA-related autoimmunity, and several environmental inhalant exposures and lung diseases have been associated with RA risk. There is additional evidence that immune and microbial dysregulation of other mucosal sites, including the oral and gastrointestinal mucosa, may contribute to the development of RA. Epidemiologic evidence linking mucosal exposures to various environmental insults as risk determinants in RA will be reviewed.

Although there is a substantial body of literature focused on understanding noninhalational risk-factors for rheumatoid arthritis, the data are mixed and often conflicting. Given the other health benefits for certain lifestyle modifications, it seems reasonable for clinicians to promote healthy lifestyle habits related to diet, exercise, maintenance of health weight, and maintenance of good dental hygiene. Overall, however, these lifestyle modifications may be expected to have modest benefit, and other strategies to prevent rheumatoid arthritis in high-risk patients are needed.

Spondyloarthropathies, also known as spondyloarthritis, encompasses a spectrum of diseases classified by it's axial and peripheral musculoskeletal manifestations. Extra-articular features are common in SpA making these systemic rheumatologic diseases involve the skin, eye, gut, and other organ systems.Research has identified risk factors for the development of spondyloarthritis, particularly regarding genetic susceptibility and the strong association with HLA-B27. Multiple studies have elucidated clinical risk factors associated with SpA disease activity and severity. In this review, we aim to explore the environmental risk factors for spondyloarthritis.

Systemic lupus erythematosus (SLE) is a complex, chronic autoimmune disease. The etiology of SLE is multifactorial and includes potential environmental triggers, which may occur sequentially (the "multi-hit" hypothesis). This review focuses on SLE risk potentially associated with environmental factors including infections, the microbiome, diet, respirable exposures (eg, crystalline silica, smoking, air pollution), organic pollutants, heavy metals, and ultraviolet radiation.

There is an increasing body of literature suggesting a relationship between environmental factors and the development of systemic sclerosis (SSc). These include occupational exposures, chemical materials, medications, alterations in the microbiome, and dysbiosis. Environmental exposures may impact epigenetic regulation thereby triggering an aberrant immune response resulting in the clinical and serologic phenotype that we diagnose as SSc. Screening and studying putative triggers will not only improve our understanding of the pathogenesis of SSc but also inform the institution for protective measures.

This is an up-to-date review on external environmental factors for adult-onset idiopathic inflammatory myopathies (IIMs). Environmental factors with suggestive evidence including ultraviolet radiation, smoking, infectious agents (viruses in particular), pollutants, medications (ie, statin) and vitamin D deficiency are discussed. We also discuss the potential implications of environmental factors in IIM development, identify current challenges, and provide insight into future investigations.

Guy Katz and Zachary S. Wallace

Systemic vasculitides are autoimmune diseases characterized by vascular inflammation. Most types of vasculitis are thought to result from antigen exposure in genetically susceptible individuals, suggesting a likely role for environmental triggers in these conditions. Seasonal and geographic variations in incidence provide insight into the potential role of environmental exposures in these diseases. Many data support infectious triggers in some vasculitides, whereas other studies have identified noninfectious triggers, such as airborne pollutants, silica, smoking, and heavy metals. We review the known and suspected environmental triggers in giant cell arteritis, Takayasu arteritis, polyarteritis nodosa, Kawasaki disease, and antineutrophil cytoplasmic antibody-associated vasculitis.

Lindsay N. Helget and Ted R. Mikuls

Gout is the most prevalent type of inflammatory arthritis worldwide and environmental factors contribute to hyperuricemia and risk for gout flare. Causes of hyperuricemia include increased purine consumption from meat, alcohol, and high fructose corn syrup as well as medications such as cyclosporine, low-dose aspirin, or diuretics. Triggers for gout flares include increased purine consumption and medication use such as urate lowering therapy and diuretics. Environmental exposures including lead exposure, particulate matter exposure, temperature fluctuations, and physiologic stress have been found to trigger flares. In the right clinical scenario, these factors should be considered when treating gout patients.

David M. Werner, Yvonne M. Golightly, Matthew Tao, Austin Post, and Elizabeth Wellsandt

Osteoarthritis is a debilitating chronic condition involving joint degeneration, impacting over 300 million people worldwide. This places a high social and economic burden on society. The knee is the most common joint impacted by osteoarthritis. A common cause of osteoarthritis is traumatic joint injury, specifically injury to the anterior cruciate ligament. The purpose of this review is to detail the non-modifiable and modifiable risk factors for osteoarthritis with particular focus on individuals after anterior cruciate ligament injury. After reading this, health care providers will better comprehend the wide variety of factors linked to osteoarthritis.

Kevin D. Deane

Targeting environmental factors can be an important way to reduce the incidence of rheumatic diseases (RDs). Such approaches may be at population levels; furthermore, an emerging ability to identify an individual who is at very high risk for the development of a future RD can allow for personalized approaches to environmental modification for prevention. In this article, we will discuss challenges and opportunities to targeting environmental factors for the prevention of RDs.

Environmental Triggers for Rheumatic Diseases

RHEUMATIC DISEASE CLINICS OF NORTH AMERICA

THE CLINICS ARE AVAILABLE ONLINE!
Access your subscription at:
www.theclinics.com

Foreword
Environmental Triggers for Rheumatic Diseases

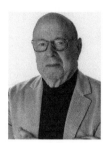

Michael H. Weisman, MD
Consulting Editor

Bryant has done a remarkable job putting together this state-of-the-art issue on environmental triggers for Rheumatic Disease. In the current issue, there is a heavily annotated and critical emphasis on the methodological aspects of how to investigate this important part of our diseases. Association and causation are different things, and our article writers are quick to point out that observations need to be examined in a variety of ways to make sure we do not rush to judgment. Different study designs are emphasized in these contributions, and each has its own benefits and shortcomings. Many of our diseases suffer from challenges in classification and long latency periods from a modifiable exposure to clinical manifestations. The good news for the field is the potential impact of mendelian randomization studies that can mimic randomized controlled trials whereby observational studies can provide evidence for an actual causation from an identifiable risk factor.

Our contributors point out that these advances in understating the environmental risk for our diseases are not quite to the point of individual patient counselling. However, we may be close to changing our view of rheumatic diseases from challenge to opportunity with true prevention studies that are being carried out currently. If our future public health system can address air pollution, dietary ingredients, common infections, and workplace exposures, perhaps we will run ourselves out of business.

Michael H. Weisman, MD
Division of Immunology and Rheumatology
Stanford University

E-mail address:
weisman@cshs.org

Rheum Dis Clin N Am 48 (2022) xi
https://doi.org/10.1016/j.rdc.2022.07.001
0889-857X/22/© 2022 Published by Elsevier Inc.

rheumatic.theclinics.com

Preface

Environmental Triggers for Rheumatic Disease: From "Why Did I Get This?" to "How Can We Prevent This?"

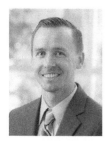

Bryant R. England, MD, PhD
Editor

Receiving the news of a new diagnosis of rheumatic disease can be overwhelming to patients. After discussing the natural history, treatment options, and initial treatment plan during such a clinic visit, many of us providers ask, "What questions do you have?" Routinely, it is not a clarifying question about the diagnosis or treatment plan, but rather the question, "Why did I get this?," the patient asks. Unfortunately, this question that is simple to ask is impossible to answer. We often respond by discussing the heritability of rheumatic diseases, but the majority of rheumatic disease risk is not related to genetics. Next, we move to environmental triggers where we may search the medical record and collect a detailed medical and social history to identify possible risk factors. Even when found, these risk factors are not typically necessary or sufficient causes, according to Rothman's Sufficient-Component Cause model. More likely, these risk factors are one of many possible component causes. And then to ensure that patients are completely overwhelmed before leaving their visit, we may introduce the concept of gene-environment interactions.

In this issue of *Rheumatic Disease Clinics of North America*, the environmental triggers for several of the most frequently encountered rheumatic diseases are reviewed. This issue begins with the methodological considerations for studying environmental risk factors for rheumatic diseases because understanding the strengths and limitations of different study designs and data sources is crucial as we interpret relevant epidemiologic and translational studies of environmental risk factors. Subsequently, the environmental triggers for rheumatoid arthritis, spondyloarthropathy, systemic lupus erythematosus, systemic sclerosis, inflammatory myositis, vasculitis, gout, and

Rheum Dis Clin N Am 48 (2022) xiii–xiv
https://doi.org/10.1016/j.rdc.2022.07.002
0889-857X/22/© 2022 Published by Elsevier Inc.

osteoarthritis are reviewed in detail. Through these articles we gain an appreciation for the wide array of possible environmental triggers of rheumatic disease that have been identified to date, including various inhalants, infections, lifestyle habits, occupational exposures, medications, and microbiome alterations.

With the evidence summarized in this issue, we are be better positioned to respond to the common patient question of "Why did I get this?" However, our ultimate goal is not to answer only the "Why did I get this?" question but also to develop answers to another question: "How can we prevent this?" Therefore, this issue concludes with a look into the future on how we could harness an understanding of environmental triggers for rheumatic disease to prevent rheumatic disease onset. After all, our best chance of answering the "Why did I get this?" question is preventing it in the first place!

Bryant R. England, MD, PhD
Division of Rheumatology & Immunology
Department of Internal Medicine
VA Nebraska-Western Iowa Health Care System
University of Nebraska Medical Center
986270 Nebraska Medicine
Omaha, NE 68198-6270, USA

E-mail address:
Bryant.england@unmc.edu

Epidemiologic Opportunities and Challenges in Studying Environmental Risk Factors for Rheumatic Diseases

Vanessa L. Kronzer, MD, MSCI[a],*, John M. Davis III, MD, MS[a],
Cynthia S. Crowson, PhD[a,b]

KEYWORDS

- Epidemiology • Environment • Rheumatology • Study design

KEY POINTS

- Heritability of rheumatic diseases ranges from only 12% to 35%, meaning environmental factors account for most of the risk for rheumatic diseases.
- Smoking, obesity, and silica exposure are associated with increased risk of many rheumatic diseases.
- To assess quality of the evidence for associations between environmental risk factors and rheumatic diseases, clinicians should evaluate rheumatic disease data sources for case selection bias, duration of follow-up, misclassification of exposures or outcomes, sample size, and generalizability.
- An emerging study design, Mendelian randomization uses genetic variants as instrumental variables to assess for a causal relationship between environmental risk factors and rheumatic diseases.

INTRODUCTION

When diagnosed with a rheumatic disease, patients frequently want to know what "caused" it. Most of the risk for rheumatic diseases comes from environmental exposures. This article provides an overview of key environmental risk factors, data sources, and publication pitfalls that all rheumatology clinicians should know.

First, we synthesize the types of evidence and data sources in rheumatic disease research to provide a digestible overview of what we have learned so far about

[a] Division of Rheumatology, Mayo Clinic, Rochester, MN, USA; [b] Department of Quantitative Health Sciences, Mayo Clinic, Rochester, MN, USA
* Corresponding author. Division of Rheumatology, Mayo Clinic, 200 First Street Southwest, Rochester, MN 55905.
E-mail address: kronzer.vanessa@mayo.edu

Rheum Dis Clin N Am 48 (2022) 763–779
https://doi.org/10.1016/j.rdc.2022.06.001
0889-857X/22/© 2022 Elsevier Inc. All rights reserved.

rheumatic.theclinics.com

environmental risk factors for rheumatic diseases, and how. Second, we summarize the key pitfalls to know about existing research, along with their corresponding opportunities for future research moving forward.

TYPES OF EVIDENCE AND DATA SOURCES: WHAT HAVE WE LEARNED SO FAR?
Twin and Family-Based Studies

Because rheumatic diseases often co-occur in families, some of the earliest rheumatic disease studies used twins. For example, the Danish Twin Registry captures data on nearly all twin pairs born in Denmark since 1870, and demonstrated that heritability of osteoarthritis (OA) in the hip is approximately 47% (**Table 1** contains details on each mentioned data source).[1] Similarly, gout has heritability of 35%, meaning 65% of the risk comes from environmental factors.[2]

Autoimmune diseases tend to demonstrate an even lower heritability and higher environmental component. For example, concordance of monozygotic pairs for systemic lupus erythematosus (SLE) is only 24%[3] and for juvenile idiopathic arthritis (JIA) is only 15%.[4] In the Danish Twin Registry, the heritability of rheumatoid arthritis (RA) was recently estimated to be only 12%.[5] When sufficient twin data is not available, family-based studies may be performed. One such study in Sweden showed the heritability of idiopathic inflammatory myopathy (IIM) is approximately 20%.[6] Overall, the heritability of rheumatic disease ranges from only 12% to 35%, underscoring the importance of studying environmental risk factors (**Fig. 1**).

Cross-Sectional Studies

Although cross-sectional studies cannot establish causal relationships, they have reported several interesting findings. For example, in 1957, a high frequency of systemic sclerosis (SSc) was reported in gold miners exposed to mining dust containing silica, leading to the term now known as "Erasmus syndrome" to describe SSc occurring after silica exposures.[7] In 1988, a cross-sectional study noted that among 41 patients with JIA, 14 were born in 1963 when the H2N2 influenza epidemic occurred, suggesting presensitization to influenza A as an etiology.[8] Finally, in 1999, a study showed evidence of spatial clustering of IIM in Australia, again supporting the role of environmental factors in the pathogenesis of rheumatic disease.

Referral Cohorts

In contrast to population-based cohorts that include individuals based on residence in a particular geographic area, referral cohorts include individuals based on referral to a particular hospital or provider. Useful especially for the very rare diseases like IIM, SSc, and vasculitis, referral cohorts have provided numerous interesting findings in rheumatic diseases as well. One referral cohort found an elevated history of solvent exposure in patients with SSc, especially in men and those with anti–Scl-70 positive disease.[9] A referral cohort of 380 patients with IIM found ultraviolet radiation intensity in the state of residence at disease onset was associated with increased risk of dermatomyositis and anti–Mi-2 autoantibodies.[10] In vasculitis, a cohort of 484 patients with antineutrophil cytoplasmic antibody–associated vasculitis (AAV) and matched controls found smoking to be associated with AAV,[11] whereas another cohort found history of horse and farm exposure increased odds of granulomatosis with polyangiitis.[12] A major downside of referral cohorts, however, is its inherent referral bias. This form of selection bias can inflate associations and reduce generalizability due to unrepresentativeness of referral populations compared to the general population.

Table 1
Data sources for rheumatic disease research highlighted in this article

Name	Types	Diseases	Criteria	Population	Time	Data
Agricultural Health Study[37]	Prospective cohort	RA	Self-report, medications, and/or medical records	52,394 pesticide applicators in Iowa and North Carolina	1993–1997	Questionnaire
Carolina Lupus Study[24]	Registry	Lupus	ACR	>260 SLE Southeast Carolina	1995–1999	Questionnaire, laboratory
Danish National Patient Registry	Health system database	Several	Codes	Denmark	1977 – present	Clinical data, laboratory, pharmacy
Danish Twin Registry[1]	Registry	Several	Must use another source	170,000 Danish twins	1870 – present	Sex, date of birth, zygosity, date of death
EIRA[20]	Population-based cohort	RA	ACR/EULAR	>3000 RA Middle and southern Sweden	1996 – present	Questionnaire, clinical data, laboratory, pharmacy, serum, DNA
HUNT[23]	Population-based cohort	Several	Self-report and codes	Norway adults >20 y (75% in HUNT2 and 54% HUNT3)	1995–7 (HUNT2); 2006–8 (HUNT3)	Questionnaire, some clinical data and pharmacy
IWHS[89]	Prospective cohort	Several	Self-report then ACR	>68,000 postmenopausal women in Iowa	1986 – present	Questionnaire
LUMINA[76]	Registry	Lupus	ACR	>600 SLE from Texas, Puerto Rico, or Alabama	1994 – present	Questionnaire

(continued on next page)

Table 1
(continued)

Name	Types	Diseases	Criteria	Population	Time	Data
Mass General Brigham Biobank[40]	Biobank	Several	ACR	>117,000 participants in Boston area	2010 – present	Questionnaire, clinical care, laboratory, serum, DNA
Mayo Clinic Biobank[39]	Biobank	Several	Codes + medication	>56,000 participants in Olmsted County	2009 – present	Questionnaire, clinical care, laboratory, pharmacy, serum, DNA
MYOVISION[77]	Registry	Myositis	Bohan & Peter or Griggs	>1800 from Myositis Association mailing list or volunteers	2010–2012	Questionnaire
National Patient Register[46]	Health system database	Several	Codes	Sweden (99% hospitalizations, 80% outpatient visits)	1987 – present	Clinical care, laboratory, pharmacy
Norwegian Patient Registry[66]	Health system database	Several	Codes	Norway	2008 – present	Specialist clinical care and procedures
NHS[71]	Prospective cohort	Several	ACR	>230,000 female nurses aged 19–55 y from 14 states	1976 – present	Questionnaires, clinical care, laboratory
OptumHealth[67]	Claims database	Several	Codes	80 million private insured	1993 – present	Clinical codes, laboratory, pharmacy

REP[47]	Population-based cohort	Several	ACR/EULAR	>500,000 in Olmsted County, MN	1966 – present	Clinical care, laboratory, pharmacy
Taiwan's NHI Database[65]	Health system database	Several	Codes	Taiwan, 99.9% coverage	1995 – present	Surveys, clinical care, laboratory, pharmacy
THIN[64]	Health system database	Several	Codes	>11 million (6%) in UK from 650 general practices	1994 – present	Clinical care, laboratory, pharmacy
UK Biobank[41]	Biobank	Several	Self-report + medication	>500,000 randomly selected from UK aged 40–69 y	2006–2010	Questionnaires, examination, clinical care, laboratory, pharmacy, serum, DNA
VARA[36]	Registry and linked health system database	RA	ACR	>3,000 US veterans from multiple VA sites	2002 – present	Clinical care, laboratory, pharmacy, serum, DNA
WTC Health Program[27]	Registry	Several	Physician diagnosis	>15,000 WTC site-exposed workers	2001 – present	Questionnaire incl. exposure duration, clinical care, laboratory, pharmacy

Abbreviations: ACR, American College of Rheumatology; EIRA, Epidemiological Investigation of RA; HUNT, Nord-Trøndelag Health Study; IWHS, Iowa Women's Health Study; LUMINA, Lupus in Minorities: Nature vs Nurture; NHS, Nurses' Health Study; NHI, National Health Insurance; RA, rheumatoid arthritis; REP, Rochester Epidemiology Project; SLE, systemic lupus erythematosus; THIN, The Health Improvement Network; VA, Veterans Affairs; VARA, Veterans Affairs Rheumatoid Arthritis; WTC, World Trade Center.

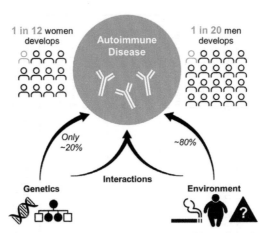

Fig. 1. Autoimmune rheumatic diseases are common, driven largely by environmental factors.

Case-Control Studies

Case-control studies have validated many findings from cross and referral cohort studies. For example, a prospective, blinded case-control study showed history of solvent and silica exposure increased risk of SSc.[13] Case-control studies have linked silica exposure with many other rheumatic diseases, including SLE,[14] RA,[15] and AAV.[16] The association between sunlight and dermatomyositis was also replicated in a case-control study within the "MYOVISION" registry. In that study, dermatomyositis was associated with sunburn in the year before diagnosis and elevated job or hobby-related sun exposure compared to polymyositis and inclusion body myositis.[17] Although the association between smoking and AAV has yet to be replicated, smoking has been associated with the development of nearly all autoimmune rheumatic diseases including IIM,[18] large vessel vasculitis (LVV),[19] RA,[20] SLE,[21] and spondyloarthropathies such as psoriatic arthritis (PsA)[22] and ankylosing spondylitis (AS) (using the population-based Nord-Trøndelag Health [HUNT] Study).[23]

As these examples show, case-control studies can take place within a cohort (a "nested case-control") such as the HUNT study or can be case-control by design such as the Epidemiological Investigation of Rheumatoid Arthritis (EIRA).[20] Nested case-control studies often have more flexibility, for example, with control selection criteria and the ability to study multiple outcomes. In contrast, designated case-control studies are often more cost-efficient and can collect more pertinent risk factor data for the disease of interest.

Similarly, some data sources cover just one disease such as the Carolina Lupus Study, which found that previous infections and family history of SLE increased the risk of SLE 2- to 3-fold.[24] These focused studies often have the advantage of verifying the rheumatic disease using validated criteria (see **Table 1**). In contrast, many data sources cover multiple autoimmune diseases. A UK medical records database called The Health Improvement Network (THIN) covers 6% of the UK population and studies many rheumatic diseases—though defines them using codes. In this database, antibiotic exposure was associated with 2-fold increased risk of JIA in a dose-dependent fashion,[25] whereas PsA was associated with obesity and pharyngitis, and PsA, RA, and AS were all inversely associated with statin exposure.[26] The World Trade Center (WTC) Health Program also studies multiple autoimmune diseases but uses physician diagnosis. This data set showed the odds for incident autoimmune disease including RA, spondyloarthritis, SLE, SSc, Sjogren's, and GPA increased by 13% for each additional month worked at the WTC site after September 11, 2001.[27]

Cohort Studies

Considered stronger than case-control studies, cohort studies have clarity of temporal sequence and avoid the possibility of match-related selection bias. The downside is mainly their financial and time costs, which are amplified for rare diseases with long latency such as many rheumatic diseases. Nevertheless, several rheumatic disease cohort studies with long follow-up do exist, establishing some of the most important environmental risk factors for rheumatic diseases. For example, many years ago, the Nurses' Health Study (NHS) showed that women with early menarche, oral contraceptive (OCP) use, and postmenopausal hormones had an increased risk of SLE.[28] More recently in RA, the NHS has shown not only cigarette smoking[29] but also passive smoke exposure,[30] proximity to a road,[31] low physical activity,[32] sugar-sweetened soda,[33] and inflammatory diet[34] are all associated with increased risk of RA. The prospective nature of these studies provides higher assurance that the exposure precedes the outcome—important for assessing causation.

Other cohorts have played an important role as well. For example, the Danish National Patient Registry showed that higher body fat percentage, waist circumference, and obesity were associated with higher risk of RA.[35] A nested study within the Veterans Affairs RA (VARA) cohort recently showed military burn pit and waste disposal exposure were associated with anti-CCP positivity in RA patients,[36] whereas the Agricultural Health Study showed that chemical fertilizers and solvents increased the risk of RA.[37] A matched longitudinal study within THIN showed that individuals with psoriasis exposed to trauma, especially bone and joint, had an increased risk of PsA.[38]

Although designed to collect biological and genetic data, biobanks have also become a source of environmental data. For example, data from the Mayo Clinic Biobank showed asthma and food allergies were associated with an increased risk of RA.[39] Studies in the Mass General Brigham[40] and UK biobanks[41] are also forming. These cohorts provide a unique opportunity to study the interaction of environmental risk factors with genetics (see **Fig. 1**). For example, both smoking,[42] and more recently textile dust exposure,[43] have been associated with strongly increased risk of RA in the presence of the shared epitope alleles.

Population-Based Studies

Population-based studies limit themselves to one geographic area and therefore may not generalize externally. However, they have an advantage over other cohorts due to lower risk of selection bias. For example, Hart and colleagues extracted data down to an individual household level in Stockholm, finding an association between gaseous air pollutants and seronegative RA.[44] Another study from EIRA recently showed respiratory diseases are associated with an increased risk of RA.[45] Preceding infections and respiratory diseases were also associated with IIM within the Swedish National Patient Register, which covers 99% of inpatient hospitalizations and 80% of outpatient visits in Sweden.[46] Another important population-based study is the Rochester Epidemiology Project (REP).[47] Using its five decades of longitudinal data, the REP revealed periodicity in the incidence of RA and LVV occurring approximately every 10 years, which significantly corresponded to solar cycles and geomagnetic effects.[48] Unfortunately, few population-based studies exist at this time.

Randomized and Randomization Studies

Although widely considered the pinnacle of study design, randomized controlled trials (RCTs) seldom study environmental risk factors for rheumatic disease. This occurs partly because rheumatic diseases are so rare, and partly because randomizing environmental risk factors is difficult. Dietary factors are one exception. For example, RCTs of vitamin D and E showed no difference in RA incidence.[49,50]

An emerging study design, Mendelian randomization studies use genetic variants as instrumental variables to draw causal inferences from observational data. They have supported the association between obesity and rheumatic diseases by demonstrating that genetically predicted BMI increased the risk of RA,[51] gout,[52] and OA.[53] Because genotypes are always randomly assigned at birth and precede disease onset, Mendelian randomization studies act just like an RCT but can be performed with observational data. Thus, Mendelian randomization has become a useful tool for rheumatic disease research.[54]

DISCUSSION: CHALLENGES AND OPPORTUNITIES

As illustrated by the challenges with RCTs and corresponding opportunities with Mendelian randomization, rheumatic disease research has faced and overcome numerous challenges. Below we describe the most common challenges (**Fig. 2**) and the most salient opportunities for future rheumatic research going forward.

Publication Bias

Before 2012, clinicians believed vitamin D reduced the risk of RA. A study within the Iowa Women's Health Study in 2004 showed an association between increased

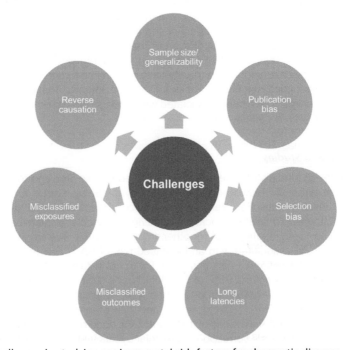

Fig. 2. Challenges in studying environmental risk factors for rheumatic diseases.

vitamin D intake and reduced risk of RA. By 2012, a meta-analysis of 11 studies showed a positive association between vitamin D and RA or RA disease activity.[55] However, the prospective NHS cohort had shown no association.[56] Indeed, in 2012, an RCT of over 36,000 women showed no association between vitamin D and risk of incident RA.[50] A subsequent Mendelian randomization study has supported this finding.[57] One reason for this discrepancy could be publication bias, which withholds negative results from publication. For example, positive studies have increased by over 20% in the last 20 years.[58] Indeed, impressive simulations by Dr Ioannidis showed that for most studies, research claims are more likely to be false than true.[59]

Three opportunities can combat this challenging bias. First, journals can strive to publish high-quality negative studies. Second, authors can write protocols prespecifying their analysis plans. Third, authors can write manuscripts following guidelines (eg, Strengthening the Reporting of Observational Studies in Epidemiology [STROBE] guidelines).[60] Because these guidelines promote high-quality research, many journals now require them. Finally, synthetization of findings across studies should include evaluation of publication bias.

Selection Bias

Defined as bias that occurs when individuals in a study differ systematically from the general population, selection bias represents a major challenge in rheumatic disease referral cohorts and registries. Biobanks have this problem as well, with participation rates often ranging from 5% to 30%.[39,61] Similarly, studies that restrict the study population only to patients with a certain outcome can find erroneous results. For example, case-control studies of patients with psoriasis found a negative association between smoking and PsA, termed the "smoking paradox."[62,63] Subsequent data in the general population have shown that in fact smoking is a risk factor for PsA,[22] and that the negative association in the previous studies resulted from selecting only participants with psoriasis.[64]

Using population-based studies like the REP or EIRA provides an opportunity to reduce selection bias.[20,47] Health system databases with high coverage rates can act in a similar fashion. For example, the Swedish National Patient Register covers 99% hospitalizations and 80% outpatient visits,[46] whereas the Taiwanese National Health Insurance (NHI) database covers 99.9% of the population in Taiwan.[65] Similarly, the Danish National Patient Registry includes data from all public hospitals since 1977, and outpatient visits since 1995,[35] whereas the Norwegian Patient Registry and Norwegian Registry for Primary Health Care represent all government-funded health care in Norway since 2017.[66] In the United States, Medicare has data on most US adults aged 65 years and older, but left censoring limits its ability to study environmental risk factors for incident disease. The OptumHealth database covers 80 million US residents, but only individuals who are privately insured.[67] Thus, for the United States and other countries without a current unified health system, forming a complete health system database represents a major opportunity for the future.

Long Latency Between Triggers, Disease, and Diagnosis

Many rheumatic diseases exhibit a long latency between environmental triggers and disease onset or clinical diagnosis. For example, respiratory tract exposures have the strongest association with RA when they occur 5 to 10 years before disease onset.[44,68] Meanwhile, many diseases have a long latency between symptom onset and clinical diagnosis. For example, in SSc, the mean latency between Raynaud's onset and clinical diagnosis is 5 years,[69] whereas in RA, autoantibodies signaling disease onset begin 5 years before clinical diagnosis.[70]

Data sources with long follow-up provide an opportunity to address this challenge. For example, the NHS began in 1976,[71] and the REP began in 1966.[47] The Danish outpatient registry, THIN, EIRA, and NHI began several decades ago in 1995 (see **Table 1**), whereas the Swedish National Patient Register began in 1987 for inpatient codes.[46] OptumHealth reports data collection since 1993, though individual members may only contribute a few years of data.[67] Overall, carefully evaluating each data source for its duration of follow-up is important.

Misclassification of Outcomes

Although health system databases may cover a large population with prolonged follow-up, they often use code-based diseases. Code-based disease definitions may suffer from "upcoding," where providers assign an inaccurate code to receive insurance coverage.[65] Even if upcoding has not occurred, codes can still be inaccurate. For example, requiring 3 outpatient or 1 inpatient diagnosis code for RA has a positive predictive value of only 78%.[72] Although researchers can increase specificity, doing so reduces sensitivity, and vice versa. Patient-reported disease may be even worse. One study showed that 71% of self-reported autoimmune diseases were incorrect, mostly OA misclassified as RA.[27] Disease onset may also be difficult to establish using codes, especially for diseases with long latency such as SSc. Using established classification criteria best addresses these challenges. Many high-quality studies use established classification criteria (see **Table 1**). If using established criteria is not possible, investigators should report the validity of the outcome assessment method used.

Misclassification of Exposures

Another major challenge for rheumatic disease research to overcome is misclassification of exposures. Recall bias, where participants do not remember previous events accurately, is particularly a concern for questionnaires assessing environmental exposures and for cross-sectional studies. To illustrate, a cross-sectional study of smoking and RA performed in 1990 claimed smoking to be *protective* against RA, with the authors speculating the mechanism for this association was due to the "anti-inflammatory effects" of smoking.[73]

Environmental exposures and their association with disease can also change over time. For example, obesity was not found to be a risk factor for RA in most studies conducted before the start of the obesity epidemic in the late 1990s.[74] Obesity appears to have a modest effect on RA (odds ratio <1.5), and earlier studies may have been underpowered to detect a modest effect for a risk factor with low prevalence (ie, 10%). Similarly, OCP use had a stronger association with RA in earlier years, as the doses of estrogens and progestins were higher at that time than now.[75]

Another issue related to misclassification is unmeasured exposures or confounders. Some exposures are intrinsically difficult to measure such as diet or periodontitis. Changes in vitamin D exposure over time might have resulted from changes in unmeasured factors such as sun exposure or sunscreen use over time. Furthermore, many data sources, especially health system databases, do not have good data on most environmental exposures or important confounders (eg, smoking). Even if a data source collects all important exposures initially, it can become outdated as the field changes. For example, the LUMINA cohort collected exposure data to satisfy the existing classification criteria for SLE, but is now outdated for the new European Alliance of Associations for Rheumatology (EULAR) lupus criteria as it does not collect certain exposures like fever.[76]

One opportunity to address misclassification of exposures is to create a new prospective cohort collecting comprehensive data. For example, in 2017, the MYORISK study began studying the genetic and environmental risk factors for myositis.[77] Non-disease cohorts can also provide opportunities. For example, the first study to show smoking was a risk factor for RA came from a prospective cohort study of OCP use in England in 1987. In this manuscript (which showed no association between OCPs and RA), the authors reported the "unexpected finding" that women with previous smoking history had a much higher rate of hospitalization for RA.[78] This association was later confirmed in the NHS[79] and EIRA,[20] and smoking remains the strongest known environmental risk factor for RA. Alternatively, investigators can link various complementary data sources to provide robust capture of exposures, confounders, and outcomes.

Reverse Causation

Even when the exposures and outcomes are properly classified, the order in which they occur can be confused, a process called reverse causation. In the cross-sectional study reporting smoking protected against RA,[73] the reverse was later shown to be true, with RA diagnosis actually leading to a reduction in smoking behavior.[80] Even prospective studies are susceptible to reverse causation, especially for diseases with a long latency between disease and diagnosis.

RCTs remove the possibility of reverse causation, though often are not feasible in environmental rheumatic disease research. Mendelian randomization studies, however, represent a major opportunity to address this shortcoming.[54] First, they can clarify controversies. One question with significant debate is whether alcohol protects against RA[81] (with proponents again suggesting an "anti-inflammatory" effect), or not.[82] In 2019, a mendelian randomization study supported the latter, showing no evidence of an association between genetically predicted alcohol use and RA.[83] Mendelian randomization studies can also generate new findings, such as the negative causal association between serum calcium levels and OA[84] or telomere length and RA.[85] These new findings merit further research. Aside from Mendelian randomization, investigators can also carefully consider latency and include an exposure-to-outcome time lag in analyses to avoid inducing reverse causation.

Sample Size and Generalizability

Although the lifetime risk of any rheumatic autoimmune disease is 1 in 12 women and 1 in 20 men, the frequency of each individual disease is relatively low.[86] As a result, rheumatic diseases commonly suffer from small sample sizes. Furthermore, many of the highest-quality data sources like the Danish National Patient Registry and REP have almost all White participants, or like the NHS have only one sex or age group (see **Table 1**). Even the highest-quality population-based prospective cohorts (eg, EIRA, REP) are by definition limited to one geographic area.

Certain opportunities can circumvent these problems. For example, the UK Biobank makes data on its >500,000 individuals publicly available for a small fee. Meanwhile, LUMINA[76] and NHS 3[87] both explicitly target racial minorities to expand generalizability. Finally, combining data sets is also possible. For example, the North American Rheumatoid Arthritis Consortium pooled genetic and questionnaire data from over 1000 RA patients and family members.[88] Indeed, collaboration benefits all researchers, populations, and individuals with rheumatic diseases.

SUMMARY

In summary, the study of environmental factors for rheumatic diseases has evolved over time. It started with twin and cross-sectional studies and now leverages study designs such as Mendelian randomization and population-based cohort studies with long-term follow-up. To address challenges such as selection bias, misclassification, reverse causation, and small sample size, it will continue to evolve. Nevertheless, creativity and collaboration will remain fundamental tenants.

CLINICS CARE POINTS

- An emerging study design, Mendelian randomization uses genetic variants as instrumental variables to assess for a causal relationship between environmental risk factors and rheumatic diseases.

DISCLOSURE

Dr J.M. Davis reports research funding from Pfizer and serving on advisory boards for Abbvie and Sanofi, all unrelated to this work.

REFERENCES

1. Skousgaard SG, Hjelmborg J, Skytthe A, et al. Probability and heritability estimates on primary osteoarthritis of the hip leading to total hip arthroplasty: a nationwide population based follow-up study in Danish twins. Arthritis Res Ther 2015;17:336.
2. Kuo CF, Grainge MJ, See LC, et al. Familial aggregation of gout and relative genetic and environmental contributions: a nationwide population study in Taiwan. Ann Rheum Dis 2015;74(2):369–74.
3. Deapen D, Escalante A, Weinrib L, et al. A revised estimate of twin concordance in systemic lupus erythematosus. Arthritis Rheum 1992;35(3):311–8.
4. Silman AJ, MacGregor AJ, Thomson W, et al. Twin concordance rates for rheumatoid arthritis: results from a nationwide study. Br J Rheumatol 1993;32(10):903–7.
5. Svendsen AJ, Kyvik KO, Houen G, et al. On the origin of rheumatoid arthritis: the impact of environment and genes–a population based twin study. PLoS One 2013;8(2):e57304.
6. Che WI, Westerlind H, Lundberg IE, et al. Familial aggregation and heritability: a nationwide family-based study of idiopathic inflammatory myopathies. Ann Rheum Dis 2021;80(11):1461–6.
7. Erasmus LD. Scleroderma in goldminers on the Witwatersrand with particular reference to pulmonary manifestations. S Afr J Lab Clin Med 1957;3(3):209–31.
8. Pritchard MH, Matthews N, Munro J. Antibodies to influenza A in a cluster of children with juvenile chronic arthritis. Br J Rheumatol 1988;27(3):176–80.
9. Nietert PJ, Sutherland SE, Silver RM, et al. Is occupational organic solvent exposure a risk factor for scleroderma? Arthritis Rheum 1998;41(6):1111–8.
10. Love LA, Weinberg CR, McConnaughey DR, et al. Ultraviolet radiation intensity predicts the relative distribution of dermatomyositis and anti-Mi-2 autoantibodies in women. Arthritis Rheum 2009;60(8):2499–504.
11. McDermott G, Fu X, Stone JH, et al. Association of Cigarette Smoking With Antineutrophil Cytoplasmic Antibody-Associated Vasculitis. JAMA Intern Med 2020; 180(6):870–6.

12. Lindberg H, Colliander C, Nise L, et al. Are Farming and Animal Exposure Risk Factors for the Development of Granulomatosis With Polyangiitis? Environmental Risk Factors Revisited: A Case-control Study. J Rheumatol 2021;48(6):894–7.

13. Marie I, Gehanno JF, Bubenheim M, et al. Prospective study to evaluate the association between systemic sclerosis and occupational exposure and review of the literature. Autoimmun Rev 2014;13(2):151–6.

14. Parks CG, Cooper GS, Nylander-French LA, et al. Occupational exposure to crystalline silica and risk of systemic lupus erythematosus: a population-based, case-control study in the southeastern United States. Arthritis Rheum 2002;46(7): 1840–50.

15. Stolt P, Källberg H, Lundberg I, et al. Silica exposure is associated with increased risk of developing rheumatoid arthritis: results from the Swedish EIRA study. Ann Rheum Dis 2005;64(4):582–6.

16. Gómez-Puerta JA, Gedmintas L, Costenbader KH. The association between silica exposure and development of ANCA-associated vasculitis: systematic review and meta-analysis. Autoimmun Rev 2013;12(12):1129–35.

17. Parks CG, Wilkerson J, Rose KM, et al. Association of Ultraviolet Radiation Exposure With Dermatomyositis in a National Myositis Patient Registry. Arthritis Care Res (Hoboken) 2020;72(11):1636–44.

18. Chinoy H, Adimulam S, Marriage F, et al. Interaction of HLA-DRB1*03 and smoking for the development of anti-Jo-1 antibodies in adult idiopathic inflammatory myopathies: a European-wide case study. Ann Rheum Dis 2012;71(6):961–5.

19. Brennan DN, Ungprasert P, Warrington KJ, et al. Smoking as a risk factor for giant cell arteritis: A systematic review and meta-analysis. Semin Arthritis Rheum 2018; 48(3):529–37.

20. Stolt P, Bengtsson C, Nordmark B, et al. Quantification of the influence of cigarette smoking on rheumatoid arthritis: results from a population based case-control study, using incident cases. Ann Rheum Dis 2003;62(9):835–41.

21. Costenbader KH, Kim DJ, Peerzada J, et al. Cigarette smoking and the risk of systemic lupus erythematosus: a meta-analysis. Arthritis Rheum 2004;50(3): 849–57.

22. Li W, Han J, Qureshi AA. Smoking and risk of incident psoriatic arthritis in US women. Ann Rheum Dis 2012;71(6):804–8.

23. Videm V, Cortes A, Thomas R, et al. Current smoking is associated with incident ankylosing spondylitis – the HUNT population-based Norwegian health study. J Rheumatol 2014;41(10):2041–8.

24. Cooper GS, Dooley MA, Treadwell EL, et al. Risk factors for development of systemic lupus erythematosus: allergies, infections, and family history. J Clin Epidemiol 2002;55(10):982–9.

25. Horton DB, Scott FI, Haynes K, et al. Antibiotic Exposure and Juvenile Idiopathic Arthritis: A Case-Control Study. Pediatrics 2015;136(2):e333–43.

26. Meer E, Thrastardottir T, Wang X, et al. Risk factors for diagnosis of psoriatic arthritis, psoriasis, rheumatoid arthritis, and ankylosing spondylitis: A set of parallel case-control studies. J Rheumatol 2021;49(1):53–9.

27. Webber MP, Moir W, Zeig-Owens R, et al. Nested case-control study of selected systemic autoimmune diseases in World Trade Center rescue/recovery workers. Arthritis Rheumatol 2015;67(5):1369–76.

28. Costenbader KH, Feskanich D, Stampfer MJ, et al. Reproductive and menopausal factors and risk of systemic lupus erythematosus in women. Arthritis Rheum 2007;56(4):1251–62.

29. Costenbader KH, Feskanich D, Mandl LA, et al. Smoking intensity, duration, and cessation, and the risk of rheumatoid arthritis in women. Am J Med 2006;119(6): 503.e1-9.

30. Yoshida K, Wang J, Malspeis S, et al. Passive Smoking Throughout the Life Course and the Risk of Incident Rheumatoid Arthritis in Adulthood Among Women. Arthritis Rheumatol 2021;73(12):2219–28.

31. Hart JE, Laden F, Puett RC, et al. Exposure to traffic pollution and increased risk of rheumatoid arthritis. Environ Health Perspect 2009;117(7):1065–9.

32. Liu X, Tedeschi SK, Lu B, et al. Long-Term Physical Activity and Subsequent Risk for Rheumatoid Arthritis Among Women: A Prospective Cohort Study. Arthritis Rheumatol 2019;71(9):1460–71.

33. Hu Y, Costenbader KH, Gao X, et al. Sugar-sweetened soda consumption and risk of developing rheumatoid arthritis in women. Am J Clin Nutr 2014;100(3): 959–67.

34. Sparks JA, Barbhaiya M, Tedeschi SK, et al. Inflammatory dietary pattern and risk of developing rheumatoid arthritis in women. Clin Rheumatol 2019;38(1):243–50.

35. Linauskas A, Overvad K, Symmons D, et al. Body Fat Percentage, Waist Circumference, and Obesity As Risk Factors for Rheumatoid Arthritis: A Danish Cohort Study. Arthritis Care Res (Hoboken) 2019;71(6):777–86.

36. Ebel AV, Lutt G, Poole JA, et al. Association of Agricultural, Occupational, and Military Inhalants With Autoantibodies and Disease Features in US Veterans With Rheumatoid Arthritis. Arthritis Rheumatol 2021;73(3):392–400.

37. Parks CG, Meyer A, Beane Freeman LE, et al. Farming tasks and the development of rheumatoid arthritis in the agricultural health study. Occup Environ Med 2019;76(4):243–9.

38. Thorarensen SM, Lu N, Ogdie A, et al. Physical trauma recorded in primary care is associated with the onset of psoriatic arthritis among patients with psoriasis. Ann Rheum Dis 2017;76(3):521–5.

39. Kronzer VL, Crowson CS, Sparks JA, et al. Investigating Asthma, Allergic Disease, Passive Smoke Exposure, and Risk of Rheumatoid Arthritis. Arthritis Rheumatol 2019;71(8):1217–24.

40. Kronzer VL, Huang W, Zaccardelli A, et al. Association of sinusitis and upper respiratory tract diseases with incident rheumatoid arthritis: A case-control study. J Rheum (In Press 2021;49(4):358–64.

41. Prisco L, Moll M, Wang J, et al. Relationship between rheumatoid arthritis and pulmonary function measures on spirometry in the UK Biobank. Arthritis Rheumatol 2021;73(11):1994–2002.

42. Kokkonen H, Brink M, Hansson M, et al. Associations of antibodies against citrullinated peptides with human leukocyte antigen-shared epitope and smoking prior to the development of rheumatoid arthritis. Arthritis Res Ther 2015;17:125.

43. Too CL, Muhamad NA, Ilar A, et al. Occupational exposure to textile dust increases the risk of rheumatoid arthritis: results from a Malaysian population-based case-control study. Ann Rheum Dis 2016;75(6):997–1002.

44. Hart JE, Källberg H, Laden F, et al. Ambient air pollution exposures and risk of rheumatoid arthritis: results from the Swedish EIRA case-control study. Ann Rheum Dis 2013;72(6):888–94.

45. Kronzer VL, Westerlind H, Alfredsson L, et al. Respiratory Diseases as Risk Factors for Seropositive and Seronegative Rheumatoid Arthritis and in Relation to Smoking. Arthritis Rheumatol 2021;73(1):61–8.

46. Svensson J, Holmqvist M, Lundberg IE, et al. Infections and respiratory tract disease as risk factors for idiopathic inflammatory myopathies: a population-based case-control study. Ann Rheum Dis 2017;76(11):1803–8.

47. St Sauver JL, Grossardt BR, Yawn BP, et al. Data resource profile: the Rochester Epidemiology Project (REP) medical records-linkage system. Int J Epidemiol 2012;41(6):1614–24.

48. Wing S, Rider LG, Johnson JR, et al. Do solar cycles influence giant cell arteritis and rheumatoid arthritis incidence? BMJ Open 2015;5(5):e006636.

49. Karlson EW, Shadick NA, Cook NR, et al. Vitamin E in the primary prevention of rheumatoid arthritis: the Women's Health Study. Arthritis Rheum 2008;59(11):1589–95.

50. Racovan M, Walitt B, Collins CE, et al. Calcium and vitamin D supplementation and incident rheumatoid arthritis: the Women's Health Initiative Calcium plus Vitamin D trial. Rheumatol Int 2012;32(12):3823–30.

51. Tang B, Shi H, Alfredsson L, et al. Obesity-related traits and the development of rheumatoid arthritis - evidence from genetic data. Arthritis Rheumatol 2020;73(2):203–11.

52. Larsson SC, Burgess S, Michaëlsson K. Genetic association between adiposity and gout: a Mendelian randomization study. Rheumatology (Oxford) 2018;57(12):2145–8.

53. Fan J, Zhu J, Sun L, et al. Causal association of adipokines with osteoarthritis: a Mendelian randomization study. Rheumatology (Oxford) 2021;60(6):2808–15.

54. Jiang X, Alfredsson L. Modifiable environmental exposure and risk of rheumatoid arthritis-current evidence from genetic studies. Arthritis Res Ther 2020;22(1):154.

55. Song GG, Bae SC, Lee YH. Association between vitamin D intake and the risk of rheumatoid arthritis: a meta-analysis. Clin Rheumatol 2012;31(12):1733–9.

56. Costenbader KH, Feskanich D, Holmes M, et al. Vitamin D intake and risks of systemic lupus erythematosus and rheumatoid arthritis in women. Ann Rheum Dis 2008;67(4):530–5.

57. Bae SC, Lee YH. Vitamin D level and risk of systemic lupus erythematosus and rheumatoid arthritis: a Mendelian randomization. Clin Rheumatol 2018;37(9):2415–21.

58. Joober R, Schmitz N, Annable L, et al. Publication bias: what are the challenges and can they be overcome? J Psychiatry Neurosci 2012;37(3):149–52.

59. Ioannidis JP. Why most published research findings are false. Plos Med 2005;2(8):e124.

60. von Elm E, Altman DG, Egger M, et al. The Strengthening the Reporting of Observational Studies in Epidemiology (STROBE) Statement: guidelines for reporting observational studies. Int J Surg 2014;12(12):1495–9.

61. Karlson EW, Boutin NT, Hoffnagle AG, et al. Building the partners healthcare biobank at partners personalized medicine: informed consent, return of research results, recruitment lessons and operational considerations. J Pers Med 2016;6(1).

62. Eder L, Shanmugarajah S, Thavaneswaran A, et al. The association between smoking and the development of psoriatic arthritis among psoriasis patients. Ann Rheum Dis 2012;71(2):219–24.

63. Pattison E, Harrison BJ, Griffiths CE, et al. Environmental risk factors for the development of psoriatic arthritis: results from a case-control study. Ann Rheum Dis 2008;67(5):672–6.

64. Nguyen UDT, Zhang Y, Lu N, et al. Smoking paradox in the development of psoriatic arthritis among patients with psoriasis: a population-based study. Ann Rheum Dis 2018;77(1):119–23.

65. Hsieh CY, Su CC, Shao SC, et al. Taiwan's National Health Insurance Research Database: past and future. Clin Epidemiol 2019;11:349–58.

66. Bakken IJ, Ariansen AMS, Knudsen GP, et al. The Norwegian Patient Registry and the Norwegian Registry for Primary Health Care: Research potential of two nationwide health-care registries. Scand J Public Health 2020;48(1):49–55.

67. Feldman SR, Zhao Y, Shi L, et al. Economic and comorbidity burden among moderate-to-severe psoriasis patients with comorbid psoriatic arthritis. Arthritis Care Res (Hoboken) 2015;67(5):708–17.

68. Kronzer VL, Huang W, Crowson CS, et al. Timing of sinusitis and other respiratory tract diseases and risk of rheumatoid arthritis. Semin Arthritis Rheum 2022;52: 151937.

69. Hudson M, Thombs B, Baron M. Time to diagnosis in systemic sclerosis: is sex a factor? Arthritis Rheum 2009;61(2):274–8.

70. Nielen MM, van Schaardenburg D, Reesink HW, et al. Specific autoantibodies precede the symptoms of rheumatoid arthritis: a study of serial measurements in blood donors. Arthritis Rheum 2004;50(2):380–6.

71. Sparks JA, Malspeis S, Hahn J, et al. Depression and subsequent risk for incident rheumatoid arthritis among women. Arthritis Care Res (Hoboken) 2020;73(1): 78–89.

72. Widdifield J, Bombardier C, Bernatsky S, et al. An administrative data validation study of the accuracy of algorithms for identifying rheumatoid arthritis: the influence of the reference standard on algorithm performance. BMC Musculoskelet Disord 2014;15:216.

73. Hazes JM, Dijkmans BA, Vandenbroucke JP, et al. Lifestyle and the risk of rheumatoid arthritis: cigarette smoking and alcohol consumption. Ann Rheum Dis 1990;49(12):980–2.

74. Crowson CS, Matteson EL, Davis JM 3rd, et al. Contribution of obesity to the rise in incidence of rheumatoid arthritis. Arthritis Care Res (Hoboken) 2013; 65(1):71–7.

75. Doran MF, Crowson CS, O'Fallon WM, et al. The effect of oral contraceptives and estrogen replacement therapy on the risk of rheumatoid arthritis: a population based study. J Rheumatol 2004;31(2):207–13.

76. Alarcón GS, Roseman J, Bartolucci AA, et al. Systemic lupus erythematosus in three ethnic groups: II. Features predictive of disease activity early in its course. LUMINA Study Group. Lupus in minority populations, nature versus nurture. Arthritis Rheum 1998;41(7):1173–80.

77. Feldon M, Farhadi PN, Brunner HI, et al. Predictors of Reduced Health-Related Quality of Life in Adult Patients With Idiopathic Inflammatory Myopathies. Arthritis Care Res (Hoboken) 2017;69(11):1743–50.

78. Vessey MP, Villard-Mackintosh L, Yeates D. Oral contraceptives, cigarette smoking and other factors in relation to arthritis. Contraception 1987;35(5):457–64.

79. Hernandez Avila M, Liang MH, Willett WC, et al. Reproductive factors, smoking, and the risk for rheumatoid arthritis. Epidemiology 1990;1(4):285–91.

80. Sparks JA, Chang SC, Nguyen UDT, et al. Smoking Behavior Changes in the Early Rheumatoid Arthritis Period and Risk of Mortality During Thirty-Six Years of Prospective Followup. Arthritis Care Res (Hoboken) 2018;70(1):19–29.

81. Källberg H, Jacobsen S, Bengtsson C, et al. Alcohol consumption is associated with decreased risk of rheumatoid arthritis: results from two Scandinavian case-control studies. Ann Rheum Dis 2009;68(2):222–7.

82. Sundström B, Johansson I, Rantapää-Dahlqvist S. Diet and alcohol as risk factors for rheumatoid arthritis: a nested case-control study. Rheumatol Int 2015;35(3): 533–9.
83. Bae SC, Lee YH. Alcohol intake and risk of rheumatoid arthritis: a Mendelian randomization study. Z Rheumatol 2019;78(8):791–6.
84. Qu Z, Yang F, Hong J, et al. Causal relationship of serum nutritional factors with osteoarthritis: a Mendelian randomization study. Rheumatology (Oxford) 2021; 60(5):2383–90.
85. Zeng Z, Zhang W, Qian Y, et al. Association of telomere length with risk of rheumatoid arthritis: a meta-analysis and Mendelian randomization. Rheumatology (Oxford) 2020;59(5):940–7.
86. Crowson CS, Matteson EL, Myasoedova E, et al. The lifetime risk of adult-onset rheumatoid arthritis and other inflammatory autoimmune rheumatic diseases. Arthritis Rheum 2011;63(3):633–9.
87. Bao Y, Bertoia ML, Lenart EB, et al. Origin, Methods, and Evolution of the Three Nurses' Health Studies. Am J Public Health 2016;106(9):1573–81.
88. Lee HS, Irigoyen P, Kern M, et al. Interaction between smoking, the shared epitope, and anti-cyclic citrullinated peptide: a mixed picture in three large North American rheumatoid arthritis cohorts. Arthritis Rheum 2007;56(6):1745–53.
89. Merlino LA, Curtis J, Mikuls TR, et al. Vitamin D intake is inversely associated with rheumatoid arthritis: results from the Iowa Women's Health Study. Arthritis Rheum 2004;50(1):72–7.

Inhalant and Additional Mucosal-Related Environmental Risks for Rheumatoid Arthritis

Brent A. Luedders, MD[a,b], Ted R. Mikuls, MD, MSPH[a,b],
Geoffrey M. Thiele, PhD[a,b], Jill A. Poole, MD[c],
Bryant R. England, MD, PhD[a,b,*]

KEYWORDS

- Rheumatoid arthritis • Autoantibodies • Anticitrullinated protein antibodies
- Autoimmunity • Mucosal inflammation

KEY POINTS

- Several inhalant exposures, including cigarette smoke, silica, and other occupational exposures, have been associated with an increased odds of developing rheumatoid arthritis (RA) in epidemiologic studies.
- Articular and lung manifestations in RA demonstrate a bidirectional temporal relationship with airway and lung parenchymal involvement most frequently developing after arthritis, although lung disease may be the initial presenting finding.
- Mucosal surfaces, particularly those within the airways and lungs, may be early sites of RA-related autoimmunity.
- Dysbiosis of the microbiome of the gut, oral, and lung mucosa has been identified in RA patients and may have a pathogenic role in RA.

INTRODUCTION

Rheumatoid arthritis (RA) is a chronic autoimmune disease with the classic clinical manifestations being symmetric inflammatory arthritis of the small joints. Extra-articular manifestations such as subcutaneous nodules, osteoporosis, cardiovascular disease, and lung disease, among others, are also common and illustrate the systematic nature of RA. The heritability of RA is estimated to be between 25% and 50%, with *HLA-DRB1* alleles accounting for the strongest genetic risk.[1,2] Many studies have

[a] Division of Rheumatology & Immunology, University of Nebraska Medical Center, 986270 Nebraska Medical Center, Omaha, NE 68198-6270, USA; [b] VA Nebraska-Western Iowa Health Care System, 4101 Woolworth Avenue, Omaha, NE 68105, USA; [c] Division of Allergy & Immunology, University of Nebraska Medical Center, 985990 Nebraska Medical Center, Omaha, NE 68198-5990, USA
* Corresponding author. 986270 Nebraska Medicine, Omaha, NE 68198-6270.
E-mail address: Bryant.england@unmc.edu

Rheum Dis Clin N Am 48 (2022) 781–798
https://doi.org/10.1016/j.rdc.2022.06.002
0889-857X/22/Published by Elsevier Inc.

been conducted to identify environmental risk factors for RA as well as their potential gene-environment interactions.[3] A growing body of evidence suggests that exposures or diseases causing inflammation of the lung, oral, or gastrointestinal mucosa may affect RA risk by affecting early tolerance loss, with the early initiation and propagation of RA-related autoimmunity occurring at these mucosal sites. This review highlights some of the recent advances in the understanding of inhalant- and other mucosal-related risk factors for RA.

INHALANTS AND THE LUNG MUCOSA
Cigarette Smoking

The association between cigarette smoking and the risk of RA is well established, serving perhaps as a prototypical link between lung mucosal and inhalant exposures with the development of RA (**Table 1**). A 2010 meta-analysis of 16 studies estimated that cigarette smoking was associated with a 2-fold higher risk of RA.[4] This effect was strongest in men and for seropositive RA.[4] A dose-response relationship between cigarette smoking and RA exists, though cigarette smoke exposure beyond 20-pack-years has little additional impact on RA risk.[5] In addition, a gene-environment interaction occurs in which cigarette smoking among individuals with *HLA-DRB1* shared epitope alleles markedly increases the risk of seropositive RA.[6] It has been estimated that smoking is responsible for 35% of cases of anticitrullinated protein antibody (ACPA)-positive RA, increasing to 55% among subjects that are dual positive for shared epitope alleles.[7] Therefore, the elimination of cigarette smoking as an environmental exposure would substantially reduce the incidence of RA, preventing up to 1 in 2 cases among those with the greatest genetic predisposition. Importantly, the elevated risk associated with cigarette smoking seems to decrease after smoking cessation, although some residual risk is still evident even 30 years after smoking cessation.[8] In contrast, studies evaluating passive (or "second-hand") cigarette smoke exposure have not consistently demonstrated clear associations between second-hand smoke exposure and disease risk,[9–11] though passive smoke exposure at certain time points in life, such as in childhood, may predispose to the development of RA in later life.[12] Beyond its impact on developing RA, cigarette smoking may increase the risk of other disease consequences including higher disease activity, poorer treatment response, and the development of RA-related lung disease, cardiovascular disease, and lung cancer.[13–15]

Occupational Exposures

In addition to cigarette smoking, other environmental and occupational exposures (**Table 2**) are thought to increase RA risk by stimulating immune responses within the respiratory mucosa. Occupational inhalation exposure to silica during work-related activities such as sand-blasting or concrete/brick sawing or drilling has consistently been implicated as a risk factor for RA. Meta-analyses of epidemiologic studies have estimated a 2-fold higher odds of developing RA among those exposed to silica, an effect that, similar to cigarette smoking, appears to be stronger for seropositive RA and among those who have ever smoked.[16,17] Bricklayers, concrete workers, material handling operators, and electrical and electronics workers were found to have an increased odds of developing RA independent of cigarette smoking and other risk factors in a Swedish Epidemiologic Investigation of Rheumatoid Arthritis (EIRA) case-control study,[18] an effect that was hypothesized to relate to noxious airborne occupational exposures other than silica. Among a population of older males residing in the Appalachian region of the United States, previous work in coal mining, an

Table 1
Association of cigarette smoking exposures with rheumatoid arthritis

Exposure Type	Evidence of Association with RA
Ever smoking	
Overall	In a meta-analysis of epidemiologic studies, ever smoking was associated with an increased risk of RA (OR 1.40) compared to never smoking. Similarly, the OR for current smoking was increased at 1.35, whereas past smoking was associated with a lower but significant OR of 1.25.[4]
Sex	Smoking seems to have a greater impact on RA risk among men compared to women. In a meta-analysis, ever smoking showed a greater association with RA among men (OR 1.89) than among women (OR 1.27).[4]
Seropositivity	The risk incurred by cigarette smoking is greatest for the development of seropositive RA. In a meta-analysis, ever smoking was more strongly associated with RF-positive RA (OR 1.66) than with all RA (OR 1.40). This increased risk was especially prominent among men (OR 3.2 for RF-positive RA vs 1.89 for all RA).[4]
Duration/intensity of smoking exposure	A meta-analysis of 3 prospective cohort and 7 case-control studies showed an increase in the risk of RA as pack-years of smoking increased, with a plateau around a 20 pack-year smoking history[5] RR for 1–10 pack-years = 1.26 (1.14, 1.39) RR for 11–20 pack-years = 1.70 (1.44, 2.01) RR for 21–30 pack-years = 1.94 (1.65, 2.27) RR for 31–40 pack years = 2.02 (1.44, 2.82) RR for > 40 pack-years = 2.07 (1.15, 3.73)
Passive smoke exposure	In case-control studies, there was no significant association between passive smoke exposure and RA.[10,11] In a French cohort, passive smoke exposure during childhood showed a borderline, but not statistically significant, increased risk of RA in adulthood both among never-smokers and ever-smokers.[9] In the NHS prospective cohort, parental smoking during childhood was associated with seropositive RA in adulthood (HR 1.41).[12]
Smoking cessation	In the NHS prospective cohort, sustained smoking cessation was associated with a lower risk of developing RA compared to current smoking or recent cessation, and was more pronounced as the duration of smoking cessation increased.[8] HR never smoker = 1 (referent) HR quit smoking 0–5 y ago = 1.57 (1.26, 1.95) HR quit smoking 5–10 y ago = 1.63 (1.30, 2.04) HR quit smoking 10–20 y ago = 1.37 (1.15, 1.64) HR quit smoking 20–30 y ago = 1.19 (0.99, 1.45) HR quit smoking >30 y ago = 1.25 (1.02, 1.53)
Gene-environment interaction	A significant gene-environment interaction exists between smoking and shared epitope alleles for seropositive RA, as illustrated by the following results from a Swedish case-control study:[81] RR for nonsmokers with 0 SE alleles = 1 (referent) RR for nonsmokers with 1 SE allele = 3.3 (1.8, 5.9) RR for nonsmokers with 2 SE alleles = 5.4 (2.7, 10.8) RR for smokers with 0 SE alleles = 1.5 (0.8, 2.6) RR for smokers with 1 SE allele = 6.5 (3.8, 11.4) RR for smokers with 2 SE alleles: = 21.0 (11.0, 40.2)

Abbreviations: HR, hazard ratio; NHS, Nurses' Health Study; OR, odds ratio; RF, rheumatoid factor; RR, relative risk; SE, shared epitope.

Table 2
Inhalant exposures associated with rheumatoid arthritis

Inhalant Exposure	Evidence	Association with Seropositive vs Seronegative Disease	Gene-Environment or Environment-Environment Interactions
Silica	Meta-analysis of 12 epidemiologic studies found silica exposure to be associated with a nearly 2-fold increased odds of RA[17]	Silica exposure most closely associated with seropositive disease (OR 1.7) although associations also observed for seronegative RA (OR 1.2) in meta-analysis of 7 studies[17]	Unknown
Coal mining	Coal mining associated with RA (OR 3.6) in random telephone survey of 973 Appalachian men aged ≥ 50 y [19]	Unknown	While exposure to silica may co-occur with exposure to coal dust, coal mining seems to be independently associated with RA risk[19]
Military exposure	Reported exposure to burn pits was associated with seropositivity among a population of known RA patients,[21] but deployment within a 3-mile radius of burn pits was not associated with a self-reported diagnosis of RA.[22] Among a sample of 438,086 veterans, inorganic dust exposure during military service estimated via military occupation codes was associated with RA (OR 1.10) defined by ICD codes.[23]	Anti-CCP antibodies were more common among US veterans with RA reporting exposure to military burn pits (OR 1.7).[21] Inorganic dust exposure was associated with seronegative (OR 1.25) but not seropositive RA.[23]	Association of burn pits with anti-CCP antibodies stronger (OR increased from 1.7 to 5.7) among those positive for shared epitope alleles[21]

Pesticides	Among a large cohort of women, a significant trend was observed with more frequent and more direct/personal application of pesticides in childhood (OR 1.8 for direct and frequent use).[25] Among women with childhood-only farm residence, RA was associated with a history of personal exposure to pesticide use on crops (OR 1.8) and livestock (OR 2.0).[25]	Unknown	Unknown
Airborne pollutants and particulate matter	Mixed findings; meta-analysis found positive associations with RA and ozone exposure (RR 1.16) and close proximity to roadway (RR 1.34), with 2 eligible studies for each respective exposure. In contrast, no association was observed between RA and particulate matter, NO_2, CO, or SO_2 (range of 2–5 studies per exposure).[27]	Fine particulate matter associated with anti-CCP antibody concentration, but not RF, in 557 veterans with established RA[29]	Unknown

Abbreviations: CCP, cyclic citrullinated peptide; CO, carbon monoxide; ICD, International Classification of Diseases; NO_2, nitrogen dioxide; OR, odds ratio; RF, rheumatoid factor; SO_2, sulfur dioxide.

occupation associated with inhalational exposures to coal, silica, and other mineral dusts, was estimated to contribute to 33% of the risk for RA after adjusting for smoking and other risk factors.[19] This was higher than the population attributable fraction estimated for silica (10%), and no interaction between coal mining and silica was observed.[19] In a study of September 11th World Trade Center rescue and recovery workers compared to controls, there were increased odds of developing autoimmune disease (of which RA was the most common diagnosis) among exposed workers, and these odds increased with longer periods of exposure.[20]

Several studies of inhalant exposures have been conducted among those who served in the military. Among a US cohort of veterans with RA, reported exposure to military burn pits was associated with 1.7-fold higher odds of anti-cyclic citrullinated peptide (CCP) antibody positivity, which was increased to 5.7-fold higher odds among those who were positive for shared epitope alleles.[21] This is in contrast to an earlier study that did not find a significant association between close proximity to burn pits and the development of RA in the Millennium Cohort Study, although this study was limited by a low number of RA cases and short duration of follow-up.[22] Finally, among a sample of US veterans serving during Iraq and Afghanistan wars, military inorganic dust exposure determined by occupational codes was associated with a small (10%), but significantly higher, rate of RA development.[23]

Occupational tasks including the application of chemical fertilizers, painting, and the use of solvents have also been associated with an increased odds of developing RA (hazard ratios ranging from 1.26 to 1.50) among pesticide applicators and their spouses.[24] In addition, the frequent direct or indirect use of pesticides at childhood residence, as well as reported exposure to pesticide use on a childhood farm, have been associated with increased odds of developing RA later in adulthood.[25] Although epidemiologic links between the aforementioned occupational exposures and the risk of developing RA are still being elucidated, it is poorly understood whether these occupational inhalant exposures are associated with disease severity or other relevant disease-related outcomes.[21]

Pollution and Particulates

Airborne pollution and particulate matter (including carbon dioxide, ozone precursors, black carbon, sulfate, nitrogen oxides, volatile organic compounds, and particulate organic material) generated from human influences such as burning fossil fuels (eg, power plants, vehicles) and biomass, as well as naturally occurring events (eg, forest fires, dust storms), have been implicated in numerous health conditions.[26] Limited studies investigating these exposures as risk factors for RA have yielded mixed results (see **Table 2**). Higher levels of ozone (O_3) exposure as well as closer proximity to roadways, a proxy for air pollution, were associated with RA in a meta-analysis of epidemiologic studies.[27] In contrast, there was no association between nitrogen dioxide (NO_2), carbon monoxide (CO), and sulfur dioxide (SO_2) exposures with RA, and there appeared to be an inverse association between exposure to fine particulate matter (<2.5 μm) and incident RA.[27] The conclusions that can be drawn from this meta-analysis are limited by the small number of eligible studies (range of 2–5 studies evaluating each individual exposure), substantial heterogeneity among the included studies, and likely bias related to confounding (eg, socioeconomic status) given the geographic variables used in some studies. Further investigations evaluating the potential roles of airborne pollutants and particulate matter with regard to RA risk are warranted.

These same exposures have been studied in at-risk and established RA populations. Among first-degree relatives of RA patients, greater exposure to particulate matter by residential zip codes and ambient air pollution monitoring data was not associated with the presence of RA-related autoantibodies or tender/swollen joint counts.[28] In contrast, particulate matter exposure (defined using the same data sources) was associated with ACPA concentration in US veterans with established RA.[29]

Biologic mechanisms underpinning the link between airborne pollutants (as well as other inhalant exposures) and RA are not well understood. In recent efforts, investigators have leveraged novel animal modeling approaches to help elucidate the mechanisms linking different inhalant exposures to RA pathogenesis and RA clinical manifestations.[30–33] These models have used the collagen-induced arthritis model in DBA/1J mice in addition to intranasal treatment with organic dust extract, an agriculture-related extract that induces airway inflammation, or lipopolysaccharide, a ubiquitous inflammatory agent found in many different environmental exposures that triggers airway inflammation. Initial findings from these models of particular importance include sex differences in disease expression following these exposures, susceptibility to lung disease, and transitions of inflammatory lung manifestations to fibrotic disease.[30–33]

Lung and Articular Disease in Rheumatoid Arthritis—A Bidirectional Relationship

The aforementioned data linking several inhalant exposures with disease risk build upon the clinical recognition that lung diseases are over-represented in RA. Pulmonary manifestations have long been recognized as a complication of RA and can include interstitial lung disease (ILD) targeting the lung parenchyma, nodules, airway inflammatory diseases, and pleural disease.[34] Although understood that RA can be responsible for the development of lung disease, there is now mounting evidence that lung disease may be a risk factor for developing RA. These findings suggest the possibility of a bidirectional relationship between the articular disease that is most characteristic of RA and the less frequent manifestation of lung disease. As an illustration of this potential bidirectionality, up to 14% of patients with RA-ILD from a population-based Danish cohort were diagnosed with ILD 1 to 5 years before being diagnosed with RA.[35]

Recent studies examining lower and upper respiratory tract disorders have suggested these conditions may also be associated with an increased risk of developing RA. In a meta-analysis, preexisting asthma was associated with a 1.4-fold higher risk of developing RA using pooled data from 6 cohort studies. Although a similar association was present among 14 case-control studies, it did not reach statistical significance.[36] There was also a high degree of heterogeneity among both the cohort and case-control studies in this meta-analysis, which may be related to differences in the classification of asthma and RA (eg, diagnostic codes vs self-report), variable confounder adjustment, and concern for publication bias of positive findings.[36] In addition to asthma, the presence of chronic obstructive pulmonary disease (COPD) was associated with a near 2-fold higher risk of developing RA in the Nurses' Health Study.[37] Similarly, a case-control study using the Swedish EIRA cohort found acute and chronic lower respiratory diseases to be associated with RA, particularly seropositive RA.[38] This same study observed a weaker association between chronic, but not acute, upper respiratory disease and RA, findings that were more pronounced among nonsmokers.[38] Findings are conflicting on whether allergic rhinitis is associated with RA risk.[39] Respiratory infections have also been suggested as risk factors for the development of RA. Using an ecological study design, incident RA was found to be more likely to develop during the weeks following peaks of respiratory viral infections including parainfluenza virus, coronavirus, and metapneumovirus.[40] Cases of new-onset RA have been reported after infection with SARS-CoV-2, the etiologic agent of COVID-19,[41] but larger epidemiologic studies are needed to determine whether a true association exists.

Lung Microbiome

Although initially thought to be a sterile mucosal site, differences in the composition of the lung microbiome in patients with various lung diseases versus healthy individuals have established that the lung microbiome exists and that lung microbial diversity may accompany or contribute to disease risk.[42] Little is known about the role of the lung microbiome in RA compared to the more commonly studied mucosal sites such as the gastrointestinal tract or oral cavity in RA. In a small cross-sectional study, patients with early DMARD-naïve RA were found to have a lower microbial diversity in fluid samples obtained via bronchoalveolar lavage (BAL) and evaluated by 16S rRNA sequencing compared to healthy controls.[43] Namely, *Actinomyces* and *Burkholderia* as well as some periodontopathic taxa (eg, *Prevotella*) were decreased in RA, findings that were similarly observed in patients with pulmonary sarcoidosis.[43] In contrast to controls and sarcoidosis patients, BAL fluid of RA patients showed increased levels of *Pseudonocardia*,[43] although little is understood about the role of this genus in RA pathogenesis. Further characterization of the lung microbiome in RA, RA-associated lung diseases, and at-risk populations is needed to better understand its potential role in the development and perpetuation of RA, which may later facilitate its use as an indicator of risk and as a potential therapeutic or preventive target.

The Lungs and Rheumatoid Arthritis-Related Autoimmunity

Several of the previously described epidemiologic studies linking inhalant exposures with RA have observed stronger associations with seropositive RA, suggesting that the lungs may be an early site of autoimmunity. Supporting these epidemiologic data, ACPAs have been detected in the sputum of established RA patients[44] as well as first-degree relatives of RA patients (ie, at-risk for RA), including some who lacked ACPAs in the serum.[44,45] Smoking, an established risk factor for RA, has been shown to increase citrullination and levels of peptidylarginine deiminase 2 (PAD-2) on BAL cells of healthy smokers relative to nonsmokers.[46] Antibodies to PAD-4, which can increase PAD-4 activity in vitro, have also been found in the sputum of RA patients,[47] suggesting that these antibodies may play a role in driving RA-related autoimmunity in the lungs. Further supporting shared immune responses in the lungs and the joints, biopsy specimens from the lungs and synovium of RA patients revealed shared citrullinated peptides, including citrullinated vimentin, at both sites.[48]

Immunoglobulin A (IgA) is the second most prevalent immunoglobulin in the serum but represents the primary immunoglobulin present at mucosal surfaces. At mucosal surfaces, IgA is present in a secretory form consisting of a dimer of 2 IgA molecules linked by a J chain and complexed with a secretory component.[49] During the development of disease-specific autoimmunity that typically precedes RA onset, rheumatoid factor (RF) IgA has been shown to be present several years before other RF isotypes in preclinical banked serum of RA patients.[50] In contrast, IgA ACPA does not appear to predate other ACPA isotypes during the evolution of preclinical autoimmunity.[50] Circulating IgA, as well as IgG, anti-malondialdehyde-acetaldehyde (MAA) antibodies also predate clinically apparent RA, but appear after RF and ACPAs.[51] Secretory IgA ACPA has been detected in the serum of a subset of early RA patients and was more likely to be present among ever smokers compared to nonsmokers.[52] Furthermore, levels of free secretory component (not bound to IgA) in the blood have been shown to be elevated in early RA patients compared to controls and associate with both ACPA and smoking,[53] These elevations in IgA antibodies and related secretory component of pre and early RA patients suggest the possibility that mucosal irritants, such as smoking or other inhalant exposures, may lead to citrullination and other post-translational protein modifications in the lungs with the potential to drive an early auto-immune response that could ultimately lead to clinically apparent RA.

The presence of RA-related autoimmunity may not only indicate a risk of developing articular features of RA, but also lung abnormalities. First-degree relatives of RA patients who were without inflammatory arthritis but positive for either ACPA and/or ≥2 RF isotypes were more likely to have high-resolution computed tomography (HRCT) abnormalities including bronchial wall thickening, air trapping, and airways disease compared to autoantibody-negative controls. These HRCT findings were similar to early RA patients within the same cohort suggesting that, like the measurement of autoantibodies, detectable airway disease may precede disease onset.[54] Similarly, in a cohort of patients with recently diagnosed RA, a higher number of ACPA fine specificities was associated with parenchymal abnormalities on HRCT.[55] The presence of serum ACPA secretory component in early RA patients has also been associated with parenchymal abnormalities on HRCT.[56]

Findings from patients with RA-associated lung disease may provide insights into RA-related autoimmunity in the lungs. Organized lymphoid aggregates were discovered on lung biopsy specimens from patients with RA-associated ILD (RA-ILD), termed inducible bronchus-associated lymphoid tissue (iBALT), but much less frequently or not at all in other lung disorders such as idiopathic pulmonary fibrosis.[57] Moreover, these iBALT aggregates had elevated levels of PAD-2, which facilitate citrullination of peptides, as well RF- and ACPA-producing plasma cells.[57] Bronchiectasis, another RA-associated lung disease,[58] has additionally been proposed as a model for the loss of immune tolerance and development of autoimmunity. In a cross-sectional study, patients with bronchiectasis and without RA were shown to have increased frequencies of ACPA when compared to healthy controls, which correlated with the presence of antibodies to related arginine-containing peptides.[59] However, among patients with bronchiectasis and RA, the autoantibody response was specific for ACPA and did not correlate with antibodies to arginine-containing peptides. It was hypothesized that chronic exposure to citrullinated peptides in the inflamed lung with bronchiectasis may facilitate epitope spreading and a citrulline-specific autoimmune response.[59] These thought-provoking findings require further validation.

ADDITIONAL MUCOSAL SITES

In addition to the lungs, evidence has accumulated supporting a role for other mucosal sites, such as the oral and gut mucosa, in RA pathogenesis. At these sites, the microbiome has been of particular interest, with dysbiosis of the oral and gut microbiota of RA patients being identified through sequencing of fecal, oral, and dental samples.[60] Given the female predominance of RA, the urogenital tract has also been speculated as a possible site of RA risk, although data on this site remain limited.[61]

Periodontal disease and the oral microbiota

Oral health has been linked to systemic diseases and RA since ancient times. A meta-analysis of 17 studies comparing RA patients to healthy controls showed a modestly (~13%) increased risk of periodontitis among RA patients, although there was a large degree of heterogeneity among the included studies.[62] In this same study, subanalyses were completed on 4 studies comparing RA and osteoarthritis (OA) patients, finding no significant difference in the prevalence of periodontitis. Again, there was substantial heterogeneity and negative findings were driven largely by a single, relatively small study.[62] Given the largely cross-sectional nature of these studies, it is difficult to determine whether the link between periodontal disease and RA is one of causality or instead related to shared risk factors (eg, cigarette smoking) or a consequence of systemic disease. Suggesting the possibility that periodontal disease predates the clinically apparent RA, ACPA-positive patients without clinical arthritis were found to have a higher prevalence of periodontal disease and increased abundance of the periodontal-related pathogen *Porphyromonas gingivalis* compared to controls.[63] In addition to being more common among RA patients, periodontitis may also be associated with a more severe RA disease course.[64]

P gingivalis has been the subject of much of the research regarding the role of the oral microbiota in the pathogenesis of RA. This is predominantly related to *P gingivalis* possessing its own unique active PAD enzymes (PPAD), which may contribute to the citrullination of human proteins.[65] However, interest has extended beyond *P gingivalis*, more broadly characterizing the oral microbiota in patients with RA. In a study of new-onset, DMARD-naïve, seropositive RA patients, subgingival biofilm samples evaluated with 16S rRNA sequencing showed no significant differences in microbial richness or diversity when compared to established RA or non-RA controls.[66] Rather, differences in microbial composition at various taxonomic levels were explained by the presence or absence of periodontal disease.[66] Similarly, the prevalence and abundance of *P gingivalis* did not correlate with the presence of RA, but rather with moderate-to severe periodontal disease in this study.[66] A subsequent case-control study of RA and OA patients again showed no compelling differences in the subgingival microbiome related to RA status, but distinctive microbial patterns based on the presence versus absence of periodontal disease.[67] In contrast, a microbiome analysis of salivary samples was performed among RA and OA patients, which was able to discriminate between diseases with high accuracy with 8 bacterial biomarkers.[68] *Aggregatibacter actinomycetemcomitans* is another pathogen in the oral cavity hypothesized to have implications in RA pathogenesis. Incubation of neutrophils with *A actinomycetemcomitans,* but not other microbial species, has been shown to induce hypercitrullination in vitro.[69] This is relevant to RA pathogenesis because the pattern of hypercitrullination in the periodontal microenvironment is similar to that in RA synovium.[69]

With several studies identifying periodontal disease as a risk factor for RA and a more severe disease course, it is possible that the treatment of periodontal disease may prevent RA onset, or if already present, leads to improved RA control. No trials have evaluated RA prevention through periodontal treatment and only a few small trials have evaluated periodontal treatment for RA control. In a meta-analysis of 9 smaller clinical trials (n $\leq$ 60), patients randomized to nonsurgical periodontal treatment had a moderately (approximately half the minimum important difference) greater improvement in clinical disease activity (disease activity score in 28 joints [DAS28]) compared to controls.[70] The impact of periodontal treatment on individual components of composite clinical measures and other inflammatory cytokines were less consistent. Tender and swollen joint counts as well as C-reactive protein (CRP) tended to improve among those receiving periodontal treatment, but no significant difference was seen for erythrocyte sedimentation rate (ESR), interleukin-6 (IL-6), or tumor necrosis factor alpha (TNF-α).[70]

Gut microbiota

Marked advances have occurred in the understanding of how the gut microbiome contributes to health and disease. Specific to RA, studies over the last decade have demonstrated differences in the microbiome of patients with RA when compared to healthy controls and other inflammatory disease states, including an over-representation of *Prevotella copri*. Through the use of 16S rRNA sequencing of stool samples, Scher and colleagues[71] demonstrated that treatment-naive, new-onset RA patients had a markedly higher rate of carriage of *P copri* in their intestinal microbiota

(77%) compared to healthy controls (21%). Similarly, in a cohort of first-degree relatives of RA patients, those with RA-related autoimmunity and/or signs/symptoms of possible RA had increased levels of *P copri* in stool samples when compared to controls lacking these characteristics.[72] Further supporting a possible pathogenic role of *P copri* in RA, a subset of patients with new-onset RA have been shown to have Th1 responses to *P copri* peptides.[73] Moreover, serum antibody responses to *P copri* have been detected in a subset of both new-onset and chronic RA patients, a finding encountered only rarely among individuals with other rheumatic diseases and healthy controls.[73] A Mendelian randomization study did not find a causal link between the gut microbiome and RA risk,[74] but there were questions regarding the degree to which genetics influence the gut microbiome and their suitability as instrumental variables.[75]

Although alterations in the microbiome may contribute to RA onset, treatment of RA with DMARDs appears to partially restore a healthy oral and gut microbiome in a subset of patients, particularly among those with a good clinical response to therapy.[60] Treatment specifically with methotrexate, the anchor drug for RA, has been demonstrated to lead to shifts in the gut microbiome.[76] Moreover, machine learning–derived models from pretreatment metagenomic gut microbiome data have shown an ability to predict methotrexate response in a small cohort of new-onset RA patients.[77] Data from healthy adults have suggested that even a single course of minocycline or other antibiotics can lead to long-lasting shifts in the composition of the intestinal microbiome, whereas the salivary microbiome was shown to be more resistant to these changes.[78] It is conceivable that the observed beneficial effects of minocycline in the treatment of RA[79] may partially be related to its impact on the microbiome of the gut or other sites (eg, oral microbiome).

DISCUSSION

Mounting evidence supports the notion that the risk of developing RA is multifactorial and impacted by many genetic and environmental factors (**Fig. 1**). Particularly among individuals who carry *HLA-DRB1* risk alleles, environmental exposures and diseases affecting the respiratory tract act as major risk factors for the development of RA, with a leading theory being that the lung mucosa may be an initial site of autoimmunity in RA. Exposures and diseases at other mucosal sites including the oral cavity and gastrointestinal tract similarly seem capable of stimulating immune responses characteristic of RA. However, the totality of the epidemiologic and translational evidence for these mucosal sites is less than for the lungs. Although this review has focused on mucosal-related triggers of RA, it is important to understand that environmental risk factors very likely influence RA risk through mechanisms beyond the mucosa. A key question moving forward is how mucosal and nonmucosal factors interact to affect RA risk as well as disease phenotype across various populations, such as in men and women or those defined by autoantibody status.

As our understanding of these risk factors has improved, a future step will be harnessing and applying this information to prevent RA. Given the many different environmental risk factors for RA, a detailed personalized risk assessment will ultimately prove valuable for identifying relevant risks at an individual level. Disclosure of these risks has the potential to motivate healthy behaviors.[80] Cigarette smoking cessation, use of an appropriate mask when exposed to noxious inhalants, good dental hygiene, and adhering to a healthy diet may eventually be recommended by clinicians as part of a personalized approach not only for minimizing RA risk and burden but also for general health benefits yielded from these indicated (and relatively low cost) interventions. Ultimately, the development and implementation of effective RA prevention strategies

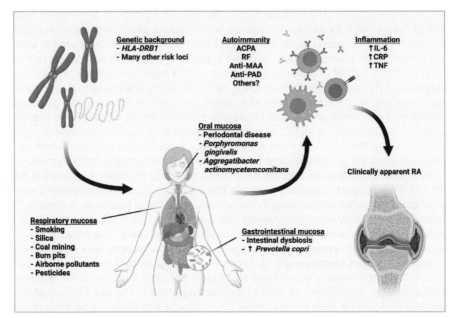

Fig. 1. Contribution of environmental exposures at mucosal surfaces to the development of clinically apparent RA. Genetic variants predispose to RA, with the most established genetic risk variant being *HLA-DRB1* shared epitope alleles. Many environmental exposures have been associated with the development of RA, with relevant exposures at respiratory, oral, and gastrointestinal mucosal sites being shown. Following environmental exposures in a genetically susceptible individual, RA-related autoimmunity and inflammation develop, frequently preceding clinically apparent RA by several years. *Created with* BioRender.com.

that target the reviewed environmental risk factors could dramatically reduce the morbidity, mortality, and exorbitant costs that accompany RA.

SUMMARY

Inhalant exposures including cigarette smoking and a variety of other occupational and environmental biohazard exposures are associated with a higher risk of developing RA. Similarly, respiratory diseases such as asthma, COPD, and infections have been linked to RA risk, though the relative contributions of these diseases versus the environmental exposures that led to these diseases largely remain to be determined. Beyond the respiratory tract, periodontal disease and alterations of the oral and gastrointestinal microbiome are more common in patients with RA and likely influence disease risk. RA-related autoimmunity occurring with or before the development of clinically apparent RA may be originating at these mucosal surfaces as a result of genetic predisposition and relevant environmental exposures.

CLINICS CARE POINTS

- Many exposures at the respiratory, oral, and gastrointestinal mucosa have been associated with the development of RA, and mitigation of these risk factors may help to decrease the individual and societal burden of RA.

- Environmental inhalant exposures may incite autoantibody responses within the lungs that predate the onset of clinically apparent RA as well as contribute to the development of RA-associated lung diseases.

- Dysregulation of the oral, gastrointestinal, and respiratory microbiome has been identified in RA patients, and elucidating the role of the microbiome in disease pathogenesis and its effects on treatment response may help guide RA management in the future.

FUNDING

B.R. England received support from the VA CSR&D (IK2 CX002203). T.R. Mikuls is supported by the VA BLR&D (I01 BX004660), the Department of Defense (PR200793), the Rheumatology Research Foundation, and the National Institute of General Medical Sciences (U54 GM115458). G.M. Thiele receives funding from the VA BLR&D (I01 BX004660), the Department of Defense (PR200793), and the NIH (R01 AR077607). J.A. Poole receives funding from the Department of Defense (PR200793) and National Institute for Occupational Safety and Health (R01OH012045 and U54OH010162).

DISCLOSURE

B.A. Luedders none. T.R. Mikuls has consulted with Pfizer, Sanofi, Gilead, Horizon and received research funding from Bristol-Myers Squibb and Horizon. G.M. Thiele serves as a speaker for unbranded information for Sanofi/Regeneron. J.A. Poole has received research grant funding from AstraZeneca. B.R. England has consulted with Boehringer-Ingelheim.

REFERENCES

1. Frisell T, Holmqvist M, Kallberg H, et al. Familial risks and heritability of rheumatoid arthritis: role of rheumatoid factor/anti-citrullinated protein antibody status, number and type of affected relatives, sex, and age. Arthritis Rheum 2013; 65(11):2773–82.
2. Raychaudhuri S, Sandor C, Stahl EA, et al. Five amino acids in three HLA proteins explain most of the association between MHC and seropositive rheumatoid arthritis. Nat Genet 2012;44(3):291–6.
3. Deane KD, Demoruelle MK, Kelmenson LB, et al. Genetic and environmental risk factors for rheumatoid arthritis. Best Pract Res Clin Rheumatol 2017; 31(1):3–18.
4. Sugiyama D, Nishimura K, Tamaki K, et al. Impact of smoking as a risk factor for developing rheumatoid arthritis: a meta-analysis of observational studies. Ann Rheum Dis 2010;69(1):70–81.
5. Di Giuseppe D, Discacciati A, Orsini N, et al. Cigarette smoking and risk of rheumatoid arthritis: a dose-response meta-analysis. Arthritis Res Ther 2014; 16(2):R61.
6. Lundström E, Källberg H, Alfredsson L, et al. Gene-environment interaction between the DRB1 shared epitope and smoking in the risk of anti-citrullinated protein antibody-positive rheumatoid arthritis: all alleles are important. Arthritis Rheum 2009;60(6):1597–603.
7. Källberg H, Ding B, Padyukov L, et al. Smoking is a major preventable risk factor for rheumatoid arthritis: estimations of risks after various exposures to cigarette smoke. Ann Rheum Dis 2011;70(3):508–11.

8. Liu X, Tedeschi SK, Barbhaiya M, et al. Impact and timing of smoking cessation on reducing risk of rheumatoid arthritis among women in the nurses' health studies. Arthritis Care Res (Hoboken) 2019;71(7):914–24.

9. Seror R, Henry J, Gusto G, et al. Passive smoking in childhood increases the risk of developing rheumatoid arthritis. Rheumatology (Oxford, England) 2019;58(7): 1154–62.

10. Hedström AK, Klareskog L, Alfredsson L. Exposure to passive smoking and rheumatoid arthritis risk: results from the Swedish EIRA study. Ann Rheum Dis 2018; 77(7):970–2.

11. Kronzer VL, Crowson CS, Sparks JA, et al. Investigating Asthma, Allergic Disease, Passive Smoke Exposure, and Risk of Rheumatoid Arthritis. Arthritis Rheumatol (Hoboken, NJ) 2019;71(8):1217–24.

12. Yoshida K, Wang J, Malspeis S, et al. Passive Smoking Throughout the Life Course and the Risk of Incident Rheumatoid Arthritis in Adulthood Among Women. Arthritis Rheumatol (Hoboken, NJ) 2021;73(12):2219–28.

13. Joseph RM, Movahedi M, Dixon WG, et al. Smoking-Related Mortality in Patients With Early Rheumatoid Arthritis: A Retrospective Cohort Study Using the Clinical Practice Research Datalink. Arthritis Care Res 2016;68(11):1598–606.

14. Gwinnutt JM, Verstappen SM, Humphreys JH. The impact of lifestyle behaviours, physical activity and smoking on morbidity and mortality in patients with rheumatoid arthritis. Best Pract Res Clin Rheumatol 2020;34(2):101562.

15. Saevarsdottir S, Wedren S, Seddighzadeh M, et al. Patients with early rheumatoid arthritis who smoke are less likely to respond to treatment with methotrexate and tumor necrosis factor inhibitors: observations from the Epidemiological Investigation of Rheumatoid Arthritis and the Swedish Rheumatology Register cohorts. Arthritis Rheum 2011;63(1):26–36.

16. Mehri F, Jenabi E, Bashirian S, et al. The association between occupational exposure to silica and risk of developing rheumatoid arthritis: a meta-analysis. Saf Health Work 2020;11(2):136–42.

17. Morotti A, Sollaku I, Franceschini F, et al. Systematic review and meta-analysis on the association of occupational exposure to free crystalline silica and rheumatoid arthritis. Clin Rev Allergy Immunol 2021;62(2):333–45.

18. Ilar A, Alfredsson L, Wiebert P, et al. Occupation and risk of developing rheumatoid arthritis: results from a population-based case-control study. Arthritis Care Res (Hoboken) 2018;70(4):499–509.

19. Schmajuk G, Trupin L, Yelin E, et al. Prevalence of arthritis and rheumatoid arthritis in coal mining counties of the United States. Arthritis Care Res 2019; 71(9):1209–15.

20. Webber MP, Moir W, Zeig-Owens R, et al. Nested case-control study of selected systemic autoimmune diseases in World Trade Center rescue/recovery workers. Arthritis Rheumatol 2015;67(5):1369–76.

21. Ebel AV, Lutt G, Poole JA, et al. Association of Agricultural, Occupational, and Military Inhalants With Autoantibodies and Disease Features in US Veterans With Rheumatoid Arthritis. Arthritis Rheumatol 2021;73(3):392–400.

22. Jones KA, Smith B, Granado NS, et al. Newly reported lupus and rheumatoid arthritis in relation to deployment within proximity to a documented open-air burn pit in Iraq. J Occup Environ Med 2012;54(6):698–707.

23. Ying D, Schmajuk G, Trupin L, et al. Inorganic dust exposure during military service as a predictor of rheumatoid arthritis and other autoimmune conditions. ACR Open Rheumatol 2021;3(7):466–74.

24. Parks CG, Meyer A, Beane Freeman LE, et al. Farming tasks and the development of rheumatoid arthritis in the agricultural health study. Occup Environ Med 2019;76(4):243–9.
25. Parks CG, D'Aloisio AA, Sandler DP. Childhood residential and agricultural pesticide exposures in relation to adult-onset rheumatoid arthritis in women. Am J Epidemiol 2018;187(2):214–23.
26. Kim KH, Kabir E, Kabir S. A review on the human health impact of airborne particulate matter. Environ Int 2015;74:136–43.
27. Di D, Zhang L, Wu X, et al. Long-term exposure to outdoor air pollution and the risk of development of rheumatoid arthritis: A systematic review and meta-analysis. Semin Arthritis Rheum 2020;50(2):266–75.
28. Gan RW, Deane KD, Zerbe GO, et al. Relationship between air pollution and positivity of RA-related autoantibodies in individuals without established RA: a report on SERA. Ann Rheum Dis 2013;72(12):2002–5.
29. Alex AM, Kunkel G, Sayles H, et al. Exposure to ambient air pollution and autoantibody status in rheumatoid arthritis. Clin Rheumatol 2020;39(3):761–8.
30. Mikuls TR, Gaurav R, Thiele GM, et al. The impact of airborne endotoxin exposure on rheumatoid arthritis-related joint damage, autoantigen expression, autoimmunity, and lung disease. Int Immunopharmacol 2021;100:108069.
31. Gaurav R, Mikuls TR, Thiele GM, et al. High-throughput analysis of lung immune cells in a combined murine model of agriculture dust-triggered airway inflammation with rheumatoid arthritis. PLoS One 2021;16(2):e0240707.
32. Poole JA, Thiele GM, Janike K, et al. Combined Collagen-Induced Arthritis and Organic Dust-Induced Airway Inflammation to Model Inflammatory Lung Disease in Rheumatoid Arthritis. J Bone Miner Res 2019;34(9):1733–43.
33. Nelson AJ, Roy SK, Warren K, et al. Sex differences impact the lung-bone inflammatory response to repetitive inhalant lipopolysaccharide exposures in mice. J Immunotoxicol 2018;15(1):73–81.
34. Yunt ZX, Solomon JJ. Lung disease in rheumatoid arthritis. Rheum Dis Clin North Am 2015;41(2):225–36.
35. Hyldgaard C, Hilberg O, Pedersen AB, et al. A population-based cohort study of rheumatoid arthritis-associated interstitial lung disease: comorbidity and mortality. Ann Rheum Dis 2017;76(10):1700–6.
36. Charoenngam N, Ponvilawan B, Rittiphairoj T, et al. Patients with asthma have a higher risk of rheumatoid arthritis: A systematic review and meta-analysis. Semin Arthritis Rheum 2020;50(5):968–76.
37. Ford JA, Liu X, Chu SH, et al. Asthma, chronic obstructive pulmonary disease, and subsequent risk for incident rheumatoid arthritis among women: a prospective cohort study. Arthritis Rheumatol (Hoboken, NJ) 2020;72(5):704–13.
38. Kronzer VL, Westerlind H, Alfredsson L, et al. Respiratory Diseases as Risk Factors for Seropositive and Seronegative Rheumatoid Arthritis and in Relation to Smoking. Arthritis Rheumatol (Hoboken, NJ) 2021;73(1):61–8.
39. Charoenngam N, Ponvilawan B, Rittiphairoj T, et al. The association between allergic rhinitis and risk of rheumatoid arthritis: A systematic review and meta-analysis. J Evid Based Med 2021;14(1):27–39.
40. Joo YB, Lim YH, Kim KJ, et al. Respiratory viral infections and the risk of rheumatoid arthritis. Arthritis Res Ther 2019;21(1):199.
41. Derksen V, Kissel T, Lamers-Karnebeek FBG, et al. Onset of rheumatoid arthritis after COVID-19: coincidence or connected? Ann Rheum Dis 2021;annrheumdis-2021:219859.

42. Moffatt MF, Cookson WO. The lung microbiome in health and disease. Clin Med (Lond) 2017;17(6):525–9.
43. Scher JU, Joshua V, Artacho A, et al. The lung microbiota in early rheumatoid arthritis and autoimmunity. Microbiome 2016;4(1):60.
44. Willis VC, Demoruelle MK, Derber LA, et al. Sputum autoantibodies in patients with established rheumatoid arthritis and subjects at risk of future clinically apparent disease. Arthritis Rheum 2013;65(10):2545–54.
45. Demoruelle MK, Harrall KK, Ho L, et al. Anti-Citrullinated Protein Antibodies Are Associated With Neutrophil Extracellular Traps in the Sputum in Relatives of Rheumatoid Arthritis Patients. Arthritis Rheumatol (Hoboken, NJ) 2017;69(6): 1165–75.
46. Makrygiannakis D, Hermansson M, Ulfgren AK, et al. Smoking increases peptidyl-larginine deiminase 2 enzyme expression in human lungs and increases citrullination in BAL cells. Ann Rheum Dis 2008;67(10):1488–92.
47. Demoruelle MK, Wang H, Davis RL, et al. Anti-peptidylarginine deiminase-4 antibodies at mucosal sites can activate peptidylarginine deiminase-4 enzyme activity in rheumatoid arthritis. Arthritis Res Ther 2021;23(1):163.
48. Ytterberg AJ, Joshua V, Reynisdottir G, et al. Shared immunological targets in the lungs and joints of patients with rheumatoid arthritis: identification and validation. Ann Rheum Dis 2015;74(9):1772–7.
49. Woof JM, Kerr MA. The function of immunoglobulin A in immunity. J Pathol 2006; 208(2):270–82.
50. Kelmenson LB, Wagner BD, McNair BK, et al. Timing of Elevations of Autoantibody Isotypes Prior to Diagnosis of Rheumatoid Arthritis. Arthritis Rheumatol (Hoboken, NJ) 2020;72(2):251–61.
51. Mikuls TR, Edison J, Meeshaw E, et al. Autoantibodies to Malondialdehyde-Acetaldehyde Are Detected Prior to Rheumatoid Arthritis Diagnosis and After Other Disease Specific Autoantibodies. Arthritis Rheumatol (Hoboken, NJ) 2020;72(12):2025–9.
52. Roos K, Martinsson K, Ziegelasch M, et al. Circulating secretory IgA antibodies against cyclic citrullinated peptides in early rheumatoid arthritis associate with inflammatory activity and smoking. Arthritis Res Ther 2016;18(1):119.
53. Martinsson K, Roos Ljungberg K, Ziegelasch M, et al. Elevated free secretory component in early rheumatoid arthritis and prior to arthritis development in patients at increased risk. Rheumatology (Oxford, England) 2020;59(5):979–87.
54. Demoruelle MK, Weisman MH, Simonian PL, et al. Brief report: airways abnormalities and rheumatoid arthritis-related autoantibodies in subjects without arthritis: early injury or initiating site of autoimmunity? Arthritis Rheum 2012;64(6):1756–61.
55. Joshua V, Hensvold AH, Reynisdottir G, et al. Association between number and type of different ACPA fine specificities with lung abnormalities in early, untreated rheumatoid arthritis. RMD Open 2020;6(2):e001278.
56. Roos Ljungberg K, Joshua V, Skogh T, et al. Secretory anti-citrullinated protein antibodies in serum associate with lung involvement in early rheumatoid arthritis. Rheumatology (Oxford, England) 2020;59(4):852–9.
57. Rangel-Moreno J, Hartson L, Navarro C, et al. Inducible bronchus-associated lymphoid tissue (iBALT) in patients with pulmonary complications of rheumatoid arthritis. J Clin Invest 2006;116(12):3183–94.
58. Martin LW, Prisco LC, Huang W, et al. Prevalence and risk factors of bronchiectasis in rheumatoid arthritis: A systematic review and meta-analysis. Semin Arthritis Rheum 2021;51(5):1067–80.

59. Quirke AM, Perry E, Cartwright A, et al. Bronchiectasis is a Model for Chronic Bacterial Infection Inducing Autoimmunity in Rheumatoid Arthritis. Arthritis Rheumatol 2015;67(9):2335–42.

60. Zhang X, Zhang D, Jia H, et al. The oral and gut microbiomes are perturbed in rheumatoid arthritis and partly normalized after treatment. Nat Med 2015;21(8): 895–905.

61. Wilson TM, Trent B, Kuhn KA, et al. Microbial Influences of Mucosal Immunity in Rheumatoid Arthritis. Curr Rheumatol Rep 2020;22(11):83.

62. Fuggle NR, Smith TO, Kaul A, et al. Hand to Mouth: A Systematic Review and Meta-Analysis of the Association between Rheumatoid Arthritis and Periodontitis. Front Immunol 2016;7:80.

63. Mankia K, Cheng Z, Do T, et al. Prevalence of Periodontal Disease and Periodontopathic Bacteria in Anti-Cyclic Citrullinated Protein Antibody-Positive At-Risk Adults Without Arthritis. JAMA Netw Open 2019;2(6):e195394.

64. Hussain SB, Botelho J, Machado V, et al. Is there a bidirectional association between rheumatoid arthritis and periodontitis? A systematic review and meta-analysis. Semin Arthritis Rheum 2020;50(3):414–22.

65. Wegner N, Wait R, Sroka A, et al. Peptidylarginine deiminase from Porphyromonas gingivalis citrullinates human fibrinogen and α-enolase: implications for autoimmunity in rheumatoid arthritis. Arthritis Rheum 2010;62(9):2662–72.

66. Scher JU, Ubeda C, Equinda M, et al. Periodontal disease and the oral microbiota in new-onset rheumatoid arthritis. Arthritis Rheum 2012;64(10):3083–94.

67. Mikuls TR, Walker C, Qiu F, et al. The subgingival microbiome in patients with established rheumatoid arthritis. Rheumatology (Oxford, England) 2018;57(7): 1162–72.

68. Chen B, Zhao Y, Li S, et al. Variations in oral microbiome profiles in rheumatoid arthritis and osteoarthritis with potential biomarkers for arthritis screening. Scientific Rep 2018;8(1):17126.

69. Konig MF, Abusleme L, Reinholdt J, et al. Aggregatibacter actinomycetemcomitans-induced hypercitrullination links periodontal infection to autoimmunity in rheumatoid arthritis. Sci Transl Med 2016;8(369):369ra176.

70. Sun J, Zheng Y, Bian X, et al. Non-surgical periodontal treatment improves rheumatoid arthritis disease activity: a meta-analysis. Clin Oral Investig 2021;25(8): 4975–85.

71. Scher JU, Sczesnak A, Longman RS, et al. Expansion of intestinal Prevotella copri correlates with enhanced susceptibility to arthritis. Elife 2013;2:e01202.

72. Alpizar-Rodriguez D, Lesker TR, Gronow A, et al. Prevotella copri in individuals at risk for rheumatoid arthritis. Ann Rheum Dis 2019;78(5):590–3.

73. Pianta A, Arvikar S, Strle K, et al. Evidence of the Immune Relevance of Prevotella copri, a Gut Microbe, in Patients With Rheumatoid Arthritis. Arthritis Rheumatol 2017;69(5):964–75.

74. Inamo J. Non-causal association of gut microbiome on the risk of rheumatoid arthritis: a Mendelian randomisation study. Ann Rheum Dis 2021;80(7):e103.

75. Alpizar Rodriguez D, Lesker TR, Gilbert B, et al. Response to: 'Non-causal association of gut microbiome on the risk of rheumatoid arthritis: a Mendelian randomisation study' by Inamo. Ann Rheum Dis 2021;80(7):e104.

76. Nayak RR, Alexander M, Deshpande I, et al. Methotrexate impacts conserved pathways in diverse human gut bacteria leading to decreased host immune activation. Cell Host Microbe 2021;29(3):362–77, e311.

77. Artacho A, Isaac S, Nayak R, et al. The Pretreatment Gut Microbiome Is Associated With Lack of Response to Methotrexate in New-Onset Rheumatoid Arthritis. Arthritis Rheumatol (Hoboken, NJ) 2021;73(6):931–42.
78. Zaura E, Brandt BW, Teixeira de Mattos MJ, et al. Same Exposure but Two Radically Different Responses to Antibiotics: Resilience of the Salivary Microbiome versus Long-Term Microbial Shifts in Feces. mBio 2015;6(6):e01693–715.
79. O'Dell JR, Haire CE, Palmer W, et al. Treatment of early rheumatoid arthritis with minocycline or placebo: results of a randomized, double-blind, placebo-controlled trial. Arthritis Rheum 1997;40(5):842–8.
80. Sparks JA, Iversen MD, Yu Z, et al. Disclosure of personalized rheumatoid arthritis risk using genetics, biomarkers, and lifestyle factors to motivate health behavior improvements: a randomized controlled trial. Arthritis Care Res (Hoboken) 2018;70(6):823–33.
81. Klareskog L, Stolt P, Lundberg K, et al. A new model for an etiology of rheumatoid arthritis: smoking may trigger HLA-DR (shared epitope)-restricted immune reactions to autoantigens modified by citrullination. Arthritis Rheum 2006;54(1):38–46.

Lifestyle, Hormonal, and Metabolic Environmental Risks for Rheumatoid Arthritis

Nancy Desai, MD[a], Lydia Federico, BA[a],
Joshua F. Baker, MD, MSCE[a,b,c],*

KEYWORDS

- Rheumatoid arthritis • Environmental exposure • Risk factors • Coffee • Diet
- Alcohol drinking/drug effects • Reproductive health • Periodontitis

KEY POINTS

- Although inhalational exposures are well-accepted environmental risk factors for rheumatoid arthritis (RA), noninhalational exposures are more controversial.
- A lower risk of RA is observed among thinner people with better dietary, physical activity, and dental hygiene habits although confounding and other forms of bias may be present.
- Although the promotion of healthy lifestyle habits may be of value in at-risk patients, the benefits are likely to be modest in terms of preventing RA.

INTRODUCTION

The interaction between smoking and genetic risk for rheumatoid arthritis (RA) has illustrated the clear relevance of gene–environment interactions in the development of the disease. Chronic inflammation of many types and origins may lead to protein modifications that can lead to the presentation of these modified self-peptides to the immune system. Environmental exposures that may increase the risk of chronic inflammation, or dysregulation of the response to it, may contribute to an increased risk of the disease. A plethora of epidemiologic research has been performed to explore risk factors for the development of RA; however, there remains a significant lack of clarity regarding the relative contribution of noninhalational exposures to the development of the disease. This is in part due to limitations in the ability of large

Funding: Dr J.F. Baker is supported by a Veterans Affairs Clinical Science Research and Development Merit Award (I01 CX001703) and Rehabilitation Research and Development Merit Award (I01 RX003644).
[a] Division of Rheumatology, University of Pennsylvania, 3400 Spruce Street, 5 White Building, Philadelphia, PA 19104, USA; [b] Philadelphia VA Medical Center, 3900 Woodland Avenue, Philadelphia, PA 19104, USA; [c] Department of Epidemiology and Biostatistics, University of Pennsylvania, 423 Guardian Drive, Philadelphia, PA 19104 USA
* Corresponding author. 5th Floor White Building, 3600 Spruce Street, Philadelphia, PA 19104.
E-mail address: Joshua.baker@pennmedicine.upenn.edu

studies to consider and adjust for confounding and in accurately classifying incident disease. This review will discuss literature on noninhalational exposures such as diet, exercise, obesity, dental hygiene, and hormonal exposures (**Fig. 1**).

DIET

As a potentially modifiable environmental risk factor, it is important to establish the role of healthy eating in RA prevention for patients with arthralgias or in preclinical phases of disease.[1] Several studies have evaluated different dietary patterns. For example, in the prospective Nurses' Health Study cohort, a proinflammatory diet pattern was associated with an increased risk of seropositive RA with onset before 55 years of age, suggesting that adherence to "anti-inflammatory" dietary patterns may help in early RA prevention.[2] However, the lack of association with other subgroups of RA suggests that this finding is not very robust. Because it is not typically possible to randomize people to receive a particular diet, the literature is limited by the potential for confounding related to other behaviors. These data should therefore be interpreted with that in mind.

MEDITERRANEAN DIET

The Mediterranean diet consists of high consumption of olive oil, cereals, fruits and vegetables, fish, and moderate amounts of dairy, meat, and wine, making it high in bioactive compounds such as antioxidants and omega-3 fatty acids. Because the Mediterranean diet has been observed to be associated with a lower risk of cardiovascular disease, cancer, and overall mortality,[3,4] its association with RA risk is a natural topic for investigation.

Results from studies addressing the role of the Mediterranean diet have been mixed. In a case-control study from the Swedish Epidemiologic Investigation of RA, researchers observed an inverse association between Mediterranean diet score and RA, although results were only significant among men and for seropositive disease.[5] Further, in a large prospective cohort study of French women, researchers observed a statistically significant 9% decrease in RA risk per 1-point increase in Mediterranean diet adherence score among ever-smokers but not among never-smokers.[4] However, 2 large prospective cohorts of women from the Nurses' Health Study found no association between a Mediterranean dietary pattern and incident RA.[6]

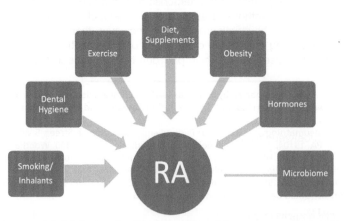

Fig. 1. Environmental risk factors for RA. The width of the arrows represents the authors' interpretation of the strength of the body of evidence for each respective risk factor.

Overall, results are inconclusive but hint that adherence to a Mediterranean diet might reduce the risk of RA for some clinical populations. Additional study is warranted to further elucidate any associations specific to sex or to patient subgroups at higher risk, such as smokers or those with positive RA antibodies.

FISH AND OMEGA-3 FATTY ACIDS

Associations between fish consumption and RA risk have been studied because omega-3 fatty acids found in certain fish have been hypothesized to have anti-inflammatory properties.[7] In a recent systematic review and meta-analysis of animal protein sources and RA risk, Asoudeh and colleagues found an inverse association between fish consumption and RA risk independent of other known risk factors. In that study, 100 g/d increment in fish intake was observed to be associated with a 15% reduction in RA risk, with the lowest risk at a moderate fish intake of 20 to 30 g/d.[7] Research specifically focused on the relationship between RA risk and omega-3 fatty acids from a wide variety of food sources have shown mixed results. For example, in the Swedish Mammography Cohort, researchers observed an inverse association between both fish and omega-3 fatty acid consumption and risk of developing RA, whereas researchers in the Women's Health Initiative Observational Study and Clinical Trials cohort found no association.[8,9]

In a recent small prospective study of anti-citrullinated peptide antibody (ACPA)-positive patients without RA, a one-standard deviation higher level of omega-3 fatty acids measured red blood cell membranes was associated with a significantly decreased risk of incident RA.[10,11] Considered together, there is moderate evidence to support fish and omega-3 fatty acids as beneficial in protecting against the development of RA, although further research is needed to elucidate the mechanism by which omega-3 fatty acids might play a role in the pathophysiology of the disease.

RED MEAT, POULTRY, AND DAIRY PRODUCTS

There are limited and conflicting data to support associations between other sources of animal protein and RA risk. A recent systematic review and meta-analysis by Asoudeh and colleagues summarizes existing data on this topic.[7] This group found no significant association between consumption of red meat, poultry, or dairy products and risk of developing RA.[7] In a recent cross-sectional study, Jin and colleagues observed higher red meat intake ($\geq$100g red meat per day) to be associated with earlier age of onset RA.[12] However, because this study was cross-sectional among patients with established disease, it is difficult to infer a causal relationship.

ALCOHOL

Associations between alcohol consumption and incident RA risk have been widely studied. Between 8% and 12% of RA risk has been previously attributed to less than moderate alcohol intake.[13,14] In a meta-analysis of prospective studies evaluating the relationship between alcohol consumption and RA risk, Jin and colleagues found that low to moderate alcohol consumption during at least 10 years was associated with a 17% decrease in incident RA risk, compared with no alcohol consumption.[15] Scott and colleagues also found a protective effect of alcohol consumption on RA risk in a meta-analysis of case-control/cohort studies, although the effect was limited to ACPA-positive subjects.[16] In a more recent study in the Nurses' Health Study cohort, long-term moderate alcohol consumption was observed to be associated with a 22% lower RA risk. When the analysis was restricted to seropositive RA, the association strengthened further.[17] Evidence thus points to an inverse association between long-term moderate alcohol consumption and RA risk.

It has been proposed that this association may be attributable to alcohol-induced downregulation of the immune response and decreased production of proinflammatory cytokines.[18,19] However, another interpretation is that a confounding or even a reverse causal effect may be driving the association, because those who abstain completely from alcohol consumption often do so in the context of chronic illness and poor health status.[18] Before we make recommendations for patients to increase alcohol consumption, it is important to establish a better mechanistic understanding of this relationship given the potential adverse health consequences of excess alcohol use.

COFFEE

Coffee is one of the most consumed beverages worldwide and has been studied as a risk factor in a variety of disease states. For example, recent evidence suggests coffee may be associated with an increased risk of osteoarthritis,[20] whereas moderate consumption may be protective against other conditions such as cardiovascular disease.[21]

Not surprisingly, evidence in RA has been inconsistent. In a 2014 meta-analysis evaluating the association between coffee intake and RA risk, Lee and colleagues observed a positive association between high rates of coffee consumption and incident RA but this association was observed only in seropositive RA.[22] Indeed, in the cross-sectional Mini-Finland Health Survey, Heliövaara and colleagues found that the number of cups of coffee subjects consumed daily was directly proportional to their RF titer. However, the linear trend was not significant after adjusting for smoking, highlighting smoking as an important confounder in the assessment of associations between coffee and RA risk.[23] Furthermore, in both a recent large prospective study in the Women's Health Initiative Observational Study cohort and a cross-sectional analysis of the Korea National Health and Nutrition Examination Survey, investigators found no independent association between coffee consumption and incident RA.[24,25]

Overall, the current evidence for coffee intake as a risk factor for RA is weak and further research is needed to clarify this relationship, its associated mechanisms, and to account for potential confounding with other known risk factors such as smoking.

VITAMIN D

Vitamin D has been shown to have immunomodulatory effects through a variety of mechanisms including IL-2 inhibition, lymphocyte proliferation, and antibody production. In addition, it binds to nuclear vitamin D receptors, which are expressed on most immune cell types that play a role in innate and adaptive immunity.[26]

Although hypovitaminosis D and low levels of vitamin D intake have been suggested as risk factors for autoimmune diseases, including RA,[27] epidemiologic data have not been consistent. Two studies published using Nurses' Health Study I and II data did not identify a significant association between levels of vitamin D intake and the risk of adult-onset RA.[28,29] However, a meta-analysis performed by Song and colleagues showed that participants with the highest total vitamin D intake had a 24.2% lower risk of developing RA compared with those in the lowest quintile group.[30] Data recently presented from the Vitamin D and Omega 3 Trial (VITAL) suggested that those randomized to vitamin D had a lower risk of autoimmune diseases.[31] However, overall, the epidemiologic data supporting the use of vitamin D supplementation in RA is less compelling in comparison to the data available for other autoimmune diseases such as multiple sclerosis, systemic lupus erythematosus (SLE), and systemic sclerosis (SSc).[32]

ANTIOXIDANT SUPPLEMENTATION

Increased oxidation secondary to free oxygen radicals along with proinflammatory cytokines has been proposed as one of the mediators of tissue damage in RA.[33,34] Low serum antioxidant levels have been correlated with an increased risk of RA,[35] and patients with inflammatory arthritis have been observed to report lower dietary vitamin C levels (OR 3.3).[36] Several larger studies have investigated this further, including a study by Costenbader and colleagues.[37] This group did not find any association between cumulatively averaged vitamins A, C, E, or intake of other antioxidants, such as a-carotenoid, ß-carotenoid, ß-cryptoxanthin, lycopene, and lutein, and the risk of developing RA.[38] Using data from the Iowa Women's Health Study cohort, Cerhan and colleagues[39] found a weak inverse association between total and supplemental intake of vitamins C and E and the risk of RA that was not significant. A case-control study within a Finnish cohort[40] suggested an inverse relationship between serum selenium and occurrence of seronegative RA. However, this finding was neither consistent in long-term follow-up nor when focused on seropositive disease.

Overall, there is scarce evidence to support the use of antioxidants in the form of vitamin or trace mineral supplementation to prevent RA. Inconsistencies between epidemiologic studies likely stem from confounding related to other health behaviors.

PHYSICAL ACTIVITY

Physical activity is associated with reduced risk of a variety of disease states, such as cancer, cardiovascular disease, and all-cause mortality. One mechanism by which moderate-vigorous physical activity may produce health benefits seems to be via the reduction of chronic low-grade inflammation.[41] Physical activity may also reduce rates of joint pain and decrease symptoms of arthritis.[42]

There have been some conflicting results in this area of research across multiple large prospective cohort studies. In the Iowa Women's Health Study, researchers found no association between quartiles of physical activity and RA risk.[43] However, in the Nurse's Health Study II, higher levels of physical activity were observed to be associated with decreased RA risk independent of dietary and body mass index (BMI) history, with a 33% risk reduction in women who exercised $\geq$7 h/wk compared with those who exercised less than 1 h/wk.[44] Similarly, results from the Swedish Mammography Cohort suggested that women who participated in daily walking/bicycling greater than 20 minutes per day and weekly exercise for greater than 1 hour were at 35% lower RA risk independent of BMI.[45]

In a recent meta-analysis of physical activity and RA risk, Sun and colleagues converted reported physical activity to standardized metabolic equivalent task (MET)-hours to enable comparison of the effect of exercise across studies using different assessments. An inverse association was observed between physical activity and subsequent risk of developing RA in both categorical and dose–response analyses, suggesting a risk reduction of 7% per additional 10 MET-hours per week.[46]

In general, evidence suggests that physical activity is likely to be beneficial. Although the best form of physical activity is not characterized in these studies, it does seem that even modest amounts of daily exercise may be beneficial. Notably, most research on this topic has been observational and conducted in women cohorts of predominantly European ancestry, potentially limiting generalizability. In addition, additional research is needed to improve the understanding of the mechanisms by which physical activity might help to reduce RA risk in different populations.

OBESITY

Because obesity is a chronic inflammatory state, it has been hypothesized as a potential environmental trigger for the loss of tolerance of self-peptides and the development of RA. Strong associations have been observed between metabolic obesity and psoriasis/psoriatic arthritis with a lowering of risk among those that undergo bariatric surgery and lose weight.[47] For this reason, several studies have evaluated obesity as a potential risk factor for RA, and this study has been summarized in reviews and meta-analyses.[48] Overall, the results are not consistent. These data support a modest risk attributable to obesity, although there is substantial statistical heterogeneity among published studies.

Some evidence suggests that obesity is associated primarily with the development of seronegative disease, suggesting either a phenotypic difference in the disease versus differential misclassification of obese patients.[49] In a recent study, investigators found no association between obesity and the development of seropositive RA among men or women.[50] However, among women, there was a significant association between obesity and the development of seronegative RA. This study supports several prior studies.[51,52]

Another recent study evaluated abdominal obesity as a risk factor for RA from the Nurses' Health Study.[53] This study demonstrated significant associations between waist circumference and the risk of RA; however, this was not independent of the previously described associations with BMI described in this cohort, suggesting that abdominal obesity may not be the most important aspect of obesity that drives the risk of the disease.

A recent study by Ye and colleagues[13] evaluated lifestyle factors associated with RA and determined the population attributable risk for obesity based on the prevalence of risk factors in the US population and the pooled estimates of the excess risk based on prior epidemiologic studies (27% increase in risk). The investigators note that excess weight might account for 15% of all RA cases in the population. Although this number is not inconsequential and suggests an important public health impact of obesity on the incidence of RA, it relies on risk estimates from only 4 heterogeneous studies.

A limitation of studies in this area is the concern for confounding by other behaviors that are associated with obesity. Furthermore, these studies do not address whether weight loss in an individual might reduce their risk of RA. An interesting study by Maglio and colleagues addressed this question in a novel way by studying patients who underwent bariatric surgery for their obesity. They observed no evidence for a reduction in the risk of RA among patient undergoing bariatric surgery compared with obese patients who did not undergo surgery.[47]

Although, overall, there does seem to be a modest increase in the risk of being diagnosed with RA among obese individuals that could have a significant impact at a population level, it is important to acknowledge that differential misclassification of RA may be an important source of bias. Because obesity is associated with higher rates of amplified pain, osteoarthritis, and other musculoskeletal conditions, it is possible that it may lead to misdiagnosis of RA even among experienced rheumatologists. It is difficult to assess this risk of bias and determine its potential impact and therefore the question remains unanswered.

DENTAL HYGIENE

It has been proposed that RA and gingival disease are driven by a comparable pathogenesis with similarities in underlying inflammatory profile.[54] Periodontal disease is driven by oral bacterial biofilm that results in the subsequent destruction of tooth-supporting structures including alveolar bone and has been associated with other systemic diseases due to its chronic inflammatory nature.[55]

Several clinical studies have investigated the relationship between periodontitis and the risk of developing RA without clear consensus.[56,57] However, a recently published longitudinal cohort study used data from a national Korean insurance database found that the people with periodontitis were 10% more likely to develop RA.[58] This relationship may be inflated[59] because underlying environmental risk factors are shared by both disease processes.

Overall, given the plausible pathophysiology and suggestive clinical data, it seems likely that prevention of periodontitis would modestly reduce the risk of developing RA.

HORMONAL EXPOSURE

The higher incidence of RA in women has led to the suggestion that hormonal or reproductive factors may influence risk. Several large studies investigated the role of reproductive factors such as age of menarche and pregnancy in RA. A study from the Nurses' Health Study found an increased risk of developing seropositive RA with early age ($\leq$10 years) at menarche (adjusted RR 1.6).[60] In contrast, no association with age at menarche was noted in an analysis using data from the Third National Health and Nutrition Survey.[61] This same study found that women who experienced menopause before 40 years had increased risk of developing postmenopausal RA (OR 2.52). Overall, findings do not seem to support a link between the duration of hormone exposure and the risk of disease. A large Mendelian randomization study in patients of European ancestry also did not find convincing evidence of a causal relationship between the genetics underlying age of menarche or age at menopause and the development of RA.[62]

The available data investigating the relationship between oral contraceptives (OCPs) and the risk of RA is also conflicting. Several early studies implicated a protective effect of OCP use, including a case-control study by Vandenbroucke and colleagues, which found a 42% decreased risk of RA compared with never users of OCPs.[63,64] There have been several meta-analysis and systematic reviews since, finding no conclusive association between OCP use and risk of RA.[65,66] A recently published meta-analysis by Qi and colleagues of 12 case-control and 5 cohort studies again failed to find an association between OCP and RA risk.[67]

There are few studies looking at incidence of RA in relation to postmenopausal hormone replacement therapy (HRT) with varied results. Data from the ESPOIR cohort suggested a protective association between HRT and HLADRB1*01 and/or *04 alleles, which that have been linked as a risk factors for RA,[68] and subsequent reduction of anti-cyclic citrullinated peptide (CCP) antibodies.[69] On the contrary, a recent large study of the Korean National Health Insurance Service database demonstrated a 25% increase in risk among people who used HRT for 5 or more years compared with never users.[70] Other prior studies have not found statistically significant or consistent associations between the risk of developing RA and HRT use.[71,72]

Overall, an association between hormonal exposure and the risk of RA seems to be weak and inconsistent.

PREGNANCY

Pregnancy has also been extensively studied as a possible risk factor in the development of RA as well as other connective tissue diseases. Although evidence has suggested that disease activity in RA is often reduced during pregnancy,[73] the relationship between pregnancy and the risk of developing RA is less clear. A few studies have suggested an increased risk of RA incidence within 0 to 3 months postpregnancy[74,75] but no significant associations were found in a meta-analysis when looking up to 12 months postpartum.[76]

Several studies have looked at parity as a risk factor for RA and noted a trend toward risk reduction in women with multiple pregnancies.[77,78] A study looking at a population of North American Natives, a population with high fertility rates and high prevalence of RA, found that women with 6 or more births had significant reduced risk for RA development in comparison with women who had 1 to 2 births (OR 0.43).[77] Other studies, have not identified an association between parity and risk of developing RA,[60,79,80] and a meta-analysis by Chen and colleagues did not find a significant association of developing RA with either gravity or parity.[76]

There are few studies looking at age of women at first pregnancy and the risk of RA. A case-control study in Sweden noted that younger age at first birth, defined as less than 23 years, was associated with an increased risk of ACPA-negative RA (adjusted OR 2.5) but not ACPA-positive RA.[81] Peschken and colleagues also noted that women who gave birth after the age of 20 had significantly reduced risk of developing RA (OR 0.33) in comparison to women who had their first pregnancy at $\leq$ 17 years.[77] In contrast, an older retrospective case-control study found that when compared with nulliparous women, the estimated risk of developing RA was lowest among those that had their first pregnancy between 16 and 19 years of age.[82]

PREGNANCY COMPLICATIONS

Adverse outcomes during pregnancy such as preterm birth, low birth weight, pregnancy associated hypertensive disorders, and hyperemesis have also been studied. Jørgensen and colleagues found that the risk of RA was significantly increased in women with prior history of pregnancy complicated by hyperemesis, gestational hypertension, and pre-eclampsia.[83] Self-reported "poor" pregnancy courses by patients were also found to have a 3-fold risk of RA in comparison to women who reported "very good" pregnancy health in the same cohort.[78] It is difficult to differentiate whether the association of pregnancy complications is a risk factor in the development of RA or reflection of common risk factors for both outcomes.

SUMMARY

Although smoking has been accepted as a clear and important risk factor for the development of RA, the relevance of noninhalational exposures has been less clearly defined. It is an easy recommendation to suggest that physicians should recommend a healthy diet, exercise, maintenance of a healthy weight, and maintenance of good dental hygiene in the hope of reducing the long-term risk of RA in someone with a strong family history. However, epidemiologic studies may be limited in establishing causal relationships on their own, and a focus on developing a mechanistic understanding of the epidemiologic links will be of value.

CLINICS CARE POINTS

- A Mediterranean diet rich in fish may help reduce risk of RA in addition to other potential health benefits.
- Regular exercise, even modest exercise, may lower the risk of RA and other types of arthritis.
- Weight reduction and maintenance of healthy weight may prevent RA in addition to other forms of arthritis.

- Regular dental visits and attention to dental hygiene may help reduce risks.
- There is insufficient evidence to recommend the use of alcohol, particular health supplements, avoidance of coffee, or avoidance of hormonal exposures such as estrogens to reduce the risk of RA.

ACKNOWLEDGMENTS

Dr J.F. Baker would like to acknowledge funding through a Veterans Affairs Clinical Science Research & Development Career Merit Award (I01 CX001703) and a Rehabilitation Research & Development Merit Award (I01 RX003644). The contents of this article do not represent the views of the Department of the Veterans Affairs or the United States Government.

CONFLICTS OF INTEREST

The authors have nothing to disclose.

REFERENCES

1. Philippou E, Nikiphorou E. Are we really what we eat? Nutrition and its role in the onset of rheumatoid arthritis. Autoimmun Rev 2018;17(11):1074–7.
2. Sparks JA, Barbhaiya M, Tedeschi SK, et al. Inflammatory dietary pattern and risk of developing rheumatoid arthritis in women. Clin Rheumatol 2019;38(1):243–50.
3. Sofi F, Macchi C, Abbate R, et al. Mediterranean diet and health status: an updated meta-analysis and a proposal for a literature-based adherence score. Public Health Nutr 2014;17(12):2769–82.
4. Nguyen Y, Salliot C, Gelot A, et al. Mediterranean Diet and Risk of Rheumatoid Arthritis: Findings From the French E3N-EPIC Cohort Study. Arthritis Rheumatol 2021;73(1):69–77.
5. Johansson K, Askling J, Alfredsson L, et al. Mediterranean diet and risk of rheumatoid arthritis: a population-based case-control study. Arthritis Res Ther 2018; 20(1):175.
6. Hu Y, Costenbader KH, Gao X, et al. Mediterranean diet and incidence of rheumatoid arthritis in women. Arthritis Care Res (Hoboken) 2015;67(5):597–606.
7. Asoudeh F, Jayedi A, Kavian Z, et al. A systematic review and meta-analysis of observational studies on the association between animal protein sources and risk of rheumatoid arthritis. Clin Nutr 2021;40(7):4644–52.
8. Krok-Schoen JL, Brasky TM, Hunt RP, et al. Dietary Long-Chain n-3 Fatty Acid Intake and Arthritis Risk in the Women's Health Initiative. J Acad Nutr Diet 2018;118(11):2057–69.
9. Di Giuseppe D, Wallin A, Bottai M, et al. Long-term intake of dietary long-chain n-3 polyunsaturated fatty acids and risk of rheumatoid arthritis: a prospective cohort study of women. Ann Rheum Dis 2014;73(11):1949–53.
10. Saidane O, Semerano L, Sellam J. Could omega-3 fatty acids prevent rheumatoid arthritis? Joint Bone Spine 2019;86(1):9–12.
11. Gan RW, Bemis EA, Demoruelle MK, et al. The association between omega-3 fatty acid biomarkers and inflammatory arthritis in an anti-citrullinated protein antibody positive population. Rheumatology (Oxford) 2017;56(12):2229–36.
12. Jin J, Li J, Gan Y, et al. Red meat intake is associated with early onset of rheumatoid arthritis: a cross-sectional study. Sci Rep 2021;11(1):5681.

13. Ye D, Mao Y, Xu Y, et al. Lifestyle factors associated with incidence of rheumatoid arthritis in US adults: analysis of National Health and Nutrition Examination Survey database and meta-analysis. BMJ Open 2021;11(1):e038137.

14. Sparks JA, Chen CY, Hiraki LT, et al. Contributions of familial rheumatoid arthritis or lupus and environmental factors to risk of rheumatoid arthritis in women: a prospective cohort study. Arthritis Care Res (Hoboken) 2014;66(10):1438–46.

15. Jin Z, Xiang C, Cai Q, et al. Alcohol consumption as a preventive factor for developing rheumatoid arthritis: a dose-response meta-analysis of prospective studies. Ann Rheum Dis 2014;73(11):1962–7.

16. Scott IC, Tan R, Stahl D, et al. The protective effect of alcohol on developing rheumatoid arthritis: a systematic review and meta-analysis. Rheumatology (Oxford) 2013;52(5):856–67.

17. Lu B, Solomon DH, Costenbader KH, et al. Alcohol consumption and risk of incident rheumatoid arthritis in women: a prospective study. Arthritis Rheumatol 2014;66(8):1998–2005.

18. Zaccardelli A, Friedlander HM, Ford JA, et al. Potential of lifestyle changes for reducing the risk of developing rheumatoid arthritis: is an ounce of prevention worth a pound of cure? Clin Ther 2019;41(7):1323–45.

19. Waldschmidt TJ, Cook RT, Kovacs EJ. Alcohol and inflammation and immune responses: summary of the 2005 Alcohol and Immunology Research Interest Group (AIRIG) meeting. Alcohol 2006;38(2):121–5.

20. Guillán-Fresco M, Franco-Trepat E, Alonso-Pérez A, et al. Caffeine, a risk factor for osteoarthritis and longitudinal bone growth inhibition. J Clin Med 2020;9(4). https://doi.org/10.3390/jcm9041163.

21. Rodríguez-Artalejo F, López-García E. Coffee consumption and cardiovascular disease: a condensed review of epidemiological evidence and mechanisms. J Agric Food Chem 2018;66(21):5257–63.

22. Lee YH, Bae SC, Song GG. Coffee or tea consumption and the risk of rheumatoid arthritis: a meta-analysis. Clin Rheumatol 2014;33(11):1575–83.

23. Heliövaara M, Aho K, Knekt P, et al. Coffee consumption, rheumatoid factor, and the risk of rheumatoid arthritis. Ann Rheum Dis 2000;59(8):631–5.

24. Lamichhane D, Collins C, Constantinescu F, et al. Coffee and tea consumption in relation to risk of rheumatoid arthritis in the women's health initiative observational cohort. J Clin Rheumatol 2019;25(3):127–32.

25. Kim SG, Kang JW, Jeong SM, et al. Is Rheumatoid Arthritis Related to Coffee Consumption in Korea? A Nationwide Cross-Sectional Observational Study. Int J Environ Res Public Health 2021;18(15). https://doi.org/10.3390/ijerph18157880.

26. Wen H, Baker JF. Vitamin D, immunoregulation, and rheumatoid arthritis. J Clin Rheumatol Mar 2011;17(2):102–7.

27. Cutolo M, Otsa K, Paolino S, et al. Vitamin D involvement in rheumatoid arthritis and systemic lupus erythaematosus. Ann Rheum Dis 2009;68(3):446–7.

28. Costenbader KH, Feskanich D, Holmes M, et al. Vitamin D intake and risks of systemic lupus erythematosus and rheumatoid arthritis in women. Ann Rheum Dis 2008;67(4):530–5.

29. Hiraki LT, Munger KL, Costenbader KH, et al. Dietary intake of vitamin D during adolescence and risk of adult-onset systemic lupus erythematosus and rheumatoid arthritis. Arthritis Care Res (Hoboken) 2012;64(12):1829–36.

30. Song GG, Bae SC, Lee YH. Association between vitamin D intake and the risk of rheumatoid arthritis: a meta-analysis. Clin Rheumatol 2012;31(12):1733–9.

31. Hahn J, Cook NR, Alexander EK, et al. Vitamin D and Marine n-3 Fatty Acid Supplementation and Prevention of Autoimmune Disease in the VITAL Randomized Controlled Trial [abstract]. BMJ 2022;376:e066452.
32. Antico A, Tampoia M, Tozzoli R, et al. Can supplementation with vitamin D reduce the risk or modify the course of autoimmune diseases? A systematic review of the literature. Autoimmun Rev 2012;12(2):127–36.
33. Choy EH, Panayi GS. Cytokine pathways and joint inflammation in rheumatoid arthritis. N Engl J Med 2001;344(12):907–16.
34. Aaseth J, Haugen M, Førre O. Rheumatoid arthritis and metal compounds–perspectives on the role of oxygen radical detoxification. Analyst 1998;123(1):3–6.
35. Heliövaara M, Knekt P, Aho K, et al. Serum antioxidants and risk of rheumatoid arthritis. Ann Rheum Dis 1994;53(1):51–3.
36. Pattison DJ, Silman AJ, Goodson NJ, et al. Vitamin C and the risk of developing inflammatory polyarthritis: prospective nested case-control study. Ann Rheum Dis 2004;63(7):843–7.
37. Costenbader KH, Kang JH, Karlson EW. Antioxidant intake and risks of rheumatoid arthritis and systemic lupus erythematosus in women. Am J Epidemiol 2010; 172(2):205–16.
38. Karlson EW, Shadick NA, Cook NR, et al. Vitamin E in the primary prevention of rheumatoid arthritis: the Women's Health Study. Arthritis Rheum 2008;59(11): 1589–95.
39. Cerhan JR, Saag KG, Merlino LA, et al. Antioxidant micronutrients and risk of rheumatoid arthritis in a cohort of older women. Am J Epidemiol 2003;157(4): 345–54.
40. Knekt P, Heliövaara M, Aho K, et al. Serum selenium, serum alpha-tocopherol, and the risk of rheumatoid arthritis. Epidemiol 2000;11(4):402–5.
41. Nimmo MA, Leggate M, Viana JL, et al. The effect of physical activity on mediators of inflammation. Diabetes Obes Metab 2013;15(Suppl 3):51–60.
42. Baillet A, Zeboulon N, Gossec L, et al. Efficacy of cardiorespiratory aerobic exercise in rheumatoid arthritis: meta-analysis of randomized controlled trials. Arthritis Care Res (Hoboken) 2010;62(7):984–92.
43. Cerhan JR, Saag KG, Criswell LA, et al. Blood transfusion, alcohol use, and anthropometric risk factors for rheumatoid arthritis in older women. J Rheumatol Feb 2002;29(2):246–54.
44. Liu X, Tedeschi SK, Lu B, et al. Long-Term physical activity and subsequent risk for rheumatoid arthritis among women: a prospective cohort study. Arthritis Rheumatol 2019;71(9):1460–71.
45. Di Giuseppe D, Bottai M, Askling J, et al. Physical activity and risk of rheumatoid arthritis in women: a population-based prospective study. Arthritis Res Ther 2015; 17:40.
46. Sun L, Zhu J, Ling Y, et al. Physical activity and the risk of rheumatoid arthritis: evidence from meta-analysis and Mendelian randomization. Int J Epidemiol 2021;50(5):1593–603.
47. Maglio C, Zhang Y, Peltonen M, et al. Bariatric surgery and the incidence of rheumatoid arthritis - a Swedish Obese Subjects study. Rheumatology (Oxford) 2020; 59(2):303–9.
48. Ohno T, Aune D, Heath AK. Adiposity and the risk of rheumatoid arthritis: a systematic review and meta-analysis of cohort studies. Sci Rep 2020;10(1):16006.
49. George MD, Baker JF. The Obesity Epidemic and Consequences for Rheumatoid Arthritis Care. Curr Rheumatol Rep 2016;18(1):6.

50. Linauskas A, Overvad K, Symmons D, et al. Body Fat Percentage, Waist Circumference, and Obesity As Risk Factors for Rheumatoid Arthritis: A Danish Cohort Study. Arthritis Care Res (Hoboken) 2019;71(6):777–86.

51. Wesley A, Bengtsson C, Elkan AC, et al. Association between body mass index and anti-citrullinated protein antibody-positive and anti-citrullinated protein antibody-negative rheumatoid arthritis: results from a population-based case-control study. Arthritis Care Res (Hoboken) 2013;65(1):107–12.

52. Lu B, Hiraki LT, Sparks JA, et al. Being overweight or obese and risk of developing rheumatoid arthritis among women: a prospective cohort study. Ann Rheum Dis 2014;73(11):1914–22.

53. Marchand NE, Sparks JA, Tedeschi SK, et al. Abdominal obesity in comparison with general obesity and risk of developing rheumatoid arthritis in women. J Rheumatol 2021;48(2):165–73.

54. Marotte H, Farge P, Gaudin P, et al. The association between periodontal disease and joint destruction in rheumatoid arthritis extends the link between the HLA-DR shared epitope and severity of bone destruction. Ann Rheum Dis 2006;65(7):905–9.

55. Badran Z, Struillou X, Verner C, et al. Periodontitis as a risk factor for systemic disease: are microparticles the missing link? Med Hypotheses 2015;84(6):555–6.

56. Ceccarelli F, Saccucci M, Di Carlo G, et al. Periodontitis and Rheumatoid Arthritis: The Same Inflammatory Mediators? Mediators Inflamm 2019;2019:6034546.

57. Khantisopon N, Louthrenoo W, Kasitanon N, et al. Periodontal disease in Thai patients with rheumatoid arthritis. Int J Rheum Dis 2014;17(5):511–8.

58. Choi YY, Lee KH. Periodontitis as a risk factor for rheumatoid arthritis: a matched-cohort study. Int Dent J 2021. https://doi.org/10.1016/j.identj.2021.01.006.

59. Samborska-Mazur J, Sikorska D, Wyganowska-Świątkowska M. The relationship between periodontal status and rheumatoid arthritis - systematic review. Reumatologia 2020;58(4):236–42.

60. Karlson EW, Mandl LA, Hankinson SE, et al. Do breast-feeding and other reproductive factors influence future risk of rheumatoid arthritis? Results from the Nurses' Health Study. Arthritis Rheum 2004;50(11):3458–67.

61. Beydoun HA, el-Amin R, McNeal M, et al. Reproductive history and postmenopausal rheumatoid arthritis among women 60 years or older: Third National Health and Nutrition Examination Survey. Menopause Sep 2013;20(9):930–5.

62. Zhu J, Niu Z, Alfredsson L, et al. Age at menarche, age at natural menopause, and risk of rheumatoid arthritis - a Mendelian randomization study. Arthritis Res Ther 2021;23(1):108.

63. Vandenbroucke JP, Valkenburg HA, Boersma JW, et al. Oral contraceptives and rheumatoid arthritis: further evidence for a preventive effect. Lancet 1982;2(8303):839–42.

64. Spector TD, Hochberg MC. The protective effect of the oral contraceptive pill on rheumatoid arthritis: an overview of the analytic epidemiological studies using meta-analysis. J Clin Epidemiol 1990;43(11):1221–30.

65. Romieu I, Hernandez-Avila M, Liang MH. Oral contraceptives and the risk of rheumatoid arthritis: a meta-analysis of a conflicting literature. Br J Rheumatol 1989;28(Suppl 1):13–7 [discussion: 18-23].

66. Pladevall-Vila M, Delclos GL, Varas C, et al. Controversy of oral contraceptives and risk of rheumatoid arthritis: meta-analysis of conflicting studies and review of conflicting meta-analyses with special emphasis on analysis of heterogeneity. Am J Epidemiol 1996;144(1):1–14.

67. Qi S, Xin R, Guo W, et al. Meta-analysis of oral contraceptives and rheumatoid arthritis risk in women. Ther Clin Risk Manag 2014;10:915–23.
68. Pedersen M, Jacobsen S, Garred P, et al. Strong combined gene-environment effects in anti-cyclic citrullinated peptide-positive rheumatoid arthritis: a nationwide case-control study in Denmark. Arthritis Rheum 2007;56(5):1446–53.
69. Salliot C, Bombardier C, Saraux A, et al. Hormonal replacement therapy may reduce the risk for RA in women with early arthritis who carry HLA-DRB1 *01 and/or *04 alleles by protecting against the production of anti-CCP: results from the ESPOIR cohort. Ann Rheum Dis 2010;69(9):1683–6.
70. Eun Y, Jeon KH, Han K, et al. Menopausal factors and risk of seropositive rheumatoid arthritis in postmenopausal women: a nationwide cohort study of 1.36 million women. Sci Rep 2020;10(1):20793.
71. Orellana C, Saevarsdottir S, Klareskog L, et al. Postmenopausal hormone therapy and the risk of rheumatoid arthritis: results from the Swedish EIRA population-based case-control study. Eur J Epidemiol 2015;30(5):449–57.
72. Walitt B, Pettinger M, Weinstein A, et al. Effects of postmenopausal hormone therapy on rheumatoid arthritis: the women's health initiative randomized controlled trials. Arthritis Rheumatism 2008;59(3):302–10.
73. Jethwa H, Lam S, Smith C, et al. Does Rheumatoid arthritis really improve during pregnancy? A systematic review and metaanalysis. J Rheumatol 2019;46(3):245–50.
74. Silman A, Kay A, Brennan P. Timing of pregnancy in relation to the onset of rheumatoid arthritis. Arthritis Rheum 1992;35(2):152–5.
75. Lansink M, de Boer A, Dijkmans BA, et al. The onset of rheumatoid arthritis in relation to pregnancy and childbirth. Clin Exp Rheumatol 1993;11(2):171–4.
76. Chen WMY, Subesinghe S, Muller S, et al. The association between gravidity, parity and the risk of developing rheumatoid arthritis: A systematic review and meta-analysis. Semin Arthritis Rheum 2020;50(2):252–60.
77. Peschken CA, Robinson DB, Hitchon CA, et al. Pregnancy and the risk of rheumatoid arthritis in a highly predisposed North American Native population. J Rheumatol 2012;39(12):2253–60.
78. Jørgensen KT, Harpsøe MC, Jacobsen S, et al. Increased risk of rheumatoid arthritis in women with pregnancy complications and poor self-rated health: a study within the Danish National Birth Cohort. Rheumatology (Oxford) 2014;53(8):1513–9.
79. Heliövaara M, Aho K, Reunanen A, et al. Parity and risk of rheumatoid arthritis in Finnish women. Br J Rheumatol 1995;34(7):625–8.
80. Pedersen M, Jacobsen S, Klarlund M, et al. Environmental risk factors differ between rheumatoid arthritis with and without auto-antibodies against cyclic citrullinated peptides. Arthritis Res Ther 2006;8(4):R133.
81. Orellana C, Wedrén S, Källberg H, et al. Parity and the risk of developing rheumatoid arthritis: results from the Swedish Epidemiological Investigation of Rheumatoid Arthritis study. Ann Rheum Dis 2014;73(4):752–5.
82. Hazes JM, Dijkmans BA, Vandenbroucke JP, et al. Pregnancy and the risk of developing rheumatoid arthritis. Arthritis Rheum 1990;33(12):1770–5.
83. Jørgensen KT, Pedersen BV, Jacobsen S, et al. National cohort study of reproductive risk factors for rheumatoid arthritis in Denmark: a role for hyperemesis, gestational hypertension and pre-eclampsia? Ann Rheum Dis 2010;69(2):358–63.

Environmental Risks for Spondyloarthropathies

Yvette Farran, MD, John Reveille, MD, Mark Hwang, MD, MS*

KEYWORDS

- Ankylosing spondylitis • Spondyloarthritis • Psoriatic arthritis • Reactive arthritis
- Risk factors

KEY POINTS

- Infections, microbiome, comorbidities, mechanical stress, and smoking are among the environmental risk factors associated with spondyloarthropathies/spondyloarthritis.
- Environmental risk factors are both shared and disease specific for psoriatic arthritis, ankylosing spondylitis, and reactive arthritis.
- Some environmental risk factors are modifiable and warrant patient discussion.

INTRODUCTION

Spondyloarthropathies, also known as spondyloarthritis (SpA), encompasses a spectrum of diseases classified by it's axial and peripheral musculoskeletal manifestations.[1,2] Extra-articular features are common in SpA making these systemic rheumatologic diseases involve the skin, eye, gut and other organ systems.[3,4]

Research has identified risk factors for the development of spondyloarthritis, particularly regarding genetic susceptibility and the strong association with HLA-B27.[5,6] Multiple studies have elucidated clinical risk factors associated with SpA disease activity and severity. In this review, we aim to explore the environmental risk factors for spondyloarthritis.

Infection

Reactive arthritis

Reactive arthritis (ReA) is an exemplar of an infectious trigger for spondyloarthritis. In ReA, various articular, entheseal, mucocutaneous, and ocular symptoms occur after a gastrointestinal, respiratory, or genitourinary infection. A variety of musculoskeletal manifestations are seen in viral diseases such as parvovirus B19 infection, HIV,

The authors report no financial disclosures relevant to this article.

Division of Rheumatology, Department of Internal Medicine, John P. and Kathrine G. McGovern School of Medicine at The University of Texas Health Science Center at Houston, 6431 Fannin MSB 5.270, Houston, TX 77030, USA

* Corresponding author.

E-mail address: Mark.C.Hwang@uth.tmc.edu

chikungunya, Lyme disease, Whipple's disease, streptococcal infections, and more recently, COVID-19 infection. These are occasionally grouped as reactive arthritis, but in general they are not included in the spectrum of spondyloarthritis and are not associated with HLA-B27.[7,8]

Microorganisms implicated in ReA share common biologic features: (1) they can invade mucosal surfaces and replicate intracellularly and (2) they contain lipopolysaccharide in their outer membrane. The most frequent type of ReA in developed countries is due to urogenital infections arising from infections with *Chlamydia trachomatis*.[9] Chlamydia are intracellular bacteria that can infect human cell types such as muscle cells and immune cells such as macrophages and monocytes.[10] *Chlamydia pneumonia* can also cause ReA by itself, albeit uncommonly.[11] Other microorganisms implicated in urogenital ReA include *Mycoplasma genitalium* and *Ureaplasma urealyticum*, although less common than *Chlamydia*.[12,13] There are also case reports of HLA-B27-associated ReA following *Gardnerella vaginalis* infections.[14]

Post-dysenteric ReA follows various *Shigella*, *Salmonella* (esp. *typhimurium* and *enteriditis*), *Campylobacter* and *Yersinia* species infections. Among the *Shigella* species, *S flexneri* is most implicated and *S dysenteriae* and *S sonnei* are less frequently involved.[15] In *Salmonella*-triggered ReA, the presence of HLA-B27 has been found to modulate the intracellular growth of *Salmonella*, allowing its persistence.[16,17] HLA-B27 expression can enhance *Salmonella* replication by reducing the threshold of endoplasmic reticulum stress induction and unfolded protein response-associated HLA-B27 misfolding.[18] Of note, antigens from *Salmonella*, *Shigella*, *Campylobacter*, *Yersinia*, and *Chlamydia* have been found in synovial tissues and fluids of patients with ReA and other types of SpA.[19,20] However, *Mycobacterum tuberculosis* DNA was also found in some samples, and *Chlamydia* nucleic acids were even in the joints of patients with osteoarthritis, raising concerns about the specificity of this testing.[21]

Campylobacter jejuni is the most common cause of human bacterial enteritis, although *Campylobacter coli*, *Campylobacter lari* and possibly *Campylobacter fetus* have also been implicated.[22–24] A population-based study of *Campylobacter*-associated ReA did not find an association with HLA-B27, although one review suggested that the incidence of *Campylobacter*-associated ReA may occur in 1% to 5% of those infected.[25,26]

Several other microorganisms that commonly cause infections, such as *beta-hemolytic Streptococci* and *Escherichia coli,* have been implicated in the pathogenesis of ReA and are listed in **Table 1**.[27]

Axial spondyloarthritis/ankylosing spondylitis

Specific pathogens have been implicated in the development of axial spondyloarthritis (axSpA). Patients with Candida infection have a 1.77-fold incidence of ankylosing spondylitis (AS) in comparison with the general population.[28] *Mycoplasma pneumonia* infection is also a risk factor for developing AS.[29] Tonsillitis, periodontitis, appendicitis, and respiratory tract infections have also been implicated.[30,31] In contrast to ReA, childhood enteric and urogenital infections were not found to be associated with the development of AS.[31]

Viral infections have also been associated with AS development. Patients with HPV had a 1.329 times higher risk of AS as compared with subjects without HPV.[32] Population studies looked at the incidence of AS in patients with HIV/AIDS, finding a lower incidence rate as compared with the general population.[33]

The role of *Klebsiella* in the AS pathogenesis has been well studied. In the 1970s, it was discovered that patients with "active" disease had increased fecal carriage of *Klebsiella* and there was lower in vitro lymphocyte responsiveness to *Klebsiella*

Table 1
Infectious agents associated with spondyloarthritis

	Pathogen	Study	Study Design
ReA	Blastocytosis	27	Systematic review
	Campylobacter	25	Cohort study
	Chlamydia trachomatis	9	Systematic review
	Clostridium difficile	27	Systematic review
	Cryptosporidium	27	Systematic review
	Cyclospora cayetanensis	27	Systematic review
	Entamoeba histolytica/dispar	27	Systematic review
	Escherichia coli	27	Systematic review
	Gardnerella vaginalis	14	Case report
	Giardia lamblia	27	Systematic review
	Hafnia alvei	27	Systematic review
	Mycobacterium bovis bacillus Calmette-Guerin	27	Systematic review
	Mycobacterium tuberculosis	27	Systematic review
	Mycoplasma genitalium	12	Case report
	Mycoplasma pneumoniae	27	Systematic review
	Neisseria meningitidis	27	Systematic review
	Rickettsia rickettsia	27	Systematic review
	Salmonella	16,17	Case series
	Shigella	15	Systematic review
	Staphylococcus lugdunensis	27	Systematic review
	beta-hemolytic Streptococci	27	Systematic review
	Strongyloides stercoralis	27	Systematic review
	Ureaplasma urealyticum	13	Cohort study
	Yersinia enterocolitica	15	Systematic review
AxSpA	Candida	28	Cohort study
	HIV	33	Cohort study
	HPV	32	Cohort study
	Klebsiella	34	Cohort study, basic science
	Mycoplasma pneumonia	29	Cohort study
PsA	Hepatitis B and C	45	Case–control

antigens in patients with HLA-B27 positivity.[34] Subsequent research showed an increased frequency of antibodies to a homologous region shared by HLA-B27 and Klebsiella nitrogenase as compared with HLA-B27–positive controls.[34] However, neither these findings nor any other specific Klebsiella pneumoniae antibody responses were confirmed by others. In fact, patients with active AS and acute anterior uveitis have been shown to have elevated IgA antibodies to a variety of gut bacteria independent of HLA-B27 status.[34–40] Similarly, a report suggesting alteration of MHC-associated gene products by a Klebsiella plasmid-derived soluble cell wall factor was not validated by other groups.[41–43] The strongest evidence against Klebsiella having a significant role in AxSpA pathogenesis comes from studies of the gut microbiome, where its presence was not found to be AS associated.[44]

Psoriatic arthritis
When evaluating the development of psoriatic arthritis (PsA) in patients with psoriasis, a significant association was found with history of infections that required antibiotic treatment. The types of infections reported included respiratory, urinary tract, skin/soft tissue, and sinus infections as well as infections with hepatitis B or C.[45]

Microbiome

Axial spondyloarthritis/ankylosing spondylitis/reactive arthritis

The gut microbiome has a role in the pathogenesis of spondyloarthritis. Many studies have identified differences in the composition of the gut microbiome in AS and PsA patients (**Table 2**).

Genetic background may influence gut microbiota composition. Changes in the microbiome composition seen in AS are partially due to effects of HLA-B27 and HLA-DRB1 on the gut microbiome.[46] Stool and intestinal biopsy samples in patients that were HLA-B27 positive demonstrated reduced carriage of *Bacterioides ovatus, Blautia obeum,* and *Dorea formicigenerans* and increased carriage of a *Roseburia* species and family Neisseriaceae.[46] When comparing risk associations with other HLA-B alleles, only B27 showed a statistically significant association with microbiome profile.[46] Significant differences in microbiota composition were also detected between HLA-B27 positive and HLA-B27 negative siblings.[47]

Compared with healthy controls, ReA patients had stool samples with an increased abundance of *Campylobacter* and *Erwinia* and decreased *Blautia, Caprococcus,*

Table 2
Microbiome composition data

	Pathogen	Study	Study Design
ReA	*Blautia*	48	Case–control
	Campylobacter	48	Case–control
	Collinsella	48	Case–control
	Coprococcus	48	Case–control
	Dialister	48	Case–control
	Erwinia	48	Case–control
	Roseburia	48	Case–control
	Ruminococcaceae	48	Case–control
AxSpa	Actinobacteria	50	Cohort study
	Actinomyces	50	Cohort study
	Actinomycetales	50	Cohort study
	Bacillis	50	Cohort study
	Bacteroides family	50	Cohort study
	Bacteroides fragilis	49	Case–control
	Bacterioides ovatus	46	Cohort study
	Bifidobacterium	50	Cohort study
	Blautia obeum	46	Cohort study
	Coriobacteriaceae family	50	Cohort study
	Dorea formicigenerans	46	Cohort study
	Erysipelotrichaceae	50	Cohort study
	F prausnitzii A2-165 strain	49	Case–control
	Firmicutes	52	Animal study
	Lactobacillales	52	Animal study
	Lactobacillus mucosae LM1	50	Cohort study
	Micrococcaceae	50	Cohort study
	Neisseriaceae	46	Cohort study
	Nocardiaceae	50	Cohort study
	Peptococcus	50	Cohort study
	Roseburia	46	Cohort study
	Ruminococcus gnavus	47	Case–control
PsA	*Akkermansia*	53	Case–control
	Pseudobutyrivibrio	53	Case–control
	Ruminococcus	53	Case–control

Roseburia, and *Collinsella.*[48] In this same group of ReA patients, those with uveitis had higher abundance of *Erwinia* and those with radiographic sacroiliitis had abundance of unclassified *Ruminococcaceae* and both were enriched in *Dialister.*[48] When comparing stool samples from children with treatment-naïve enthesitis-related arthritis and adults with SpA, both groups had decreased abundance of *Faecalibacterium prausnitzii* A2-165 strain that is reported to be anti-inflammatory.[49] In contrast, adults with SpA were found to have diminished *Bacteroides fragilis,* whereas children had in abundance.[49]

Differences are found in the microbiota in both patients with AS and healthy controls in relation to tobacco use and diet. In AS patients, *Peptococcus* at the genus level was significantly correlated with smoking whereas in health controls, *Bifidobacterium* and *Actinomyces* at the genus level were correlated with smoking.[50] Diet also had a strong influence on the gut microbiota and the composition of the microbiome was different among different diet groups.[50] Diet and its interaction with the gut microbiome influence both development and disease severity in AS.

The influence of the microbiota and its association with disease activity have also been studied. Correlation between disease activity and gut microbiota at the class level revealed a positive correlation between the genus *Bacillis* and Bath Ankylosing Spondylitis Disease Activity Index (BASDAI), *Actinomycetales* with Bath Ankylosing Spondylitis Functional Index (BASFI) and Ankylosing Spondylitis Disease Activity Score-CRP (ASDAS-CRP), *Micrococcaceae* with BASFI, *Nocardiaceae* with BASDAI and ASDAS-CRP, *Erysipelotrichaceae* with BASDAI, BASFI, and ASDAS-CRP, and *Lactobacillus mucosae LM1* with BASDAI, BASFI, and ASDAS-CRP.[50] In this study sample, AS patients had an increase in species from the *Bacteroidaceae* and *Coriobacteriaceae* families.[50] One theory proposed by the authors of this study is that *Actinobacteria*, which are more abundant in AS patients, may modulate the ubiquitination of NF-kB, which in turn activates pro-inflammatory factors in AS.[50]

In mouse models, the diversity of the intestinal microbiome decreased as AS progressed.[51] In ReA and SpA, there was less biodiversity of the microbiome as compared with healthy controls and in SpA, there was twofold to threefold increased abundance of *Ruminococcus gnavus* that was also found to correlate positively with disease activity in patients having a history of inflammatory bowel disease.[47]

The effect of rifaximin on the gut microbiome and disease progression was studied in AS mouse models. Stool studies in rifaximin treated mice showed increased abundance in *Bacteroidetes* and *Lactobacillales* and decreased *Firmicutes* .[52] In the rifaximin-treated mice, it was observed that there was less intestinal barrier breakdown and there was down-regulation of inflammatory factors.[52] This suggests that rifaximin may be beneficial in both the suppression of disease progression and regulation of the gut microbiome.

Psoriatic arthritis

When comparing patients with psoriasis and PsA to healthy controls, the gut microbiome was less diverse in the psoriasis and PsA patients. PsA patients were found to have significant reduction in *Akkermansia, Ruminococcus,* and *Pseudobutyrivibrio.*[53]

Comorbidities

Inflammatory bowel disease

Inflammatory bowel disease (IBD) patients have been shown to have an increased risk of SpA, with the prevalence of SpA in IBD of 21%.[54] Female sex, having Crohn's disease and history of treatment with at least one immunosuppressive or biologic drug are risk factors for SpA in IBD patients.[55] IBD in SpA patients are associated with higher BASDAI scores.[56] Patients with disease onset of IBD at less than 40 years and on anti-TNFα therapy have higher rates of uveitis and AS.[57]

Uveitis

Uveitis is commonly associated with SpA and PsA. In many cases, uveitis precedes the diagnosis of SpA, suggesting a bidirectional association. SpA patients with radiographic damage and longer disease duration have an increased risk for uveitis.[58] HLA-B27 positivity and family history of SpA are also associated with uveitis.[58,59] Uveitis is less prevalent in psoriasis and PsA patients.[58,59] When comparing AS with non-radiographic axSpA, AS patients are more likely to have uveitis.[60] Acute anterior uveitis has an association with risk of developing AS (hazard ratio 2.71 (2.25–3.25)).[61]

Uveitis is also associated with AS disease severity and joint involvement. In one study, the incidence rate for hip-joint lesions and number of peripheral joints involved was higher for patients with uveitis than the nonuveitis group.[62] Uveitis is associated with IBD and infliximab, independently reverse-causation may explain the infliximab association.[63]

In PsA and uveitis, the incidence rate per 10 000 person-years for PsA in patients with uveitis was 4.25, and the adjusted analysis confirmed an increased risk for PsA in patients with uveitis(3.77 [2.66–5.34]).[64] They also found an increased risk for uveitis in PsA patients.[64]

Psoriasis-for psoriatic arthritis

Severe psoriasis, presence of nail pitting, low level of education, and uveitis are predictive of the development of PsA.[65] In addition, the duration of cutaneous symptoms in patients with psoriasis is associated with an increased risk of PsA.[66] The most common types of psoriasis associated with spondyloarthropathies are plaque, scalp, palmoplantar pustulosis, and nail psoriasis.[67] In a prospective observational multicenter study of patients with psoriasis, the prevalence of PsA was 13.1%.[68]

Hyperlipidemia

Hyperlipidemia is associated with an increased risk of PsA. In US women, hypercholesterolemia was associated with elevated risks of incident psoriasis (hazard ratio (HR) 1.25 [95% CI 1.04–1.50]) and psoriasis with PsA (HR 1.58 [95% CI 1.13–2.23]).[69] It was also found that subjects with hypercholesteremia for more than 7 years had a higher risk of developing both psoriasis and PsA.[69] In this same study, there was no association between cholesterol-lowering medication use and the risk of psoriasis and psoriasis with PsA.[69] The causal link between hyperlipidemia and PsA remains unclear.

Mechanical Stress

Axial spondyloarthritis/ankylosing spondylitis

Mechanical stress is linked to the development of AS and PsA. The trauma theory states that mechanical stress at insertional locations causes enthesitis was elucidated in the 1950s.[70] Patients with AS recalled entheseal symptoms starting greater than 2 years before the onset of back pain and 44% of these patients recalled prior trauma that they felt triggered their disease.[71] Mouse models show mechanical strain drives both entheseal inflammation and new bone formation in SpA. Mice with chronic and deregulated TNF production were used to assess the development of entheseal inflammation. In these mice, the first signs of inflammation were found at the entheses and weight-bearing sites, such as the hind limbs. In addition, new bone formation was seen at entheseal sites that was promoted by biomechanical stress.[72] In observational cohorts, BASDAI and BASFI scores independently are associated with higher lifetime occupational physical activity.[73]

Psoriatic arthritis

Patients with psoriasis exposed to physical trauma, specifically bone and joint trauma, are at an increased risk of developing PsA.[74] Occupational physical activity including lifting heavy weights, recurrent squatting and pushing heavy weight, were more common in patients with PsA as compared with patients with psoriasis alone.[45] Lifting cumulative loads of at least 100 pounds/h (Odds Ratio (OR) 2.8) was significantly associated with PsA.[45] The Koebner phenomenon, in which a lesion erupts secondary to trauma of the skin, is well described in psoriasis. Microtrauma at sites of high physical stress and the resulting inflammation has been called the "Deep Koebner" phenomena. In patients with PsA, flexor tendon pulleys (an area of high physical stress), especially those with dactylitis history, were found to be thicker by ultrasonography as compared with patients with RA and healthy controls.[75] A case report of identical twins with longstanding psoriasis described the development of post-trauma dactylitis supporting mechanical stress triggering PsA in genetically susceptible patients.[76]

Smoking

Axial spondyloarthritis/ankylosing spondylitis

Smoking is a known risk factor for AS. The risk for developing AS in current smokers was increased (OR 1.99) however being a former smoker did not have a significant risk.[77] The risk of having the active disease was higher in patients who smoked at least 15 cigarettes per day or 15 pack-years (OR = 1.74 [1.06, 2.84] and 2.89 [1.56, 5.35], respectively), with an increasing number of cigarettes per day and pack-years.[78] Smokers had an increased risk of functional impairment.[78] A multivariate analysis found that smoking was associated with an earlier onset of inflammatory back pain (IBP), higher disease activity (ASDAS, BASDAI), worse functional status (BASFI), more frequent MRI inflammation of the sacroiliac joints (OR 1.57, P = .02) and spine (OR 2.33, P < .001), more frequent MRI structural lesions of the sacroiliac joints (OR 1.54, P = .03) and spine (OR 2.02, P = .01), and higher modified stoke ankylosing spondylitis spine score (MSASSS) reflecting radiographic structural damage of the spine.[79]

Psoriatic arthritis

The association between smoking and development of PsA is unclear. Multiple studies have shown that smoking is inversely associated with PsA.[45,80,81] In US women who smoke, smoking was associated with an elevated risk of incident PsA with relative risk (RR) of 1.54 for past smokers (95% CI: 1.06–2.24), and 3.13 for current smokers (95% CI: 2.08–4.71) as compared with nonsmokers.[82] However, another study found that smoking was associated with an increased risk of PsA in the general population (HR, 1.27; 95% CI: 1.19–1.36) and decreased risk among psoriasis patients (HR 0.91; 95% CI: 0.84 to 0.99).[81] In mediation analysis, the effect of smoking on PsA was mediated through its effect on psoriasis.[81] Future studies that account for the complex relationship between smoking, psoriasis and PsA are needed to estimate the effect of smoking on PsA incidence.

Obesity

Obesity seems to increase risk of PsA. Adiposity is associated with an increased risk of incident PsA.[83] Compared with individuals of normal weight, obese individuals had an HR of 2.46 (95% CI 1.65, 3.68), and overweight individuals had an HR of 1.41 (95% CI 1.00, 1.99).[83] When comparing PsA with psoriasis, the mean body mass index (BMI) for individuals with PsA was 1.80 kg/m^2 (95% CI 0.61, 2.99 kg/m^2) higher than that for those with psoriasis, and the odds of obesity were increased by 61% among individuals with PsA compared with psoriasis (95% CI 1.10, 2.37) after adjustments for covariables.[84] In patients with psoriasis, PsA incidence rates increased with BMI (RR of 1.48 in patients with BMI ≥35.0).[85] In patients without a diagnosis of psoriasis, BMI was associated with an increased risk of incident PsA.[86] Another study found that BMI at the age of 18 years was predictive of PsA (OR 1.06, $P < .01$) and that current BMI was not a significant predictor of PsA.[87] Adiposity is associated with higher levels of inflammatory cytokines, which could increase the risk of PsA in predisposed individuals.[87]

Miscellaneous

Breastfeeding
Breastfeeding may have a protective effect on AS incidence. AS patients were found to have been breastfed less often as compared with their healthy siblings OR for AS onset of 0.53 (95% CI [0.36–0.77], P value = .<0.01).[88] In addition, breastfeeding reduced familial prevalence of AS.[88]

Toxins
Alcohol intake and its effect on developing AS is unclear. Studies have explored the association between alcohol consumption and disease activity. In one study, alcohol drinking was associated with lower disease activity (BASDAI β = − 0.83, 95% CI − 1.49, − 0.17; ASDAS β = − 0.36, 95% CI − 0.66, − 0.05) and functional impairment (BASFI β = − 1.40, 95% CI − 2.12, − 0.68).[89] However, another study showed that alcohol increased the risk of spinal structural damage as measured by MSASSS.[90] In this prospective cohort study, the alcohol drinker group showed more significant MSASSS changes (≥2 units for 2 years follow-up) and new syndesmophyte/progression of pre-existing syndesmophytes than the nondrinker group (60.7% vs 29.2%, $P < .001$, 51.5% vs 26.4%, $P < .001$, respectively).[90]

In PsA, excessive alcohol intake (defined as greater than or equal to 30 g/d) was associated with an increased risk of incident PsA in a cohort of US women.[91]

AS disease severity has been linked to chemical exposures. A cohort of AS patient with abnormal occiput-to-wall distance was found to have higher urinary cadmium, antimony, tungsten, uranium and trimethylarsine oxide concentrations.[92] In addition, people who resided in older households (<1990) had abnormal AS clinical measures compared to those who reside in new households.[92]

Medications
Isotretinoin-induced axSpA is a prevalent side effect in patients with acne vulgaris. In patients treated with isotretinoin, approximately 24% developed inflammatory back pain.[93] In these patients, MRI revealed sacroiliitis in 42% of the cases and approximately 52% fulfilled the Assessment of Spondyloarthritis International Society criteria for axSpA.[93] After isotretinoin discontinuation, MRI findings had completely resolved.[93]

Acetaminophen and NSAID use may be associated with an increased risk of PsA. In a study of US women, regular acetaminophen users had a higher risk of developing psoriasis (age-adjusted HR = 1.29, 95% CI: 1.08–1.54) or psoriasis with concomitant PsA (age-adjusted HR = 2.23, 95% CI: 1.63–3.07) when compared to nonregular users. However, only the HR of PsA associated with regular acetaminophen use remained significant in fully-adjusted models accounting for aspirin and other NSAIDs (HR = 1.78, 95% CI: 1.28–4.46).[94] Reverse causation could account for this PsA association with medication.

Diet
Diet and risk of developing PsA have been investigated separately from the effect of diet on gut microbiome. Gluten intake was not associated with the risk of incident psoriasis

or PsA.[95] A study in Japan compared the diets of patients with psoriasis who had PsA with those that did not have PsA. The PsA group had higher intake of β-carotene, vitamin A, and green and yellow vegetables than the non-PSA group; however, when logistic regression analysis was done, they failed to detect the association of these variables with PsA.[96] The association between AS and diet has been studied and there is little evidence to support diet influencing disease development or severity.[97]

Weather
Weather and clinic visits were studied in relation to AS disease severity. A relationship was suggested between high humidity events and an increase in the number of patients with AS visiting the hospital the following day or 7 days later.[98]

SUMMARY

In summary, many environmental risk factors have been identified for SpA, specifically for AxSpA, ReA, and PsA. These risk factors fit broadly into groups of infections, microbiome, comorbidities, mechanical stress, smoking, and miscellaneous risk factors. Targeting some of these environmental risk factors such as smoking, obesity, and management of comorbidities may mitigate some of the risk associated with development and severity of SpA.

CLINICS CARE POINTS

- Multiple infectious organisms are implicated as triggers for reactive arthritis, spondyloarthritis, and psoriatic arthritis (PsA)
- The gut microbiome plays a major role in the development of ankylosing spondylitis (AS) and in disease activity
- The comorbidities that are strongly associated with spondyloarthritis are Inflammatory bowel disease, uveitis, psoriasis, and to a lesser extent, hyperlipidemia
- Mechanical stress is linked to the development of AS and PsA

REFERENCES

1. Rudwaleit M, van der Heijde D, Landewé R, et al. The development of Assessment of SpondyloArthritis international Society classification criteria for axial spondyloarthritis (part II): validation and final selection. Ann Rheum Dis 2009; 68:777–83.
2. Rudwaleit M, van der Heijde D, Landewé R, et al. The Assessment of SpondyloArthritis international Society classification criteria for peripheral spondyloarthritis and for spondyloarthritis in general. Ann Rheum Dis 2011;70:25–31.
3. Taurog JD, Chhabra A, Colbert RA. Ankylosing spondylitis and axial spondyloarthritis. N Engl J Med 2016;374:2563–74.
4. Ritchlin CT, Colbert RA, Gladman DD. Psoriatic Arthritis N Engl J Med 2017;376: 957–70.
5. Hwang MC, Ridley L, Reveille JD. Ankylosing spondylitis risk factors: a systematic literature review. Clin Rheumatol 2021;40:3079–93.
6. Mulder MLM, van Hal TW, Wenink MH, et al. Clinical, laboratory, and genetic markers for the development or presence of psoriatic arthritis in psoriasis patients: a systematic review. Arthritis Res Ther 2021;23(1):168.

7. Taniguchi Y, Nishikawa H, Yoshida T, et al. Expanding the spectrum of reactive arthritis (ReA): classic ReA and infection-related arthritis including poststreptococcal ReA, Poncet's disease, and iBCG-induced ReA. Rheumatol Int 2021;41: 1387–98.

8. Kocyigit BF, Akyol A. Reactive arthritis after COVID-19: a case-based review. Rheumatol Int 2021;41:2031–9.

9. Denison HJ, Curtis EM, Clynes MA, et al. The incidence of sexually acquired reactive arthritis: a systematic literature review. Clin Rheumatol 2016;35:2639–48.

10. Zeidler H, Hudson AP. New insights into Chlamydia and arthritis. Promise of a cure? Ann Rheum Dis 2014;73:637–44.

11. Contini C, Grilli A, Badia L, et al. Detection of Chlamydophila pneumoniae in patients with arthritis: significance and diagnostic value. Rheumatol Int 2010;31: 1307–13.

12. Chrisment D, Machelart I, Wirth G, et al. Reactive arthritis associated with Mycoplasma genitalium urethritis. Diagn Microbiol Infect Dis 2013;77:278–9.

13. Horowitz S, Horowitz J, Taylor-Robinson D, et al. Ureaplasma urealyticum in Reiter's syndrome. J Rheumatol 1994;21:877–82.

14. François S, Guyadier-Souguières G, Marcelli C. Reactive arthritis due to Gardnerella vaginalis. A case-report. Rev Rhum Engl Ed 1997;64:138.

15. Ajene AN, Walker CLF, Black RE. Enteric pathogens and reactive arthritis: a systematic review of campylobacter , salmonella and shigella-associated reactive arthritis. J Health Popul Nutr 2013;31:299–307.

16. Ge S, He Q, Granfors K. HLA-B27 Modulates Intracellular Growth of Salmonella Pathogenicity Island 2 Mutants and Production of Cytokines in Infected Monocytic U937 Cells. PLoS One 2012;7:e34093.

17. Ge S, Danino V, He Q, et al. Microarray analysis of response of salmonella during the Infection of HLA-B27-Transfected Human Macrophage-Like U937 Cells. BMC genomics 2010;11:456.

18. Antoniou AN, Lenart I, Kriston-Vizi J, et al. Salmonella exploits HLA-B27 and host unfolded protein responses to promote intracellular replication. Ann Rheum Dis 2019;78:74–82.

19. Pacheco-Tena C, Alvarado de la Barrera C, López-Vidal Y, et al. Bacterial DNA in synovial fluid cells of patients with juvenile onset spondyloarthropathies. Rheumatology (Oxford) 2001;40:920–7.

20. Hill Gaston JS, Cox C, Granfors K. Clinical and experimental evidence for persistent Yersinia infection in reactive arthritis. Arthritis Rheum 1999;42:2239–42.

21. Olmez N, Wang GF, Li Y, et al. Chlamydial nucleic acids in synovium in osteoarthritis: what are the implications? J Rheumatol 2001;28:1874–80.

22. Townes JM, Deodhar AA, Laine ES, et al. Reactive arthritis following culture-confirmed infections with bacterial enteric pathogens in Minnesota and Oregon: a population-based study. Ann Rheum Dis 2008;67:1689–96.

23. Goudswaard J, Sabbe L, te Winkel W. Reactive arthritis as a complication of Campylobacter lari enteritis. J Infect 1995;31:171.

24. Urman JD. Reiter's syndrome associated with campylobacter fetus infection. Ann Intern Med 1977;86:444.

25. Hannu T, Mattila L, Rautelin H, et al. Campylobacter-triggered reactive arthritis: a population-based study. Rheumatology (Oxford, England) 2002;41:312–8.

26. Pope JE, Krizova A, Garg AX, et al. Campylobacter reactive arthritis: a systematic review. Semin Arthritis Rheum 2007;37:48–55.

27. Zeidler H, Hudson AP. Reactive arthritis update: spotlight on new and rare infectious agents implicated as pathogens. Curr Rheumatol Rep 2021;23:53.

28. Wei JC, Chou M, Huang J, et al. The association between Candida infection and ankylosing spondylitis: a population-based matched cohort study. Curr Med Res Opin 2020;36:2063–9.

29. Chu K, Chen W, Hung Y, et al. Increased risk of ankylosing spondylitis after Mycoplasma pneumonia: A Nationwide population-based study. Medicine (Baltimore) 2019;98:e15596.

30. Chao W, Lin C, Chen Y, et al. Association between tonsillitis and newly diagnosed ankylosing spondylitis: A nationwide, population-based, case-control study. PloS one 2019;14:e0220721.

31. Lindström U, Exarchou S, Lie E, et al. Childhood hospitalisation with infections and later development of ankylosing spondylitis: a national case-control study. Arthritis Res Ther 2016;18:240.

32. Wei C, Lin J, Wang Y, et al. Risk of ankylosing spondylitis following human papillomavirus infection: a nationwide, population-based, cohort study. J Autoimmun 2020;113:102482.

33. Yen Y, Chuang P, Jen I, et al. Incidence of autoimmune diseases in a nationwide HIV/AIDS patient cohort in Taiwan, 2000–2012. Ann Rheum Dis 2017;76:661–5.

34. Long F, Wang T, Li Q, et al. Association between Klebsiella pneumoniae and ankylosing spondylitis: A systematic review and meta-analysis. Int J Rheum Dis 2022;4:422–32.

35. Stebbings S, Munro K, Simon MA, et al. Comparison of the faecal microflora of patients with ankylosing spondylitis and controls using molecular methods of analysis. Rheumatology (Oxford, England) 2002;41:1395–401.

36. de Vries DD, Dekker-Saeys AJ, Gyodi E, et al. Absence of autoantibodies to peptides shared by HLA-B27.5 and Klebsiella pneumoniae nitrogenase in serum samples from HLA-B27 positive patients with ankylosing spondylitis and Reiter's syndrome. Ann Rheum Dis 1992;51:783–9.

37. Stone MA, Payne U, Schentag C, et al. Comparative immune responses to candidate arthritogenic bacteria do not confirm a dominant role for Klebsiella pneumonia in the pathogenesis of familial ankylosing spondylitis. Rheumatology (Oxford, England) 2004;43:148–55.

38. Sprenkels SH, Van Kregten E, Feltkamp TE. IgA antibodies against Klebsiella and other Gram-negative bacteria in ankylosing spondylitis and acute anterior uveitis. Clin Rheumatol 1996;15(Suppl 1):48–51.

39. Kijlstra A, Luyendijk L, van der Gaag R, et al. IgG and IgA immune response against klebsiella in HLA-B27-associated anterior uveitis. Br J Ophthalmol 1986;70:85–8.

40. Mäki-Ikola O, Lehtinen K, Nissilä M, et al. IgM, IgA and IgG class serum antibodies against Klebsiella pneumoniae and Escherichia coli lipopolysaccharides in patients with ankylosing spondylitis. Br J Rheumatol 1994;33:1025–9.

41. Geczy AF, Alexander K, Bashir HV, et al. Characterization of a factor(s) present in Klebsiella culture filtrates that specifically modifies an HLA-B27-associated cell-surface component. J Exp Med 1980;152:331s–40S.

42. Trapani JA, McKenzie IF. Klebsiella 'modifying factor': binding studies with HLA-B27+ and B27- lymphocytes. Ann Rheum Dis 1985;44:169–75.

43. Ngo KY, Rochu D, D'Ambrosio AM, et al. Klebsiella plasmid K21 is not involved in the aetiology of ankylosing spondylitis. Exp Clin Immunogenet 1984;1:140–4.

44. Puccetti A, Dolcino M, Tinazzi E, et al. Antibodies Directed against a Peptide Epitope of a Klebsiella pneumoniae-Derived Protein Are Present in Ankylosing Spondylitis. PLoS one 2017;12:e0171073.

45. Eder L, Law T, Chandran V, et al. Association between environmental factors and onset of psoriatic arthritis in patients with psoriasis. Arthritis Care Res 2011;63: 1091–7.

46. Asquith M, Sternes PR, Costello M, et al. HLA Alleles associated with risk of ankylosing spondylitis and rheumatoid arthritis influence the gut microbiome. Arthritis Rheumatol 2019;71:1642–50.

47. Breban M, Tap J, Leboime A, et al. Faecal microbiota study reveals specific dysbiosis in spondyloarthritis. Ann Rheum Dis 2017;76:1614–22.

48. Manasson J, Shen N, Garcia Ferrer HR, et al. Gut Microbiota Perturbations in Reactive Arthritis and Postinfectious Spondyloarthritis. Arthritis Rheumatol (Hoboken, N.J.). 2018;70:242–54.

49. Stoll ML, Weiss PF, Weiss JE, et al. Age and fecal microbial strain-specific differences in patients with spondyloarthritis. Arthritis Res Ther 2018;20:14.

50. Zhang L, Han R, Zhang X, et al. Fecal microbiota in patients with ankylosing spondylitis: correlation with dietary factors and disease activity. Clinica Chim Acta 2019;497:189–96.

51. Liu G, Ma Y, Yang Q, et al. Modulation of inflammatory response and gut microbiota in ankylosing spondylitis mouse model by bioactive peptide IQW. J Appl Microbiol 2020;128:1669–77.

52. Yang L, Liu B, Zheng J, et al. Rifaximin alters intestinal microbiota and prevents progression of ankylosing spondylitis in mice. Front Cell Infect Microbiol 2019; 9:44.

53. Scher JU, Ubeda C, Artacho A, et al. Decreased bacterial diversity characterizes the altered gut microbiota in patients with psoriatic arthritis, resembling dysbiosis in inflammatory bowel disease. Arthritis Rheumatol (Hoboken, N.J.). 2015;67: 128–39.

54. Evans J, Sapsford M, McDonald S, et al. Prevalence of axial spondyloarthritis in patients with inflammatory bowel disease using cross-sectional imaging: a systematic literature review. Ther Adv Musculoskelet Dis 2021;13. 1759720X21996973. London (UK): SAGE Publications.

55. Ribaldone DG, Vernero M, Parisi S, et al. Risk factors of suspected spondyloarthritis among inflammatory bowel disease patients. Scand J Gastroenterol 2019;54:1233–6.

56. Wendling D, Guillot X, Prati C, et al. Effect of gut involvement in patients with high probability of early spondyloarthritis: data from the DESIR Cohort. J Rheumatol 2020;47:349–53.

57. Herzog D, Fournier N, Buehr P, et al. Age at disease onset of inflammatory bowel disease is associated with later extraintestinal manifestations and complications. Eur J Gastroenterol Hepatol 2018;30:598–607.

58. Yaşar Bilge NŞ, Kalyoncu U, Atagündüz P, et al. Uveitis-related Factors in Patients With Spondyloarthritis: TReasure Real-Life Results. Am J Ophthalmol 2021;228:58–64.

59. Gevorgyan O, Riad M, Sarran RD, et al. Anterior uveitis in patients with spondyloarthropathies in a single US academic center: a retrospective study. Rheumatol Int 2019;39:1607–14.

60. Hong C, Kwan YH, Leung Y, et al. Comparison of ankylosing spondylitis and non-radiographic axial spondyloarthritis in a multi-ethnic Asian population of Singapore. Int J Rheum Dis 2019;22:1506–11.

61. Yen J, Hsu C, Hsiao S, et al. Acute anterior uveitis as a risk factor of ankylosing spondylitis-A National Population-Based Study. Int J Environ Res Public Health 2017;14:107.

62. Sun L, Wu R, Xue Q, et al. Risk factors of uveitis in ankylosing spondylitis: an observational study. Medicine (Baltimore) 2016;95:e4233.
63. Keck K, Choi D, Savage L, et al. Insights Into Uveitis in Association With Spondyloarthritis From a Large Patient Survey. J Clin Rheumatol 2014;20:141–5.
64. Egeberg A, Khalid U, Gislason GH, et al. Association of Psoriatic Disease With Uveitis: A Danish Nationwide Cohort Study. JAMA Dermatology (Chicago, Ill.) 2015;151:1200–5.
65. Eder L, Haddad A, Rosen CF, et al. The Incidence and Risk Factors for Psoriatic Arthritis in Patients With Psoriasis: A Prospective Cohort Study. Arthritis Rheumatol (Hoboken, N.J.). 2016;68:915–23.
66. Egeberg A, Skov L, Zachariae C, et al. Duration of psoriatic skin disease as risk factor for subsequent onset of psoriatic arthritis. Acta Derm Venereol 2018;98: 546–50.
67. Roure F, Elhai M, Burki V, et al. Prevalence and clinical characteristics of psoriasis in spondyloarthritis: a descriptive analysis of 275 patients. Clin Exp Rheumatol 2016;34:82–7.
68. Vanaclocha F, Crespo-Erchiga V, Jiménez-Puya R, et al. Immune-mediated inflammatory diseases and other comorbidities in patients with psoriasis: baseline characteristics of patients in the AQUILES Study. Actas Dermosifiliogr 2014;106: 35–43.
69. Cava GL. Enthesitis-traumatic disease of insertions. J Am Med Assoc 1959;169: 254–5.
70. Wu S, Li W, Han J, et al. Hypercholesterolemia and Risk of Incident Psoriasis and Psoriatic Arthritis in US Women. Arthritis Rheumatol (Hoboken, N.J.), 66 2014;304–10.
71. Ansell RC, Shuto T, Busquets-Perez N, et al. The role of biomechanical factors in ankylosing spondylitis: the patient's perspective. Reumatismo 2015;67:91–6.
72. Jacques P, Lambrecht S, Verheugen E, et al. Proof of concept: enthesitis and new bone formation in spondyloarthritis are driven by mechanical strain and stromal cells. Ann Rheum Dis 2014;73:437–45.
73. Ward MM, Weisman MH, Davis JC, et al. Risk factors for functional limitations in patients with long-standing ankylosing spondylitis. Arthritis Rheum 2005;53: 710–7.
74. Thorarensen SM, Lu N, Ogdie A, et al. Physical trauma recorded in primary care is associated with the onset of psoriatic arthritis among patients with psoriasis. Ann Rheum Dis 2017;76:521–5.
75. Tinazzi I, McGonagle D, Aydin SZ, et al. 'Deep Koebner' phenomenon of the flexor tendon-associated accessory pulleys as a novel factor in tenosynovitis and dactylitis in psoriatic arthritis. Ann Rheum Dis 2018;77:922–5.
76. Ng J, Tan AL, McGonagle D. Unifocal psoriatic arthritis development in identical twins following site specific injury: evidence supporting biomechanical triggering events in genetically susceptible hosts. Ann Rheum Dis 2015;74:948–9.
77. Videm V, Cortes A, Thomas R, et al. Current smoking is associated with incident ankylosing spondylitis - The HUNT population- based Norwegian health study. J Rheumatol 2014;41:2041–8.
78. Zhang H, Wan W, Liu J, et al. Smoking quantity determines disease activity and function in Chinese patients with ankylosing spondylitis. Clin Rheumatol 2018;37: 1605–16.
79. Chung HY, Machado P, van der Heijde D, et al. Smokers in early axial spondyloarthritis have earlier disease onset, more disease activity, inflammation and

damage, and poorer function and health-related quality of life: results from the DESIR cohort. Ann Rheum Dis 2012;71:809–16.

80. Eder L, Shanmugarajah S, Thavaneswaran A, et al. The association between smoking and the development of psoriatic arthritis among psoriasis patients. Ann Rheum Dis 2012;71:219–24.

81. Nguyen UDT, Zhang Y, Lu N, et al. Smoking paradox in the development of psoriatic arthritis among patients with psoriasis: a population-based study. Ann Rheum Dis 2018;77:119–23.

82. Li W, Han J, Qureshi AA. Smoking and risk of incident psoriatic arthritis in US women. Ann Rheum Dis 2012;71:804–8.

83. Thomsen RS, Nilsen TIL, Haugeberg G, et al. Adiposity and physical activity as risk factors for developing psoriatic arthritis: longitudinal data from a Population-Based Study in Norway. Arthritis Care Res (2010) 2021;73:432–41.

84. Bhole VM, Choi HK, Burns LC, et al. Differences in body mass index among individuals with PsA, psoriasis, RA and the general population. Rheumatology (Oxford, England) 2012;51:552–6.

85. Love T, Zhu Y, Zhang Y, et al. Obesity and the risk of psoriatic arthritis: a population-based study. Ann Rheum Dis 2012;71:1273–7.

86. Li W, Han J, Qureshi AA. Obesity and risk of incident psoriatic arthritis in US women. Ann Rheum Dis 2012;71:1267–72.

87. Soltani-Arabshahi R, Wong B, Feng B, et al. Obesity in early adulthood as a risk factor for psoriatic arthritis. Arch dermatology (1960) 2010;146:721–6.

88. Montoya J, Matta NB, Suchon P, et al. Patients with ankylosing spondylitis have been breast fed less often than healthy controls: a case–control retrospective study. Ann Rheum Dis 2016;75:879–82.

89. Zhao S, Thong D, Duffield SJ, et al. Alcohol and disease activity in axial spondyloarthritis: a cross-sectional study. Rheumatol Int 2018;38:375–81.

90. Min HK, Lee J, Ju JH, et al. Alcohol consumption as a predictor of the progression of spinal structural damage in axial spondyloarthritis: data from the Catholic Axial Spondyloarthritis COhort (CASCO). Arthritis Res Ther 2019;21:187.

91. Wu S, Cho E, Li W, et al. Alcohol intake and risk of incident psoriatic arthritis in women. J Rheumatol 2015;42:835–40.

92. Shiue I. Relationship of environmental exposures and ankylosing spondylitis and spinal mobility: US NHAENS, 2009-2010. Int J Environ Health Res 2015;25:322–9.

93. Elnady B, Elkhouly T, Dawoud NM, et al. New onset of axial spondyloarthropathy in patients treated with isotretinoin for acne vulgaris: incidence, follow-up, and MRI findings. Clin Rheumatol 2020;39:1829–38.

94. Wu S, Han J, Qureshi AA. Use of aspirin, non-steroidal anti-inflammatory drugs, and acetaminophen (paracetamol), and risk of psoriasis and psoriatic arthritis: a cohort study. Acta dermato-venereologica. 2015;95:217–23.

95. Drucker AM, Qureshi AA, Thompson JM, et al. Gluten intake and risk of psoriasis, psoriatic arthritis, and atopic dermatitis among United States women. J Am Acad Dermatol 2020;82:661–5.

96. Yamashita H, Morita T, Ito M, et al. Dietary habits in Japanese patients with psoriasis and psoriatic arthritis: Low intake of meat in psoriasis and high intake of vitamin A in psoriatic arthritis. J Dermatol 2019;46:759–69.

97. Macfarlane TV, Abbood HM, Pathan E, et al. Relationship between diet and ankylosing spondylitis: a systematic review. Eur J Rheumatol 2018;5(1):45–52.

98. Xin L, Liu J, Zhu Y, et al. Exposure-lag-response associations between weather conditions and ankylosing spondylitis: a time series study. BMC Musculoskelet Disord 2021;22:1–641.

Systemic Lupus Erythematosus Risk
The Role of Environmental Factors

Jia Li Liu, MD[a], Jennifer M.P. Woo, PhD[b], Christine G. Parks, PhD[b],
Karen H. Costenbader, MD[c], Søren Jacobsen, MD[d],
Sasha Bernatsky, MD[e],*

KEYWORDS

- Systemic lupus erythematosus • Environmental triggers • Pollution • Microbiome
- Smoking • Infections

KEY POINTS

- Genetic risk factors only account for about one-third of heritability among individuals with a family history of SLE; a large portion of the remaining risk may be attributable to environmental exposures.
- SLE has been potentially associated with specific viral infections (eg, Epstein-Barr), with no established association with vaccinations.
- SLE has also been associated with low vitamin D and diets high in carbohydrates and low in monosaturated fatty acids, saturated fats, and trans fatty acids. SLE patients have different gut microbiomes, which may be related to SLE pathogenesis.
- The literature also supports positive associations between SLE and current smoking, organic pollutants, and occupational exposure to crystalline silica.

Systemic lupus erythematosus (SLE) is a chronic autoimmune disease with multisystemic and heterogeneous presentations.[1] It is associated with important immune dysregulation, such as self-reactive lymphocytes and loss of immune tolerance. SLE mainly affects females, as 90% of SLE cases are in females, and diagnosis is often made during reproductive years.[2] The incidence of SLE is higher in certain populations including African American/Black and American Indian/First Nation women.[3-9] The

[a] McGill University, Montreal, Quebec, Canada; [b] Epidemiology Branch, Department of Health and Human Services, National Institutes of Environmental Health Sciences, National Institutes of Health, Research Triangle Park, NC, USA; [c] Division of Rheumatology, Inflammation and Immunity, Brigham and Women's Hospital, Harvard Medical School, Boston, MA, USA; [d] Copenhagen Lupus and Vasculitis Clinic, Rigshospitalet, Copenhagen University Hospital, Denmark; [e] Centre for Outcomes Research and Evaluation, Research Institute of the McGill University Health Centre, Montreal, Quebec, Canada
* Corresponding author.
E-mail address: sasha.bernatsky@mcgill.ca

Rheum Dis Clin N Am 48 (2022) 827–843
https://doi.org/10.1016/j.rdc.2022.06.005
0889-857X/22/© 2022 Elsevier Inc. All rights reserved.

incidence of SLE ranges from 4 to 7 per 100,000 in the United States and Canada, 1 to 5 per 100,000 in European populations, 3 to 8 per 100,000 in East Asian populations, and 5 to 9 per 100,000 in Hispanic/South American cohorts.[10–12]

SLE has complex pathogenesis and multifactorial etiology, with its heterogeneous nature stemming from both genetic and environmental factors[13] ranging from physical, chemical, and other potentially modifiable exogenous exposures.[14,15]

Environmental factors that initiate and propagate the development of autoimmunity may act sequentially. There is a "first hit" genetic or environmental exposure that induces an initial break of tolerance, leading to initiation of autoantibody production. When a "second hit" environmental exposure occurs, the initially limited autoimmune response becomes more florid, with inflammation developing in target organs, and the onset of clinical disease.

This review will provide an updated overview primarily based on epidemiologic studies of various chemical and physical exposures and SLE risk in adults (**Table 1**), including infections and microbial influences, vaccinations, diet, respiratory exposures (respirable silica, air pollution, smoking, etc.), and other factors (chemicals, organic pollutants, heavy metals, and ultraviolet radiation).

INFECTIONS

Infections have been associated with triggering autoimmune diseases, such as SLE. There may be different infections, such as those acquired in early life or latent viral infections.[16,17] In infections acquired in early life, immune response tendencies could increase susceptibility to SLE later in life.[17]

Epstein-Barr virus (EBV) seropositivity was elevated in adults and children with SLE compared to age-matched controls in cross-sectional studies.[18] In contrast, EBV seropositivity, infectious mononucleosis, or severe infectious mononucleosis requiring hospital admission were not shown to be associated with SLE risk in different studies.[19,20] A meta-analysis in patients with SLE compared to healthy individuals demonstrated higher seroprevalence of anti-viral capsid antigen immunoglobulin g (IgG) and antibodies to EBV early antigen diffuse in patients with SLE;[21] however, there was publication bias and the meta-analysis included suboptimal cross-sectional

Table 1
Physical and chemical environment exposures associated with SLE

Exposure Category	Infections	Respiratory Exposures	Chemicals, Organic Pollutants, Heavy Metals	Vaccines
Specific exposures	• EBV • CMV • HTLV-1 • HIV • *PVB19* • HCV • Influenza • COVID-19 • Disrupted gut microbiome	• Crystalline silica dust • Air pollution • Current cigarette smoking	• Residential and agricultural pesticides • Household products containing solvents (eg, nail polish remover, paint thinners) • Uranium	• COVID-19 (only a few case studies; requires further evaluation in larger studies)

Abbreviations: CMV, cytomegalovirus; COVID-19, coronavirus disease 19; EBV, Epstein-Barr virus; HCV, hepatitis C virus; HIV, human immunodeficiency virus; HTLV, human T-cell lymphotropic virus; PVB19, parvovirus B19.

designs. In a recent study in family members of SLE patients, baseline levels of IgG to EBV-viral capsid antigen and early antigen showed an association with SLE risk over 6 years.[22]

Cytomegalovirus (CMV) has also been associated with SLE in case reports[23,24] and significantly higher CMV antibody titers were present in SLE patients compared to healthy controls.[25,26] Another study with 74 SLE patients demonstrated that all had CMV antigenemia; however, nearly all were on immunosuppressants.[27] Conversely, other studies have found no association between CMV and SLE.[28,29]

Human T-cell lymphotropic virus (HTLV-1), a human endogenous retrovirus associated with adult T-cell leukemia/lymphoma, has had a controversial association with SLE, with reports linking the virus to SLE manifestations,[30,31] while other studies did not.[32–34] Human immunodeficiency virus (HIV) may be associated with SLE through similar mechanisms as HTLV-1, such as T helper lymphocytes apoptotic dysregulation.[35] A recent review identified 29 case reports of SLE diagnosis in the context of known HIV, mainly in women and African-American/Black patients, with 7 patients on antiretroviral therapy (ART).[36] A cohort study found higher SLE prevalence in HIV-1–positive patients than in HIV-negative population studies.[37] However, clinical and laboratory presentations between both diseases may overlap, and simultaneous presentations of HIV and SLE could result from ART initiation.[38]

The role of parvovirus B19 (PVB19) in SLE has been suggested in case studies without a proven direct role, as with other viruses, many features of PVB19 overlap with SLE.[39,40] The presence of antiphospholipid antibodies was found in one study on recent PVB19 infection.[41] A recent meta-analysis studying the prevalence of hepatitis B (HBV) and hepatitis C (HCV) in SLE patients found a higher prevalence of HCV in SLE than in controls, with both current and past HBV infection lower in SLE patients than in the control population.[42]

Influenza infection has been associated with SLE flares requiring hospitalization within 7 days of infection, in a South Korean study.[43]

Other infections, bacterial and parasitic, have been less studied in SLE. Nonetheless, *Helicobacter pylori*, a gram-negative bacillus found in the human stomach, has been suggested to decrease SLE risk in a study showing a low rate of specific *H pylori* antibodies in an SLE cohort.[44] *Toxoplasma gondii*, an intracellular parasitic protozoan, prevented the progression to lupus nephritis in a mouse model through decrease in interferon-γ and interleukin-10.[45] Antibodies to *T gondii* were higher in rheumatoid arthritis patients but not in SLE patients compared to the general population in a European study.[46]

The global pandemic caused by severe acute respiratory syndrome coronavirus 2 (SARS-CoV-2) leading to coronavirus disease 2019 (COVID-19) caused over 296 million cases and 5 million deaths worldwide since its onset.[47] SARS-CoV-2 has been associated with autoimmune markers, including antinuclear antibody (ANA), with positivity ranging from 35.6% to 50% in patients hospitalized for this infection.[48,49] There have been a few case reports of new SLE diagnosis in the setting of confirmed SARS-CoV-2 infection, with predominantly renal and hematological involvement.[50–55] Of note, most SLE cases began during the acute phase of COVID-19 infection, and many symptoms (eg, fever) and laboratory findings (eg, hematological findings such as lymphopenia) overlap between both SLE and COVID-19 infection. SARS-CoV-2 may trigger autoimmunity through molecular mimicry as similarities were found between the virus' epitope and human proteins[56] or by accumulation of activated lymphocytes in tissues.[57,58] COVID-19 also shares immunologic pathologies with SLE, including antiphospholipid antibodies (aPL). A systematic review found 46.8% pooled prevalence for one or more aPL in COVID-19 patients, with lupus anticoagulant most frequently found.[59] As SARS-CoV-2 is a relatively new infection, pathogenic studies are necessary to elucidate the likelihood in which this infection may serve a meaningful role in SLE etiology.

VACCINATIONS

Vaccinations have been suggested to trigger SLE onset by stimulating antigen-specific immune responses, but epidemiologic studies did not support this hypothesis.[19] There was no association between any vaccination administered within 24 months, including against diphtheria, tetanus, pertussis, and poliomyelitis, with onset of SLE.[60] Vaccination for HPV was associated with localized lupus erythematosus, not SLE, in a recent large population-based study in females in Denmark.[61] Recent case reports described SLE onset associated with mRNA COVID-19 vaccinations, ranging from 1 to 2 weeks after vaccination, with the most severe case presenting as stage V lupus nephritis.[62–64] One case report described a transition from cutaneous to systemic lupus 10 days after vaccination.[65] A hypothesis regarding the mechanism includes the mRNA vaccination causing increased production of type I interferon (IFN) and multiple proinflammatory cytokines, with dysregulation of the type I IFN involved in SLE pathogenesis.[66] In an early study, the risk of SLE flare was low within 3 days of receiving a vaccine dose among an international sample of patients with SLE.[67] On the contrary, recent case reports have described relapse of lupus nephritis[68] and cutaneous flares.[69] Overall, however, the body of evidence linking vaccines to SLE risk is weak, and therefore withholding vaccines to minimize SLE risk is not recommended.

MICROBIOME

The *gut microbiome* represents the ensemble of organisms living in the human gastrointestinal system. Its role in SLE has been a focus of research for the past few years. The available research has not specifically focused on whether specific microbial exposures trigger SLE, as this would be difficult to prove. However, a recent review has described microbiome differences in both lupus-prone mice and lupus patients compared to controls.[70] An experimental model with lupus-prone mice showed increased gut *Clostridiaceae* and *Lachnospiraceae*, bacteria with inflammatory properties.[71] In one human study, gut microbiome differences were demonstrated, as organisms like *Clostridium* species ATCC BAA-442 were abundant at SLE diagnosis but diminished after treatment.[72] Another potential pathway by which the microbiome may trigger SLE is abnormal intestinal translocation of bacteria and bacterial products, which can cause immune system activation. These events have been shown in mice prone to autoimmunity, with the identification of the gut pathobiont *Enterococcus Gallinarum* as a potential culprit for immune system activation through altering T helper cell differentiation and causing autoantigens and cytokines production.[73] Liver biopsies of 3 SLE patients were positive for *Enterococcus Gallinarum,* which was not isolated in healthy liver transplant donors.[73] Its presence in the liver may signify translocation from the gastrointestinal tract into the systemic circulation. Another mouse model demonstrated that ANA production was influenced by a different commensal gut microbiome, particularly in the presence of increased segmented filamentous bacteria and interleukin-17 receptor signaling.[74] Two human studies demonstrated that immune cells and cytokine regulation could be affected by epigenetic modification induced by microbes and their metabolites.[75,76] The gut microbiome affects many autoimmune diseases and exerts different effects in patients with SLE who are untreated, compared to healthy subjects;[72,77] however, direct associations with SLE onset have not been concluded.

The microbiome may be affected by environmental exposures such as diet, and its consequences on environment-SLE effects need to be further studied.[78,79] Despite the suggested role of microbiome in SLE risk, no dietary interventions have been found to modify it in a way that decreases SLE risk. More discussion of diet is featured in the following section.

DIET

Diet is a potentially important environmental exposure. A diet with low fiber was associated with obesity, immune dysregulation, and increased autoantibody production in lupus-prone mice.[80] In SLE patients, these findings were only partially reproduced.[80] Western dietary pattern score or prudent dietary patterns including a diet rich in vegetables, fruit, legumes, whole grains, and seafood,[81] or other assessments of diet quality,[82] was not associated with SLE risk upon evaluation of the US Nurses Health Studies. There was an association between a diet high in carbohydrates and low in monosaturated fatty acids, saturated fats, and trans fatty acids, and risk of SLE in the Black Women's Health Study.[83]

The active form of vitamin D3, $1\alpha,25(OH)2D3$, has immunosuppressive properties,[84] which theoretically could reduce SLE risk.[85] Case-control studies have shown higher 25-hydroxyvitamin D [25(OH)D], a different vitamin D3 metabolite, concentrations in controls compared to SLE patients, but this is true of many chronic inflammatory diseases and does not address causation.[86] Research from the Nurses' Health Studies showed no clear protective effect related to vitamin D intake from foods or supplements (in adult or adolescent years) and delay in SLE onset.[85,87]

CRYSTALLINE SILICA DUST

Silicates are a combination of silicon-based minerals with metal ions, commonly found in rocks. When transformed into dust (such as in quarry work or sandblasting), they can be inhaled and cause adverse health effects. Crystalline silica (quartz) dust represents the most common silicate exposure and is a recognized risk factor for systemic autoimmune disease onset.[88,89] This may be because workers in trades that generate high respirable silica exposures have traditionally been male, who have a much lower baseline SLE risk than females. However, findings of association with SLE risk observed in a cohort of male construction workers[90] have been reproduced in population-based studies.[91–95] Dose-response associations with increasing intensity or duration have also been noted.[89,92,96]

Basic research has tried to elucidate the underlying mechanisms explaining the relationship between crystalline silica dust and SLE.[97] Once inhaled, particulates interact with immune cells such as lymphocytes, triggering apoptosis, antigen release, stimulation of proinflammatory cytokines, oxidative stress, and decrease in regulatory T-cells.[98] Additional autoantibodies are generated from post-translational modification of self-antigens in tertiary lymphoid structures. In lupus-prone mice exposed to silica, there was an increase in autoantibodies and immune complexes leading to glomerulonephritis[99] and systemic autoimmunity.[100]

Respirable silica associated with SLE risk is mainly studied in North America, and a few case series and cohort studies have been performed globally.[73,89,90,93,101] There have also been studies on other silicates and their associations with risk of SLE, such as asbestos, with limited evidence in humans.[97] The effect of different respirable silicates on SLE needs to be studied in different populations.[102]

AIR POLLUTION

Particulate air pollution is a complex mixture of chemical and physical components originating from natural (eg, forest fires) or anthropogenic sources (eg, traffic, industrial emissions). Particle size determines the degree to which air pollution may enter the distal respiratory tract be absorbed into the systemic circulation, with subsequent adverse health effects[103] including immune system activation. Particulate matter with a diameter less than 2.5 μm ($PM_{2.5}$) is well-known to have detrimental effects on respiratory and cardiovascular disease[103] but has also been associated with the development of SLE and other autoimmune diseases. One study, using population-based administrative data from the Canadian provinces of Quebec and Alberta, studied $PM_{2.5}$ exposures based on ambient air monitoring within residential postal code regions; they demonstrated that the odds of systemic autoimmune disease, including SLE, correlated with increasing $PM_{2.5}$ levels.[104] The same authors found similar findings using administrative health data between 1993 and 2007 (but assigning $PM_{2.5}$ exposures based on land-use regression models) in Calgary, Alberta.[105] Moreover, in a Taiwan cohort, elevated ambient $PM_{2.5}$ was associated with greater SLE risk.[106] $PM_{2.5}$ has also been associated with SLE disease activity, including renal activity (renal casts, anti–double-stranded DNA antibody).[107] Another study demonstrated spatio-temporal relationships between organ-specific SLE flares whereby joint, renal, and neurologic flares became less temporally significant after adjusting for individual and environmental such as $PM_{2.5}$, suggesting some of those factors drove the flare.[108] In univariate analysis, $PM_{2.5}$ was associated with mild increase in joint and rash flares.[108] A recent retrospective cohort study from Korea showed no association between high $PM_{2.5}$ and SLE incidence; however, it could have been limited by selection bias.[109] Mechanisms by which autoimmune diseases can be triggered by air pollution include oxidative stress generating reactive oxygen species, and inflammatory cytokines activation.[110]

CIGARETTE SMOKING

Positive associations between *cigarette smoking* and overall SLE risk and organ involvement have been shown in several studies. A meta-analysis showed that SLE development has been associated with current smokers compared to never smokers, without an association with past smoking history.[111] An updated meta-analysis, including 3 more studies, found that current smoking (odds ratio [OR] 1.54, 95% confidence interval [CI] 1.06–2.25) and potentially past smoking (OR 1.39, 95% CI 0.95–2.08) increased SLE risk compared to never smokers.[112] Within a cohort of African American women, there was also a trend for higher SLE risk among current smokers compared to never smokers (hazard ratio [HR] 1.45, 95% CI 0.97–2.18).[113]

Smoking may influence physical manifestations of SLE. In a Danish cohort of SLE patients, smoking was associated with neuropsychiatric lupus, discoid rash, and photosensitivity, with arthritis, hematological and renal disorders more common in nonsmokers.[114] A large cohort of US women showed associations between current smoking and double-stranded DNA-positive SLE, particularly noticeable in those with more than a 10-pack-year smoking history, versus never smokers.[115] The higher SLE risk in current smokers compared to prior smokers, especially those who quit over 4 to 5 years ago[112,115,116] suggests that the biological mechanisms through which cigarette smoking confers SLE risk could attenuate over time. Mechanisms relating cigarette smoke and its toxic chemicals to SLE include oxidative stress and alteration of immune cell function.[113,114,117]

OTHER RESPIRATORY EXPOSURES

Other respiratory exposures and complex mixtures also represent relevant triggers of SLE in the population. Following the September 11 World Trade Center (WTC) disaster, a resulting dust cloud has been associated with multiple diseases, including respiratory and autoimmune diseases such as SLE, among rescue and clean-up workers, with high onset among workers exposed to the highest levels of dust.[118] Female mice exposed to air samples from the September 11 disaster developed oxidative stress, epigenetic changes, and pulmonary inflammation.[119] Different types of dust which likely included respirable silica, silicates, and carbon nanotubes have been found in both lung biopsy of patients exposed to the WTC disaster and dust specimens from the site.[101,120] Years after the September 11 disaster, there were markers of increased systemic inflammation in a volunteer cohort of symptomatic individuals.[120] Upon a recently expanded analysis of 118 patients with systemic autoimmune diseases in lower Manhattan, higher composite dust exposure among the September 11 disaster emergency responders was identified and associated with elevated risk, as opposed to community members.[121]

Military exposures including burn pits (in which open-air waste combustion occurs) have well-documented adverse respiratory effects, but no clear link with SLE was found at 2.8 years of follow-up in a large US cohort. This finding could be affected by insufficient power to examine SLE, a short follow-up period of 1.3 years, or outcome ascertainment error, given that SLE was identified with electronic medical records instead of with clinical confirmation.[122,123] A recent study using a military job exposure matrix surprisingly reported an inverse association with inorganic dust exposure and SLE risk among US Veterans Affairs medical care beneficiaries.[124]

CHEMICALS, ORGANIC POLLUTANTS, AND HEAVY METALS

Exposure to *residential and agricultural pesticide* exposure has been associated with SLE risk in adult[125–127] and children[128] populations in the United States. Recall bias and potential inaccuracy of self-reported pesticide exposure represent key limitations of these studies. A study of insecticide uses in a postmenopausal female cohort showed stronger associations with SLE onset among those who lived or worked on a farm.[125] However, these studies could have been plagued by confounding, since it is likely that exposures to pesticides (which generally is greater in rural areas), often occur with multiple other exposures which may simultaneously lead to the observed increase in SLE including silica, solvents, ultraviolet light. In 2 lupus-prone mouse models, chlordecone, a persistent organic pollutant previously used in pesticides, was found to have estrogenic properties.[129] However, although estrogen was shown to decrease transitional B cells and increase marginal zone B cells, chlordecone did not have this effect, suggesting a more complex mode of action.[130]

Other chemical exposures, which may represent SLE risk factors, include common household products containing solvents (eg, nail polish remover, oil-based paints and paint thinners, solvent-based perfumes). Occupations involving solvent exposure showed increased SLE risk in some,[78,125] but not all[121,125] studies. Trichloroethylene (TCE), a widely used industrial solvent, was linked to murine lupus risk, but not conclusively in humans.[131,132] Recent experimental data on mice found TCE-induced altered gut microbiome was associated with increased ANA and systemic inflammatory changes, suggesting a pathway whereby TCE may trigger SLE.[133]

Experimental studies in animal models suggest that heavy metals may increase autoimmunity; however, evidence in human populations is sparse.[134] In human studies, there was increased SLE onset in those residing near a uranium processing plant.[135] Important association was demonstrated between estimated yearly uranium-contaminated drinking water and antichromatin and anti-dsDNA antibody levels in the Navajo Nation. Urinary arsenic markers were, however, inversely associated with autoantibodies to native DNA or chromatin.[136] Although this study was likely limited by selection bias, mechanisms of action of arsenic include inhibition of interferon-g synthesis shown in vitro,[137] decreased anti–double-stranded DNA and peripheral IgG levels as demonstrated in lupus-prone mice,[138] or inflammasome inhibition.[139] Animal models have suggested association between exposure to mercury and autoimmunity; however, the evidence in humans is limited,[140] including self-reported occupational mercury exposure in retrospective studies on SLE patients.[50,98] Gold miners with mercury exposure had elevated ANA levels.[141] This ANA elevation with mercury, or other heavy metals, was not reproduced in a general population study; however, power issues may have contributed.[142] In the Seychelles Islands, a study demonstrated association between hair mercury levels and ANA. The association was only established after adjusting for dietary long-chain polyunsaturated fatty acids, found in fish, as it is associated with decreased inflammatory markers (eg, C-reactive protein).[143] Mercury may also exist in personal products such as skin lightening cream,[144] which has widespread global use among women of color; however, these agents have not been studied as a potential trigger of SLE.

ULTRAVIOLET RADIATION

Ultraviolet light (UV) radiation may cause SLE flares; however, it has not been clearly associated with SLE risk,[145] due to limited number of studies. It could potentially cause autoimmunity by inducing reactive oxygen species with subsequent DNA damage,[146] increasing autoantigen and autoreactive T cells numbers,[147,148] and modifying T cells and cytokine production.[149] A recent review also described elevation in the production of type I interferons from UV exposure.[150] These findings result from case-control studies, therefore could be limited by recall bias.[78,150]

SUMMARY

Available evidence supports the complex and multifactorial nature of SLE. The identification of environmental risk factors for SLE, particularly those that are potentially modifiable, could theoretically support the development of disease prevention strategies.

Infections and the microbiome are areas of great interest. Viral infections including EBV and potentially others have been associated with SLE, whereas bacterial and parasitic infections are less studied. Vaccinations have not had established associations with SLE. Although there are case reports of SLE diagnosis after COVID-19 vaccination, this will require rigorously designed, larger follow-up studies, and withholding vaccines to minimize SLE risk is not recommended. Patients with SLE may have different gastrointestinal flora compared to healthy controls, and abnormal bacterial translocation across the gastrointestinal tract could lead to subsequent activation of inflammatory cascades, increasing SLE risk. Diets high in carbohydrates and low in monosaturated fatty acids, saturated fats, and trans fatty acids, and low vitamin D may be associated with SLE.

Crystalline silica (quartz) has a positive dose-response association with SLE risk in both population-based and occupational settings. Particulate air pollution, specifically $PM_{2.5}$, has been shown to increase odds of autoimmune disease, including SLE, with an additional role in SLE disease activity. Current cigarette smoking has been associated with SLE risk, compared to smokers who quit and never-smokers. Solvents, organic pollutants, and pesticides may also increase the risk of SLE. Residential proximity to a uranium processing plant was associated with SLE onset in humans. Ultraviolet radiation, which is believed to exacerbate SLE symptoms, was not clearly associated with SLE onset.

The main challenge to identifying environmental triggers of SLE remain design and analytical challenges and statistical power issues. Most of the existing literature on environmental triggers of SLE study a single exposure. Given the heterogeneity of SLE and the modest associations between individual exposures and SLE risk, its onset is likely affected by a multitude and interaction of exposures, which needs to be further studied to allow for better interventions to address the risk of SLE, particularly among vulnerable populations.

CLINICS CARE POINTS

- Many SLE patients want to know "what caused my lupus"? The answer is far from simple; though genetic factors are important, many environmental factors (infections/microbiome, respirable exposures, and others) appear to play roles.
- One theory is that multiple environmental "hits," particularly in genetically susceptible individuals, are responsible for SLE onset.
- Discussion of these factors with our patients represents an opportunity to highlight global strategies to optimize health, including avoidance of tobacco exposure.

DISCLOSURE

The authors have nothing to disclose.

REFERENCES

1. Petri M, Orbai AM, Alarcon GS, et al. Derivation and validation of the Systemic Lupus International Collaborating Clinics classification criteria for systemic lupus erythematosus. Arthritis Rheum 2012;64:2677–86.
2. Furst DE, Clarke AE, Fernandes AW, et al. Incidence and prevalence of adult systemic lupus erythematosus in a large US managed-care population. Lupus 2013;22:99–105.
3. Izmirly PM, Wan I, Sahl S, et al. The incidence and prevalence of systemic lupus erythematosus in New York County (Manhattan), New York: the manhattan lupus surveillance program. Arthritis Rheumatol 2017;69:2006–17.
4. Dall'Era M, Cisternas MG, Snipes K, et al. The incidence and prevalence of systemic lupus erythematosus in san francisco county, california: the california lupus surveillance project. Arthritis Rheumatol 2017;69:1996–2005.
5. Ferucci ED, Johnston JM, Gaddy JR, et al. Prevalence and incidence of systemic lupus erythematosus in a population-based registry of American Indian and Alaska Native people, 2007-2009. Arthritis Rheumatol 2014;66:2494–502.

6. Somers EC, Marder W, Cagnoli P, et al. Population-based incidence and prevalence of systemic lupus erythematosus: the Michigan Lupus Epidemiology and Surveillance program. Arthritis Rheumatol 2014;66:369–78.

7. Lim SS, Bayakly AR, Helmick CG, et al. The incidence and prevalence of systemic lupus erythematosus, 2002-2004: The Georgia Lupus Registry. Arthritis Rheumatol 2014;66:357–68.

8. McDougall C, Hurd K, Barnabe C. Systematic review of rheumatic disease epidemiology in the indigenous populations of Canada, the United States, Australia, and New Zealand. Semin Arthritis Rheum 2017;46:675–86.

9. Peschken CA, Esdaile JM. Systemic lupus erythematosus in North American Indians: a population based study. J Rheumatol 2000;27:1884–91.

10. Rees F, Doherty M, Grainge MJ, et al. The worldwide incidence and prevalence of systemic lupus erythematosus: a systematic review of epidemiological studies. Rheumatology (Oxford) 2017;56:1945–61.

11. Stojan G, Petri M. Epidemiology of systemic lupus erythematosus: an update. Curr Opin Rheumatol 2018;30:144–50.

12. Fatoye F, Gebrye T, Svenson LW. Real-world incidence and prevalence of systemic lupus erythematosus in Alberta, Canada. Rheumatol Int 2018;38:1721–6.

13. Kuo CF, Grainge MJ, Valdes AM, et al. Familial aggregation of systemic lupus erythematosus and coaggregation of autoimmune diseases in affected families. JAMA Intern Med 2015;175:1518–26.

14. Leffers HCB, Lange T, Collins C, et al. The study of interactions between genome and exposome in the development of systemic lupus erythematosus. Autoimmun Rev 2019;18:382–92.

15. Parks CG, de Souza Espindola Santos A, Barbhaiya M, et al. Understanding the role of environmental factors in the development of systemic lupus erythematosus. Best Pract Res Clin Rheumatol 2017;31:306–20.

16. Qiu CC, Caricchio R, Gallucci S. Triggers of Autoimmunity: The Role of Bacterial Infections in the Extracellular Exposure of Lupus Nuclear Autoantigens. Front Immunol 2019;10:2608.

17. Bach JF. The hygiene hypothesis in autoimmunity: the role of pathogens and commensals. Nat Rev Immunol 2018;18:105–20.

18. James JA, Kaufman KM, Farris AD, et al. An increased prevalence of Epstein-Barr virus infection in young patients suggests a possible etiology for systemic lupus erythematosus. J Clin Invest 1997;100:3019–26.

19. Cooper GS, Dooley MA, Treadwell EL, et al. Risk factors for development of systemic lupus erythematosus: allergies, infections, and family history. J Clin Epidemiol 2002;55:982–9.

20. Ulff-Moller CJ, Nielsen NM, Rostgaard K, et al. Epstein-Barr virus-associated infectious mononucleosis and risk of systemic lupus erythematosus. Rheumatology (Oxford) 2010;49:1706–12.

21. Hanlon P, Avenell A, Aucott L, et al. Systematic review and meta-analysis of the sero-epidemiological association between Epstein-Barr virus and systemic lupus erythematosus. Arthritis Res Ther 2014;16:R3.

22. Jog NR, Young KA, Munroe ME, et al. Association of Epstein-Barr virus serological reactivation with transitioning to systemic lupus erythematosus in at-risk individuals. Ann Rheum Dis 2019;78:1235–41.

23. Pérez-Mercado AE, Vilá-Pérez S. Cytomegalovirus as a trigger for systemic lupus erythematosus. J Clin Rheumatol 2010;16(7):335–7.

24. Yamazaki S, Endo A, Iso T, et al. Cytomegalovirus as a potential trigger for systemic lupus erythematosus: a case report. BMC Res Notes 2015;8:487.

25. Chen J, Zhang H, Chen P, et al. Correlation between systemic lupus erythematosus and cytomegalovirus infection detected by different methods. Clin Rheumatol 2015;34(4):691–8.
26. Newkirk MM, van Venrooij WJ, Marshall GS. Autoimmune response to U1 small nuclear ribonucleoprotein (U1 snRNP) associated with cytomegalovirus infection. Arthritis Res 2001;3(4):253–8.
27. Takizawa Y, Inokuma S, Tanaka Y, et al. Clinical characteristics of cytomegalovirus infection in rheumatic diseases: multicentre survey in a large patient population. Rheumatology (Oxford) 2008;47(9):1373–8.
28. James JA, Neas BR, Moser KL, et al. Systemic lupus erythematosus in adults is associated with previous Epstein-Barr virus exposure. Arthritis Rheum 2001; 44(5):1122–6.
29. Parks CG, Cooper GS, Hudson LL, et al. Association of Epstein-Barr virus with systemic lupus erythematosus: effect modification by race, age, and cytotoxic T lymphocyte-associated antigen 4 genotype. Arthritis Rheum 2005;52(4): 1148–59.
30. Olsen RG, Tarr MJ, Mathes LE, et al. Serological and virological evidence of human T-lymphotropic virus in systemic lupus erythematosus. Med Microbiol Immunol 1987;176(2):53–64.
31. Ito H, Harada R, Uchida Y, et al. Lupus nephritis with adult T cell leukemia. Nephron 1990;55(3):325–8.
32. Lipka K, Tebbe B, Finckh U, et al. Absence of human T-lymphotrophic virus type I in patients with systemic lupus erythematosus. Clin Exp Dermatol 1996;21(1): 38–42.
33. Boumpas DT, Popovic M, Mann DL, et al. Type C retroviruses of the human T cell leukemia family are not evident in patients with systemic lupus erythematosus. Arthritis Rheum 1986;29(2):185–8.
34. Shirdel A, Hashemzadeh K, Sahebari M, et al. Is there any Association Between Human Lymphotropic Virus Type I (HTLV-I) Infection and Systemic Lupus Erythematosus? An Original Research and Literature Review. Iran J Basic Med Sci 2013;16(3):252–7.
35. Esposito S, Bosis S, Semino M, et al. Infections and systemic lupus erythematosus. Eur J Clin Microbiol Infect Dis 2014;33(9):1467–75.
36. Carugati M, Franzetti M, Torre A, et al. Systemic lupus erythematosus and HIV infection. a whimsical relationship. Reports of two cases and review of the literature. Clin Rheumatol 2013;32(9):1399–405.
37. Naovarat BS, Reveille JD, Salazar GA, et al. Systemic lupus erythematosus in the setting of HIV-1 infection: a longitudinal analysis. Clin Rheumatol 2020; 39(2):413–8.
38. Mody GM, Patel N, Budhoo A, et al. Concomitant systemic lupus erythematosus and HIV: case series and literature review. Semin Arthritis Rheum 2014;44(2): 186–94.
39. Chabert P, Kallel H. Simultaneous Presentation of Parvovirus B19 Infection and Systemic Lupus Erythematosus in a Patient: Description and Review of the Literature. Eur J Case Rep Intern Med 2020;7(12):001729.
40. Sève P, Ferry T, Koenig M, et al. Lupus-like presentation of parvovirus B19 infection. Semin Arthritis Rheum 2005;34(4):642–8.
41. Loizou S, Cazabon JK, Walport MJ, et al. Similarities of specificity and cofactor dependence in serum antiphospholipid antibodies from patients with human parvovirus B19 infection and from those with systemic lupus erythematosus. Arthritis Rheumatol 1997;40:103–8.

42. Wang S, Chen Y, Xu X, et al. Prevalence of hepatitis B virus and hepatitis C virus infection in patients with systemic lupus erythematosus: a systematic review and meta-analysis. Oncotarget 2017;8(60):102437–45.

43. Joo YB, Kim KJ, Park KS, et al. Influenza infection as a trigger for systemic lupus erythematosus flares resulting in hospitalization. Sci Rep 2021;11(1):4630.

44. Sawalha AH, Schmid WR, Binder SR, et al. Association between systemic lupus erythematosus and Helicobacter pylori seronegativity. J Rheumatol 2004;31(8): 1546–50.

45. Chen M, Aosai F, Norose K, et al. Toxoplasma gondii infection inhibits the development of lupus-like syndrome in autoimmune (New Zealand Black x New Zealand White) F1 mice. Int Immunol 2004;16(7):937–46.

46. Fischer S, Agmon-Levin N, Shapira Y, et al. Toxoplasma gondii: bystander or cofactor in rheumatoid arthritis. Immunol Res 2013;56(2–3):287–92.

47. Who coronavirus (COVID-19) dashboard. World Health Organization. Available at: https://covid19.who.int/. Accessed January 7, 2022.

48. Zhou Y, Han T, Chen J, et al. Clinical and Autoimmune Characteristics of Severe and Critical Cases of COVID-19. Clin Transl Sci 2020;13(6):1077–86.

49. Gazzaruso C, Carlo Stella N, Mariani G, et al. High prevalence of antinuclear antibodies and lupus anticoagulant in patients hospitalized for SARS-CoV2 pneumonia. Clin Rheumatol 2020;39(7):2095–7.

50. Bonometti R, Sacchi MC, Stobbione P, et al. The first case of systemic lupus erythematosus (SLE) triggered by COVID-19 infection. Eur Rev Med Pharmacol Sci 2020;24(18):9695–7.

51. Slimani Y, Abbassi R, El Fatoiki FZ, et al. Systemic lupus erythematosus and varicella-like rash following COVID-19 in a previously healthy patient. J Med Virol 2021;93(2):1184–7.

52. Zamani B, Moeini Taba SM, Shayestehpour M. Systemic lupus erythematosus manifestation following COVID-19: a case report. J Med Case Rep 2021; 15(1):29.

53. Gracia-Ramos AE, Saavedra-Salinas MÁ. Can the SARS-CoV-2 infection trigger systemic lupus erythematosus? A case-based review. Rheumatol Int 2021;41(4): 799–809.

54. Hali F, Jabri H, Chiheb S, et al. A concomitant diagnosis of COVID-19 infection and systemic lupus erythematosus complicated by a macrophage activation syndrome: A new case report. Int J Dermatol 2021;60(8):1030–1.

55. Mantovani Cardoso E, Hundal J, Feterman D, et al. Concomitant new diagnosis of systemic lupus erythematosus and COVID-19 with possible antiphospholipid syndrome. Just a coincidence? A case report and review of intertwining pathophysiology. Clin Rheumatol 2020;39(9):2811–5.

56. Lyons-Weiler J. Pathogenic priming likely contributes to serious and critical illness and mortality in COVID-19 via autoimmunity. J Transl Autoimmun 2020; 3:100051.

57. Ehrenfeld M, Tincani A, Andreoli L, et al. Covid-19 and autoimmunity. Autoimmun Rev 2020;19(8):102597.

58. Podolska MJ, Biermann MH, Maueröder C, et al. Inflammatory etiopathogenesis of systemic lupus erythematosus: an update. J Inflamm Res 2015;8:161–71.

59. Taha M, Samavati L. Antiphospholipid antibodies in COVID-19: a meta-analysis and systematic review. RMD Open 2021;7:e001580.

60. Grimaldi-Bensouda L, Le Guern V, Kone-Paut I, et al. The risk of systemic lupus erythematosus associated with vaccines: an international case-control study. Arthritis Rheumatol 2014;66:1559–67.

61. Hviid A, Svanstrom H, Scheller NM, et al. Human papillomavirus vaccination of adult women and risk of autoimmune and neurological diseases. J Intern Med 2018;283:154–65.
62. Patil S, Patil A. Systemic lupus erythematosus after COVID-19 vaccination: A case report. J Cosmet Dermatol 2021;20(10):3103–4.
63. Nune A, Iyengar KP, Ish P, et al. The Emergence of new-onset SLE following SARS-CoV-2 vaccination. QJM 2021;114(10):739–40.
64. Zavala-Miranda MF, González-Ibarra SG, Pérez-Arias AA, et al. New-onset systemic lupus erythematosus beginning as class V lupus nephritis after COVID-19 vaccination. Kidney Int 2021;100(6):1340–1.
65. Kreuter A, Burmann SN, Burkert B, et al. Transition of cutaneous into systemic lupus erythematosus following adenoviral vector-based SARS-CoV-2 vaccination. J Eur Acad Dermatol Venereol 2021;35(11):e733–5.
66. Teijaro JR, Farber DL. COVID-19 vaccines: modes of immune activation and future challenges. Nat Rev Immunol 2021;21(4):195–7.
67. Felten R, Kawka L, Dubois M, et al. Tolerance of COVID-19 vaccination in patients with systemic lupus erythematosus: the international VACOLUP study. Lancet Rheumatol 2021;3(9):e613–5.
68. Tuschen K, Bräsen JH, Schmitz J, et al. Relapse of class V lupus nephritis after vaccination with COVID-19 mRNA vaccine. Kidney Int 2021;100(4):941–4.
69. Joseph AK, Chong BF. Subacute cutaneous lupus erythematosus flare triggered by COVID-19 vaccine. Dermatol Ther 2021;34(6):e15114.
70. Battaglia M, Garrett-Sinha LA. Bacterial infections in lupus: Roles in promoting immune activation and in pathogenesis of the disease. J Transl Autoimmun 2021;4:100078.
71. Zhang H, Liao X, Sparks JB, et al. Dynamics of gut microbiota in autoimmune lupus. Appl Environ Microbiol 2014;80(24):7551–60.
72. Chen BD, Jia XM, Xu JY, et al. An Autoimmunogenic and Proinflammatory Profile Defined by the Gut Microbiota of Patients With Untreated Systemic Lupus Erythematosus. Arthritis Rheumatol 2021;73:232–43.
73. Manfredo Vieira S, Hiltensperger M, Kumar V, et al. Translocation of a gut pathobiont drives autoimmunity in mice and humans. Science 2018;359(6380):1156–61.
74. Van Praet JT, Donovan E, Vanassche I, et al. Commensal microbiota influence systemic autoimmune responses. EMBO J 2015;34(1):466–74.
75. Chen B, Sun L, Zhang X. Integration of microbiome and epigenome to decipher the pathogenesis of autoimmune diseases. J Autoimmun 2017;83:31–42.
76. Azzouz D, Omarbekova A, Heguy A, et al. Lupus nephritis is linked to disease-activity associated expansions and immunity to a gut commensal. Ann Rheum Dis 2019;78:947–56.
77. Wu WH, Zegarra-Ruiz DF, Diehl GE. Intestinal Microbes in Autoimmune and Inflammatory Disease. Front Immunol 2020;11:597966.
78. Cooper GS, Wither J, Bernatsky S, et al. Occupational and environmental exposures and risk of systemic lupus erythematosus: silica, sunlight, solvents. Rheumatology (Oxford) 2010;49:2172–80.
79. Khan MF, Wang H. Environmental exposures and autoimmune diseases: contribution of gut microbiome. Front Immunol 2019;10:3094.
80. Schafer AL, Eichhorst A, Hentze C, et al. Low dietary fiber intake links development of obesity and lupus pathogenesis. Front Immunol 2021;12:696810.
81. Tedeschi SK, Barbhaiya M, Sparks JA, et al. Dietary patterns and risk of systemic lupus erythematosus in women. Lupus 2020;29:67–73.

82. Barbhaiya M, Tedeschi S, Sparks JA, et al. Association of dietary quality with risk of incident systemic lupus erythematosus in the nurses' health studies. Arthritis Care Res (Hoboken) 2021;73(9):1250–8.
83. Castro-Webb N, Cozier YC, Barbhaiya M, et al. Association of macronutrients and dietary patterns with risk of systemic lupus erythematosus in the Black Women's Health Study. Am J Clin Nutr 2021;114(4):1486–94.
84. Cantorna MT, Mahon BD. Mounting evidence for vitamin D as an environmental factor affecting autoimmune disease prevalence. Exp Biol Med (Maywood) 2004;229:1136–42.
85. Costenbader KH, Feskanich D, Holmes M, et al. Vitamin D intake and risks of systemic lupus erythematosus and rheumatoid arthritis in women. Ann Rheum Dis 2008;67:530–5.
86. Islam MA, Khandker SS, Alam SS, et al. Vitamin D status in patients with systemic lupus erythematosus (SLE): a systematic review and meta-analysis. Autoimmun Rev 2019;18:102392.
87. Costenbader KH, Kang JH, Karlson EW. Antioxidant intake and risks of rheumatoid arthritis and systemic lupus erythematosus in women. Am J Epidemiol 2010;172:205–16.
88. Miller FW, Alfredsson L, Costenbader KH, et al. Epidemiology of environmental exposures and human autoimmune diseases: findings from a National Institute of Environmental Health Sciences Expert Panel Workshop. J Autoimmun 2012; 39:259–71.
89. Boudigaard SH, Schlunssen V, Vestergaard JM, et al. Occupational exposure to respirable crystalline silica and risk of autoimmune rheumatic diseases: a nationwide cohort study. Int J Epidemiol 2021;50(4):1213–26.
90. Blanc PD, Jarvholm B, Toren K. Prospective risk of rheumatologic disease associated with occupational exposure in a cohort of male construction workers. Am J Med 2015;128:1094–101.
91. Parks CG, Cooper GS, Nylander-French LA, et al. Occupational exposure to crystalline silica and risk of systemic lupus erythematosus: a population-based, case-control study in the southeastern United States. Arthritis Rheum 2002;46:1840–50.
92. Parks CG, Cooper GS. Occupational exposures and risk of systemic lupus erythematosus: a review of the evidence and exposure assessment methods in population- and clinic-based studies. Lupus 2006;15:728–36.
93. Finckh A, Cooper GS, Chibnik LB, et al. Occupational silica and solvent exposures and risk of systemic lupus erythematosus in urban women. Arthritis Rheum 2006;54:3648–54.
94. Gold LS, Ward MH, Dosemeci M, et al. Systemic autoimmune disease mortality and occupational exposures. Arthritis Rheum 2007;56:3189–201.
95. Li X, Sundquist J, Sundquist K, et al. Occupational risk factors for systemic lupus erythematosus: a nationwide study based on hospitalizations in Sweden. J Rheumatol 2012;39:743–51.
96. Parks CG, Conrad K, Cooper GS. Occupational exposure to crystalline silica and autoimmune disease. Environ Health Perspect 1999;107(Suppl 5):793–802.
97. Pollard KM. Perspective: The Lung, Particles, Fibers, Nanomaterials, and Autoimmunity. Front Immunol 2020;11:587136.
98. Pollard KM. Silica, Silicosis, and Autoimmunity. Front Immunol 2016;7:97.
99. Brown JM, Archer AJ, Pfau JC, et al. Silica accelerated systemic autoimmune disease in lupus-prone New Zealand mixed mice. Clin Exp Immunol 2003; 131:415–21.

100. Bates MA, Brandenberger C, Langohr I, et al. Silica Triggers Inflammation and Ectopic Lymphoid Neogenesis in the Lungs in Parallel with Accelerated Onset of Systemic Autoimmunity and Glomerulonephritis in the Lupus-Prone NZBWF1 Mouse. PLoS One 2015;10:e0125481.

101. Wu M, Gordon RE, Herbert R, et al. Case report: Lung disease in World Trade Center responders exposed to dust and smoke: carbon nanotubes found in the lungs of World Trade Center patients and dust samples. Environ Health Perspect 2010;118:499–504.

102. The Lancet Respiratory M. The world is failing on silicosis. Lancet Respir Med 2019;7:283.

103. Kelly FJ, Fussell JC. Size, source and chemical composition as determinants of toxicity attributable to ambient particulate matter. Atmos Environ 2012;60: 504–26.

104. Bernatsky S, Smargiassi A, Barnabe C, et al. Fine particulate air pollution and systemic autoimmune rheumatic disease in two Canadian provinces. Environ Res 2016;146:85–91.

105. Bernatsky S, Smargiassi A, Johnson M, et al. Fine particulate air pollution, nitrogen dioxide, and systemic autoimmune rheumatic disease in Calgary, Alberta. Environ Res 2015;140:474–8.

106. Jung CR, Chung WT, Chen WT, et al. Long-term exposure to traffic-related air pollution and systemic lupus erythematosus in Taiwan: A cohort study. Sci Total Environ 2019;668:342–9.

107. Bernatsky S, Fournier M, Pineau CA, et al. Associations between ambient fine particulate levels and disease activity in patients with systemic lupus erythematosus (SLE). Environ Health Perspect 2011;119(1):45–9.

108. Stojan G, Kvit A, Curriero FC, et al. A spatiotemporal analysis of organ-specific lupus flares in relation to atmospheric variables and fine particulate matter pollution. Arthritis Rheumatol 2020;72(7):1134–42.

109. Park JS, Choi S, Kim K, et al. Association of particulate matter with autoimmune rheumatic diseases among adults in South Korea. Rheumatology (Oxford) 2021; 60(11):5117–26.

110. Risom L, Møller P, Loft S. Oxidative stress-induced DNA damage by particulate air pollution. Mutat Res 2005;592(1–2):119–37.

111. Costenbader KH, Kim DJ, Peerzada J, et al. Cigarette smoking and the risk of systemic lupus erythematosus: a meta-analysis. Arthritis Rheum 2004;50: 849–57.

112. Chua MHY, Ng IAT, W L-Cheung M, et al. Association Between Cigarette Smoking and Systemic Lupus Erythematosus: An Updated Multivariate Bayesian Metaanalysis. J Rheumatol 2020;47:1514–21.

113. Cozier YC, Barbhaiya M, Castro-Webb N, et al. Relationship of Cigarette Smoking and Alcohol Consumption to Incidence of Systemic Lupus Erythematosus in a Prospective Cohort Study of Black Women. Arthritis Care Res (Hoboken) 2019;71:671–7.

114. Leffers HCB, Troldborg A, Voss A, et al. Smoking associates with distinct clinical phenotypes in patients with systemic lupus erythematosus: a nationwide Danish cross-sectional study. Lupus Sci Med 2021;8.

115. Barbhaiya M, Tedeschi SK, Lu B, et al. Cigarette smoking and the risk of systemic lupus erythematosus, overall and by anti-double stranded DNA antibody subtype, in the Nurses' Health Study cohorts. Ann Rheum Dis 2018;77:196–202.

116. Speyer CB, Costenbader KH. Cigarette smoking and the pathogenesis of systemic lupus erythematosus. Expert Rev Clin Immunol 2018;14:481–7.

117. Rogers JM. Tobacco and pregnancy. Reprod Toxicol 2009;28:152–60.
118. Webber MP, Moir W, Crowson CS, et al. Post-September 11, 2001, Incidence of Systemic Autoimmune Diseases in World Trade Center-Exposed Firefighters and Emergency Medical Service Workers. Mayo Clin Proc 2016;91:23–32.
119. Sunil VR, Vayas KN, Fang M, et al. World Trade Center (WTC) dust exposure in mice is associated with inflammation, oxidative stress and epigenetic changes in the lung. Exp Mol Pathol 2017;102:50–8.
120. Kazeros A, Zhang E, Cheng X, et al. Systemic inflammation associated with world trade center dust exposures and airway abnormalities in the local community. J Occup Environ Med 2015;57:610–6.
121. Miller-Archie SA, Izmirly PM, Berman JR, et al. Systemic autoimmune disease among adults exposed to the September 11, 2001 Terrorist Attack. Arthritis Rheumatol 2020;72:849–59.
122. Geretto M, Ferrari M, De Angelis R, et al. Occupational exposures and environmental health hazards of military personnel. Int J Environ Res Public Health 2021;18.
123. Jones KA, Smith B, Granado NS, et al. Newly reported lupus and rheumatoid arthritis in relation to deployment within proximity to a documented open-air burn pit in Iraq. J Occup Environ Med 2012;54:698–707.
124. Ying D, Schmajuk G, Trupin L, et al. Inorganic dust exposure during military service as a predictor of rheumatoid arthritis and other autoimmune conditions. ACR Open Rheumatol 2021;3:466–74.
125. Cooper GS, Parks CG, Treadwell EL, et al. Occupational risk factors for the development of systemic lupus erythematosus. J Rheumatol 2004;31:1928–33.
126. Parks CG, Walitt BT, Pettinger M, et al. Insecticide use and risk of rheumatoid arthritis and systemic lupus erythematosus in the Women's Health Initiative Observational Study. Arthritis Care Res (Hoboken) 2011;63:184–94.
127. Williams JN, Chang SC, Sinnette C, et al. Pesticide exposure and risk of systemic lupus erythematosus in an urban population of predominantly African-American women. Lupus 2018;27:2129–34.
128. Parks CG, D'Aloisio AA, Sandler DP. Early Life Factors Associated with Adult-Onset Systemic Lupus Erythematosus in Women. Front Immunol 2016;7:103.
129. Sobel ES, Gianini J, Butfiloski EJ, et al. Acceleration of autoimmunity by organochlorine pesticides in (NZB x NZW)F1 mice. Environ Health Perspect 2005;113:323–8.
130. Wang F, Roberts SM, Butfiloski EJ, et al. Acceleration of autoimmunity by organochlorine pesticides: a comparison of splenic B-cell effects of chlordecone and estradiol in (NZBxNZW)F1 mice. Toxicol Sci 2007;99:141–52.
131. Halperin W, Vogt R, Sweeney MH, et al. Immunological markers among workers exposed to 2,3,7,8-tetrachlorodibenzo-p-dioxin. Occup Environ Med 1998;55:742–9.
132. Kilburn KH, Warshaw RH. Prevalence of symptoms of systemic lupus erythematosus (SLE) and of fluorescent antinuclear antibodies associated with chronic exposure to trichloroethylene and other chemicals in well water. Environ Res 1992;57:1–9.
133. Wang H, Banerjee N, Liang Y, et al. Gut microbiome-host interactions in driving environmental pollutant trichloroethene-mediated autoimmunity. Toxicol Appl Pharmacol 2021;424:115597.
134. Parks CG, Miller FW, Pollard KM, et al. Expert panel workshop consensus statement on the role of the environment in the development of autoimmune disease. Int J Mol Sci 2014;15:14269–97.

135. Lu-Fritts PY, Kottyan LC, James JA, et al. Association of systemic lupus erythe-matosus with uranium exposure in a community living near a uranium-processing plant: a nested case-control study. Arthritis Rheumatol 2014;66: 3105–12.

136. Erdei E, Shuey C, Pacheco B, et al. Elevated autoimmunity in residents living near abandoned uranium mine sites on the Navajo Nation. J Autoimmun 2019;99:15–23.

137. Hu H, Chen E, Li Y, et al. Effects of Arsenic Trioxide on INF-gamma Gene Expression in MRL/lpr Mice and Human Lupus. Biol Trace Elem Res 2018; 184(2):391–7.

138. Xia XR, Lin SX, Zhou Y. [Effects of arsenic trioxide on the autoimmunity and sur-vival time in BXSB lupus mice]. Zhongguo Zhong Xi Yi Jie He Za Zhi 2007;27(2): 138–41.

139. Maier NK, Crown D, Liu J, et al. Arsenic trioxide and other arsenical compounds inhibit the NLRP1, NLRP3, and NAIP5/NLRC4 inflammasomes. J Immunol 2014; 192(2):763–70.

140. Pollard KM, Cauvi DM, Toomey CB, et al. Mercury-induced inflammation and autoimmunity. Biochim Biophys Acta Gen Subj 2019;1863:129299.

141. Gardner RM, Nyland JF, Silbergeld EK. Differential immunotoxic effects of inor-ganic and organic mercury species in vitro. Toxicol Lett 2010;198:182–90.

142. Dinse GE, Jusko TA, Whitt IZ, et al. Associations Between Selected Xenobiotics and Antinuclear Antibodies in the National Health and Nutrition Examination Sur-vey, 1999-2004. Environ Health Perspect 2016;124:426–36.

143. McSorley EM, van Wijngaarden E, Yeates AJ, et al. Methylmercury and long chain polyunsaturated fatty acids are associated with immune dysregulation in young adults from the Seychelles child development study. Environ Res 2020;183:109072.

144. Hamann CR, Boonchai W, Wen L, et al. Spectrometric analysis of mercury con-tent in 549 skin-lightning products: is mercury toxicity a hidden global health hazard? J Am Acad Dermatol 2014;70:281–287 e3.

145. Zamansky GB. Sunlight-induced pathogenesis in systemic lupus erythemato-sus. J Invest Dermatol 1985;85:179–80.

146. Runger TM, Epe B, Moller K. Processing of directly and indirectly ultraviolet-induced DNA damage in human cells. Recent Results Cancer Res 1995;139: 31–42.

147. Andrade F, Casciola-Rosen LA, Rosen A. Generation of novel covalent RNA-protein complexes in cells by ultraviolet B irradiation: implications for autoimmu-nity. Arthritis Rheum 2005;52:1160–70.

148. Yung R, Powers D, Johnson K, et al. Mechanisms of drug-induced lupus. II. T cells overexpressing lymphocyte function-associated antigen 1 become autor-eactive and cause a lupuslike disease in syngeneic mice. J Clin Invest 1996;97: 2866–71.

149. Aubin F. Mechanisms involved in ultraviolet light-induced immunosuppression. Eur J Dermatol 2003;13:515–23.

150. Wolf SJ, Estadt SN, Gudjonsson JE, et al. Human and murine evidence for mechanisms driving autoimmune photosensitivity. Front Immunol 2018;9:2430.

Environmental Risks for Systemic Sclerosis

Hana Alahmari, MBBS[a], Zareen Ahmad, MD, FRCPC[a],
Sindhu R. Johnson, MD, PhD, FRCPC[b],*

KEYWORDS

- Scleroderma • Systemic sclerosis • Environmental risk factors
- Occupational risk factors

KEY POINTS

- Environmental factors that have been postulated to trigger systemic sclerosis (SSc) include occupational exposures, chemicals, medications, alterations in the microbiome, and dysbiosis.
- The weight of evidence indicates that silicone implants are not associated with SSc.
- Establishment of standard precautions in the workplace with potential exposures is a crucial preventive step.

INTRODUCTION

Systemic sclerosis or scleroderma (SSc) is a systemic autoimmune rheumatic disease comprising complex pathological pathways including endothelial injury, abundant collagen and myofibroblast deposition, and autoantibody production. It is characterized by heterogenous clinical manifestations involving the skin, lungs, gastrointestinal system, joints, kidneys, and/or heart. SSc incidence, prevalence, manifestations, and outcomes (quality of life, disability, and survival[1]) are variable between sexes (women are more commonly affected[2,3]), ethnicities,[4,5] and presence of overlaping diseases.[6]

The most relevant genetic associations for SSc are human leukocyte antigen DR isotype (HLA-DR)3 and HLA-DR5. Recent genome-wide association studies showed strong associations with HLA-DRB1*11:04, HLA-DQB1*02:02, and HLA-DPB1*13:01 alleles.[7] In addition to genetic predisposition, epigenetic modifications leading to heritable phenotypes can influence and contribute to the development of SSc.[8] However, only a small proportion of the heritability of SSc has been explained.[9] Evidence of

[a] Toronto Scleroderma Program, Mount Sinai Hospital, 2nd Floor, Box 9, 60 Murray Street, Toronto, Ontario M5T 3L9, Canada; [b] Toronto Scleroderma Program, Division of Rheumatology, Department of Medicine, Toronto Western Hospital, Mount Sinai Hospital, Institute of Health Policy, Management and Evaluation, University of Toronto, Room 2-004, Box 9, 60 Murray Street, Toronto, Ontario M5T 3L9, Canada
* Corresponding author.
E-mail address: Sindhu.Johnson@uhn.ca

Rheum Dis Clin N Am 48 (2022) 845–860
https://doi.org/10.1016/j.rdc.2022.06.006
0889-857X/22/© 2022 Elsevier Inc. All rights reserved.

geographic clustering and low concordance rates in twin studies suggest the importance of environmental influences in disease initiation.[10]

There is a myriad of environmental triggers that have been postulated including occupational exposures, chemical materials, silicone implants, microorganisms, medications, and smoking (**Fig. 1**). Several case-control studies and systematic reviews with meta-analysis were conducted to assess the association between these exposures with clinical phenotype and disease-related autoantibodies.[11–16] SSc has a higher mortality in general population when compared with lung involvement contributing the highest risk of morbidity and mortality. Therefore, understanding preventive measures and the potential external risks are of high demand.

ENVIRONMENTAL FACTORS

The geographical variation in SSc prevalence suggest environmental factors may be important in the development of SSc. SSc is more prevalent in North America and Australia than in Europe or Japan and more prevalent in southern Europe than northern Europe.[16] Clusters of SSc have been reported on First Nation reserves, in miners and in London boroughs near international airports.[16] There are several theories that these potential factors trigger SSc through targeting cellular, innate, and adaptive immune system or even remodeling epigenetic methylation and histone modification.[17,18]

Occupational Triggers

Silica
There is often confusion about silica and its forms.

- *Silicon* refers to the chemical element
- *Silicate* refers to silicon bound to oxygen, SiO_2 and includes its crystalline forms: quartz, tridymite, and cristobalite
- *Silica* refers to bound silicon and oxygen and is expressed as a content, that is, 15% of silica
- *Silicone* refers to a synthetic polymer of silicon, carbon, and oxygen. It can take the form of a gel, liquid, or solid.

Silica constitutes the second most common mineral in the earth's crust and is frequently used as a construction material.[19] Two early seminal articles alerted the world's view to the potential association between silica exposure and SSc.[20] In a study conducted in South African gold miners, the cumulative lifetime silica exposure was significantly higher in the cases as compared with the controls.[20] Rodnan and colleagues[21] reported a correlation between SSc and exposure to silica dust among coal miners. Subsequent case control and cohort studies found that people who are exposed to silica, e.g., miners are predisposed to SSc development compared with unexposed groups. In a German study, the likelihood of developing SSc was found to be 25 times higher in workplaces where there is an exposure to silica.[22] Two meta-analysis[13,14] and one systemic review[23] provide a robust epidemiologic evidence (**Table 1**). Occupations with silica exposure are outlined in **Box 1**.

There are some important considerations. The temporal relationship between exposure and disease onset varies among studies.[24,25] It was highlighted that the exposure to silica may affect the disease phenotype. Studies suggest that silica exposure may predict myositis[11,12] and is a poor prognostic factor for progressive lung fibrosis.[11]

From a pathogenic viewpoint, in vivo and in vitro studies suggest that silica dust stimulates inflammation derived by NALP3 inflammasome-driven interleukin (IL)-1β

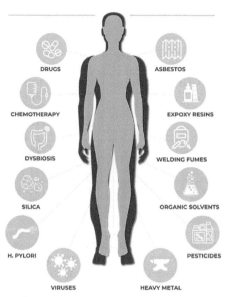

DRUGS

CHEMOTHERAPY

DYSBIOSIS

SILICA

H. PYLORI

VIRUSES

ASBESTOS

EXPOXY RESINS

WELDING FUMES

ORGANIC SOLVENTS

PESTICIDES

HEAVY METAL

Fig. 1. Environmental risk factors associated with systemic sclerosis.

activation. Binding of silica to scavenger receptors also results in apoptosis of alveolar macrophages and the release of proinflammatory cytokines resulting in lung inflammation and fibrosis[26] (**Fig. 2**). Interestingly, anti-topoisomerase I antibodies are found at increased frequency in patients exposed with silica suggesting that silica particles may be able to yield specific immune system alterations.[27,28]

Silicone implants

After the introduction of breast augmentation in 1960s, many have reported it is potential relationship with connective tissue diseases.[29] The augmentation uses silicon, paraffin, and petroleum jelly. Results of two meta-analyses indicated that there is no increased risk of connective tissue diseases associated with breast implants.[15,29] Similarly, two meta-analyses limited to SSc patients demonstrated no relationship of SSc with breast implants.[30,31] Rubio-Rivas and colleagues[14] further confirmed these findings with a meta-analysis of case-control studies reporting an risk ratio (RR) of 2.13 (95%CI 0.86–5.27). This estimate appears to have been influenced by a single study from McLaughlin and colleagues who reported an RR of 27.7 (95%CI 3.1–99.8) that is disproportionately larger than other studies. Interestingly, Rubio-Rivas and colleagues report an odds ratio (OR) of 1.68 (95%CI 1.65–1.71) from a meta-analysis of case-control studies. This estimate seems to have been influenced by a single study from Englert and colleagues who reported an OR of 1.68 (95%CI 1.65, 1.71). Despite these conflicting results, the weight of evidence suggests that silicone breast implants are not associated with an increased risk of SSc(**Table 2**).

Organic solvents. Solvents are chemical substances used for dissolving and extraction properties. They are widely used in many industries (**Box 2**). There are four meta-analyses demonstrating a correlation between solvent exposure and the risk of SSc[14,32–34] (**Table 3**). Kettaneh and colleagues[33] found that men are at higher risk than women for disease development after solvent exposure. This finding might explain that men have greater susceptibility to solvent exposure. An alternative explanation is that using solvents in household activities or hobbies is under recognized.

Table 1
Crystalline silica

Publication	Study Design	Number of Studies	Measure of Effect
McCormic 2010	Meta-analysis	16	CERR of 3.2 (95%CI 1.89–5.43) overall CERR 2.24 (95%CI 1.65–3.31) for case control studies CERR 15.49 (95%CI 4.54–52.87) for cohort studies
Rubio-Rivas 2017	Meta-analysis	19	OR of 2.81 (95%CI 1.86–4.23) RR 17.52 (95%CI 5.98–51.37) for cohort studies
Abbot 2018	Systematic review	14	OR range 3.20–25.0

Abbreviations: CERR, combined estimator of relative risk; OR, odds ratio; RR, risk ratio.

Zhao and colleagues[34] studied individual solvent exposures in their meta-analysis involving 14 studies. Some solvents had a significant relative risk over SSc including aromatic solvents, trichlorethylene (TCE), halogenated solvents, and ketones. Their study showed that subjects who had exposure to solvents for 3 months or longer had a higher risk, an OR of 2.40 (95% CI 1.48–4.03). However, assessing solvent exposures is difficult because specific solvents are often mixed in commercial products,

Box 1
Occupations and compounds with potential silica exposure

Miner

Quarryman

Sandblaster

Sandstone sculptor

Glass grinder

Cast polisher

Asphalt and roofing felt

Cement

Ceramics

Construction

Dentistry

Foundry worker

Glass and fiberglass

Steel mills

Jeweller

Ship construction

Abrasive and scouring soaps

Adapted from Rubio-Rivas M, Moreno R, Corbella X. Occupational and environmental scleroderma. Systematic review and meta-analysis. Clin Rheumatol. 2017 Mar;36(3):569-582.

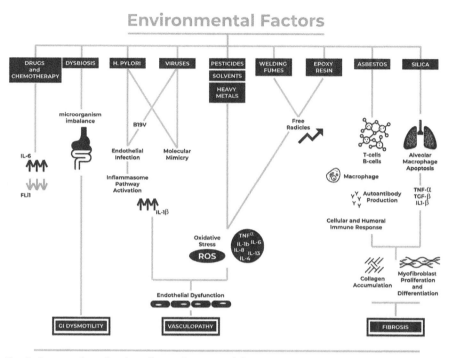

Fig. 2. Proposed mechanisms for environmental factors to trigger systemic sclerosis.

or the product has several names. A dose–response relationship is also hard to estimate. Data were based on self-report where underreporting or overreporting of exposures is possible.

Trichloroethylene exposure was observed in male patients with anti-topoisomerase I antibodies, suggesting its ability to trigger a specific autoimmune response in genetically susceptible individuals.[35] The underlying pathogenesis is suggested by experimental studies.

The production of high reactive oxygen may result in triggering of cellular inflammation.[35] Other contributors could be the induction of deoxyribonucleic acid (DNA) fragmentations and DNA hypomethylation with subsequent transcriptional changes of genes responsible for fibrosis and profibrotic cytokines production (see **Fig. 2**).

Epoxy resin, welding fumes, and pesticides. Epoxy resin is a chemical material used for adhesive purposes. It is commonly used in the construction of vehicles, bicycles, wood, and glass products. After the first reported case series in 1980, case-control studies have evaluated the link between epoxy resin exposure and disease risk.[36] Although Silman and colleagues[37] and Marie and colleagues[38] did not conclude a causal association, a meta-analysis of four case-control studies suggested a link between epoxy resin and SSc.[14] It is suspected that bis(4-amino-3-methylcyclohexyl) methane is a potential offending agent in skin sclerosis (**Table 4**).[36]

Welding fumes, a product of welding activity, may contain several metals including aluminum, arsenic, beryllium, lead, and manganese. Argon, nitrogen, carbon dioxide, carbon monoxide, and hydrogen fluoride gases often are produced during welding. The risk of welding fumes as a trigger of SSc was suggested by two case-control studies,[38,39] however further meta-analysis of four case control found no relation (**Table 4**).[14]

Box 2
Occupations and compounds associated with potential exposure to solvents

Spray painter

Mixing and blending machine operator

Building painter

Brush painter

Silk screen printer

Rotary pressman

Shoe repair: cutters, lasters, and sewers

Metal cleaner

Automobile painter

Office machine mechanic

Offset pressman

Printing pressmen

Dry cleaning machine operator

Aircraft engine mechanic

Electrical motor and generator fitter

Plastics compression, molding machine operator

Bookbinder

Organic chemist

Wooden furniture finisher

Analytical chemist

Woodworking machine operators

Time and motion study engineer

Chemistry technician

Composition tile layer

Electronics engineering technician

Adapted from Rubio-Rivas M, Moreno R, Corbella X. Occupational and environmental sclero-derma. Systematic review and meta-analysis. Clin Rheumatol. 2017 Mar;36(3):569-582.

Pesticides have been suggested as a potential causative agent for SSc in three case-control studies; however, meta-analysis did not support this (**Table 4**).

Asbestos. Asbestos is a naturally formed fibrous silicate mineral resistant to heat. It was a commonly used building material (roofing, ceiling, and insulation). Asbestos use is restricted and/or banned in some countries due to its hazardous health effect. There is growing evidence that asbestos exposure is associated with autoimmune diseases. In Montana, United States, among 6603 subjects who underwent health screening at the Center for Asbestos Related Diseases, 13.8% of them were diagnosed with an autoimmune disease (including 10 SSc cases) which was 7-fold higher than the expected prevalence.[40] As subsequent observational study had few SSc patients to make SSc-specific estimates for risk of exposure.[41] In a separate study, Gold

Table 2
Silicone implants and systemic sclerosis

Publication	Study Design	Number of Patients or Studies	Measure of Effect
Perkins 1995	Meta-analysis	3,242	RR 0.98 (95%CI 0.57–1.64)
Hochberg 1995	Meta-analysis	1,426	OR 1.04 (95%CI 0.58–1.88)
Wong 1996	Meta-analysis	2,232	OR 0.82 (95%CI 0.50–1.35) RR 1.30 (95%CI 0.86–1.96)
Whorton 1997	Meta-analysis	1,426	OR 1.02 (95%CI 0.56–1.84)
Janowsky 2000	Meta-analysis	12,445	RR 1.30 (95%CI 0.86–1.96)
Rubio-Rivas 2017	Meta-analysis	4 Case-control 5 Cohort	RR 2.13 (95%CI 0.86–5.27) for cohort studies OR 1.68 (95%CI 1.65–1.71) for case-control studies

and colleagues[42] reported an increased risk of SSc morality post-asbestos exposure with an OR of 1.2 (94%CI 1.1, 1.3).

Heavy metals. There is large case-control study by Marie and colleagues[43] evaluating heavy metal exposure and SSc. Hair samples taken from 100 patients with SSc and 300 control subjects were examined for quantification of heavy metal traces. Patients with SSc exhibited higher levels of seven heavy metals: antimony ($P = 0.001$), cadmium ($P = 0.0003$), lead ($P = 0.02$), mercury ($P = 0.02$), molybdenum ($P = 0.04$), palladium ($P = 0.001$), and zinc ($P = 0.0003$). Marie and colleagues[18] suggested a pathogenic relationship between seven common metals and SSc. Heavy metals can release radical oxygen species with DNA impairment, impaired phagocytosis, activation of T and B cells, and vascular damages by oxidative stress and none of inhibition that promote endothelial damage and fibroproliferation. Heavy metals can alter the transcription factors responsible for fibrosis by increased expression of microRNAs that are involved in oxidative stress and inflammation, altered epigenesis and hypomethylation of profibrotic genes, and by upregulation of ICAM-1 and VCAM-1 (see **Fig. 2**). Interestingly, cadmium has also been reported to be associated with higher serum

Table 3
Organic solvents and risk of systemic sclerosis

Publication	Study Design	Number of Studies	Measure of Effect
Aryal 2001	Meta-analysis	7	CERR 3.14 (95%CI 1.56–6.33) for case control studies
Kettaneh 2007	Meta-analysis	11	OR 1.76 (95%CI 1.24–2.50)
Zhao 2016	Meta-analysis	14	Combined estimator OR 2.07 (95%CI 1.55–2.78) Men > Women OR 5.2 (95%CI, 3.46–8.0) *Solvent sub-analysis* Aromatic solvents OR 2.72 (95%CI 1.21–6.09) TCE OR 2.07 (95%CI 1.34–3.17) Halogenated solvents OR 1.49 (95%CI 1.12–1.99) Ketones OR 4.20 (95% CI 2.19–8.06)
Rubio-Rivas 2017	Meta-analysis	13	OR 2.00 (95%CI 1.32–3.02; $P = 0.001$)

Abbreviations: CERR, combined estimator of relative risk; OR, odds ratio; TCE, trichloroethylene.

Table 4
Epoxy resin, welding fumes, and pesticide exposure and risk of systemic sclerosis

Publication	Study Design	Number of Studies	Measure of Effect
Rubio-Rivas 2017			
Epoxy resin	Meta-analysis	4 case-control	OR 2.97 (95%CI 2.31–3.83)
Welding fumes	Meta-analysis	4 case-control	OR 1.29 (95%CI 0.44–3.74)
Pesticides	Meta-analysis	1 mortality study	OR 1.02 (95%CI 0.78–1.32)

levels of galetin-3 that is a biomarker of myocardial fibrosis. **Box 3** outlines the occupations and compounds with potential heavy metal exposure.

Medications. Case reports and case series have suggested that several medications have been potentially linked to SSc-like skin changes or SSc disease initiation (**Table 5**). Taxanes induce production of IL-2, IL-6, and GM-SCF. Halogenated anaesthetics share physicochemical and toxicological properties with solvents. Bleomycin increases type-I procollagen synthesis in human skin and lung fibroblast cultures.[44] In a patient receiving paclitaxel, it was found that friend leukemia integration 1 (Fli1) proteins are below the detectable levels in dermal fibroblasts.[45] Fli1 is a protein that suppresses the type 1 collagen gene in dermal fibroblasts.

Whether discontinuation of the suspect medication will improve skin sclerosis depends on the patient. In the case of taxane-based agents, two cases underwent reversible changes after drug withdrawal,[46,47] and in one patient after methysergide discontinuation.[48]

Infectious triggers
An increasing body of evidence suggests that there are potential infectious triggers for SSc. Although the evidence supporting these potential associations come from case reports and case series, their detection in tissue samples, cell lines, and animal models have led to the proposed pathogenic roles of these organisms (**Table 6**).

Herpes virus family. There is growing evidence concerning human herpes viruses (HHV) and SSc, namely, Epstein–Bar virus (EBV), human cytomegalovirus (HCMV),

Box 3
Heavy metal-related occupations and compounds

Working in gold, diamond mines

Production of semi-conductors

Infrared detectors

Lead storage batteries

Solder

Sheet and pipe metal bearings

Castings

Pewter

Metal alloys

Fire-retardant formulations for plastics, rubbers, textiles, paper, paints, and explosives

Manufacturing of electronics

Table 5
Medications associated with scleroderma-like skin changes or scleroderma

Medication	Finding
Bleomycin	SSc-like lesion[49]
Taxanes	SSc or SSc-like skin changes[50]
Gemcitabine	SSc-like lesion[50]
Doxorubicin	Closer temporal relationship with the administration of chemotherapy[51]
Tryptophan	Biopsy proven fibrosis and eosinophilia[52]
L-5-hydroxytryptophan	Elevated kynurenine and serotonin in blood[53]
Letrozole	Puffy hands, centromere antibodies, and Raynaud's phenomenon[54]
Appetite suppressants	Limited SSc and morphea[55]
Pentazocine	Skin induration and woody texture[56]
Methysergide	SSc-like skin fibrosis and edema[57]
Bromocriptine	Morphea-like lesion[58]
Methylphenidate	Limited SSc, improved after discontinuation[48]
Check points inhibitors	Limited and diffused SSc with morphea[59]
Interferon-alfa	Limited SSc[60]
Vitamin A, D, E injections	Diffuse SSc[61]
Vitamin K1 injection	Morphea-like skin change[62]
Mineral oil injection	SSc-like skin fibrosis[63]
Mepivacaine	Linear morphea[64]
Inhaled halogenated anaesthetics	Raynaud's phenomenon, skin tightness, and ANA[65]
Local anesthesia	Dermatomyositis and SSc[66]
Cocaine	Scleroderma renal crisis. One case with anti-centromere and two cases with anti-Scl70 antibodies[67]

Abbreviation: ANA, anti-nuclear antibody.

and HHV-6. Several studies showed high levels of EBV load in endothelial and fibroblast cells.[68] In EBV-infected monocytes cells, it triggers immunogenicity by upregulation of toll like receptor (TLR)-8 expression and increasing interferon (IF) signature.[69]

HCMV has been postulated as a putative organism. HCMV gene transcripts were found in the endothelial cells from skin specimens of women with SSc.[70] Vitro models also demonstrated molecular mimicry between HCMV UL94 peptide and endothelial / fibroblast self-peptides. This cross-talk causes endothelial injury with inflammatory and fibrosis cascades.[71]

HHV-6 is a virus that most commonly affects children, but latent reactivation can occur. Similar to HCMV, higher levels of HHV-6 A/B DNA were measured in the peripheral blood cells of patients with SSc as compared with controls.[72] In vitro studies demonstrated that endothelial cells loaded with HHV-6 virus had released abundant amounts of profibrotic cytokines and impaired endothelial angiogenesis.[73] Both HCMV- and HHV-6A-modulated miRNA micro Ribonucleic acid (miRNA) of transforming growth factor (TGF)-ß and platelet-derived growth factor (PDGF) were reported to be involved in vivo in the pathogenesis of SSc.[74] High viral load is correlated with the presence of anti-topoisomerase antibody and extensive skin fibrosis.[72,75]

Parvovirus B19. Parvovirus B19 (PVB-19) infection has been implicated to be a potential trigger of autoimmune disorders, including SSc. PVB-19 DNA or viral

Table 6 Potential infectious triggers of systemic sclerosis	
Virus	**Finding**
Hepatitis B, C viruses	OR 2.97 (95%CI 1.92–4.53)[82]
Human papilloma virus	Adjusted hazard ratio 1.13 (95%CI 0.57–2.21)[83]
Epstein–Barr virus	Localized and diffuse SSc[84,85]
Human cytomegalovirus	Shortly after an acute episode of viral infection[70]
Coxiella burnetii	Four patients with chronic Q fever preceded or followed by diagnosis of limited SSc[86]
SARS-CoV-2	SSc with myositis 3 wk after COVID-19 infection[87]
Helicobacter pylori	H pylori infection was found more prevalent in SSc patients compared with healthy controls (OR 2.10, 95%CI 1.57–2.82)[88]
Mycosis fungoides	Coincident with the diagnosis of silicosis[89]
Toxoplasma gondii	Higher Immunoglobulin M (IgM) T gondii titer compared with controls (0.53 ± 0.48 vs. 0.3 ± 0.17, $P < 0.01$)[90]
Rhodotorula glutinis	252-fold increase in R glutinis sequences in the skin of four patients with early dcSSc comparedwith healthy controls[91]

Abbreviation: dcSSc, diffuse cutaneous systemic sclerosis.

trans-activator protein NS1 has been detected in the bone marrow, serum, and skin of patients with SSc.[76,77] The extent of PVB-19 RNA expression correlated with endothelial inflammation and TNF-α expression.[78] Several theories suggest that PBV-19 can potentiate the disease onset. Molecular mimicry with subsequent self-antigen on endothelial cells is a suggested pathway. PVB-19 can stimulate NRLP3 inflammasome pathway in monocytes, a potent IL-1b activator with subsequent inflammation and cytokines recruitment.[79]

Retrovirus. The presence of antibodies to retroviral proteins has been detected in serum specimens from patients with SSc.[80] When normal human dermal fibroblasts induced by retroviral protein, it results in the production of extracellular matrix proteins, acquiring a SSc-like phenotype.[80] A study in mice demonstrated a homology in sequence between SSc-specific autoantigens, U1 small nuclear ribonucleoprotein, Scl-70, and retroviral proteins, leading to potential cross-reactivity between the virus and these proteins.[81]

Helicobacter pylori
There are several studies suggesting a relationship between *H pylori* infection and SSc onset or progression. Meta-analysis demonstrated increased *H pylori* infection in SSc compared with healthy controls (OR 2.10).[88] However, the direction of causality remains uncertain. Gastrointestinal dysmotility in SSc might increase the association with *H pylori*[92] or increase mucosal permeability allowing bacterial shedding that elicits an immune reaction.[93] Eradication of *H pylori* may improve primary Raynaud's phenomenon.[94]

Microbiomes and dysbiosis
There is emerging evidence suggesting a role of alternations in microbial flora and autoimmune disease, with increase in pathobiont organisms and decreased commensals from gastrointestinal samples.[95] Gastrointestinal dysbiosis was found to be correlated with the severity of gastrointestinal dysmotility[96] and lung fibrosis, but not skin fibrosis.[97] SSc skin flora dysbiosis has been observed with colonization of unpredicted

species.[98] Altered molecular signature has been detected with a decrease in lipophilic organisms and increase in gram negative organisms in the skin.[98] It is difficult to establish causality as changes in the skin or gastrointestinal tract might promote the susceptibility to microorganism imbalance.[99] Whether dietary changes can improve gastrointestinal dysmotility or maldigestion through balance of the gastrointestinal microbiota remains to be understood.

SUMMARY

There is an increasing literature suggesting a relationship between SSc and environmental factors. Meta-analysis of case-control studies support organic solvents, silica, and epoxy resins as environmental triggers of SSc. Case reports and cases series suggest certain infections and medications may induce SSc or SSc-like conditions. These environmental exposures may impact epigenetic regulation as well as trigger an abhorrent immune response resulting in the clinical and serologic phenotype that we diagnose as SSc. Screening and studying putative triggers will not only improve our understanding of the pathogenesis of SSc but also guide efforts to institute protective measures.

CLINICS CARE POINTS

- Health care profesisonals play a key role in the prevention and early recognition of occupational and environmental risk factors leading to SSc.
- Recognition of occupational or environmental exposures may fasciliate access to compensation for lost income due to resultant illness and other health care benefits.
- The employer and patient's coworkers may be alerted of a potentially unhealthy work environment.

DISCLOSURES

Dr. Johnson is supported by the Gurmej Kaur Dhanda Scleroderma Research Award, Scleroderma Association of British Columbia.

REFERENCES

1. Johnson SR, Glaman DD, Schentag CT, et al. Quality of life and functional status in systemic sclerosis compared to other rheumatic diseases. J Rheumatol 2006; 33(6):1117–22.
2. Hussein H, Lee P, Chau C, et al. The effect of male sex on survival in systemic sclerosis. J Rheumatol 2014;41(11):2193–200.
3. Pasarikovski CR, Granton JT, Roos AM, et al. Sex disparities in systemic sclerosis-associated pulmonary arterial hypertension: a cohort study. Arthritis Res Ther 2016;18:30.
4. Al-Sheikh H, Ahmad Z, Johnson SR. Ethnic variations in systemic sclerosis disease manifestations, internal organ involvement, and mortality. J Rheumatol 2019;46(9):1103–8.
5. Low AH, Johnson SR, Lee P. Ethnic influence on disease manifestations and autoantibodies in Chinese-descent patients with systemic sclerosis. J Rheumatol 2009;36(4):787–93.
6. Alharbi S, Ahmad Z, Bookman AA, et al. Epidemiology and survival of systemic sclerosis-systemic lupus erythematosus overlap syndrome. J Rheumatol 2018; 45(10):1406–10.

7. Acosta-Herrera M, Kerick M, Lopéz-Isac E, et al. Comprehensive analysis of the major histocompatibility complex in systemic sclerosis identifies differential HLA associations by clinical and serological subtypes. Ann Rheum Dis 2021;80(8): 1040–7.

8. Tsou PS, Sawalha AH. Unfolding the pathogenesis of scleroderma through genomics and epigenomics. J Autoimmun 2017;83:73–94.

9. Mayes MD. The genetics of scleroderma: looking into the postgenomic era. Curr Opin Rheumatol 2012;24(6):677–84.

10. Feghali-Bostwick C, Medsger TA Jr, Wright TM. Analysis of systemic sclerosis in twins reveals low concordance for disease and high concordance for the presence of antinuclear antibodies. Arthritis Rheum 2003;48(7):1956–63.

11. Ferri C, Arcangeletti MC, Caselli E, et al. Insights into the knowledge of complex diseases: Environmental infectious/toxic agents as potential etiopathogenetic factors of systemic sclerosis. J Autoimmun 2021;124:102727.

12. Aguila LA, da Silva HC, Medeiros-Ribeiro AC, et al. Is exposure to environmental factors associated with a characteristic clinical and laboratory profile in systemic sclerosis? A retrospective analysis. Rheumatol Int 2021;41(6):1143–50.

13. McCormic ZD, Khuder SS, Aryal BK, et al. Occupational silica exposure as a risk factor for scleroderma: a meta-analysis. Int Arch Occup Environ Health 2010; 83(7):763–9.

14. Rubio-Rivas M, Moreno R, Corbella X. Occupational and environmental scleroderma. Systematic review and meta-analysis. Clin Rheumatol 2017;36(3):569–82.

15. Perkins LL, Clark BD, Klein PJ, et al. A meta-analysis of breast implants and connective tissue disease. Ann Plast Surg 1995;35(6):561–70.

16. Ouchene L, Muntyanu A, Lavoué J, et al. Toward Understanding of Environmental Risk Factors in Systemic Sclerosis. J Cutan Med Surg 2021;25(2):188–204.

17. Altorok N, Kahaleh B. Epigenetics and systemic sclerosis. Semin Immunopathol 2015;37(5):453–62.

18. Marie I. Systemic sclerosis and exposure to heavy metals. Autoimmun Rev 2019; 18(1):62–72.

19. Mora GF. Systemic sclerosis: environmental factors. J Rheumatol 2009;36(11): 2383–96.

20. Sluis-Cremer GK, Hessel PA, Nizdo EH, et al. Silica, silicosis, and progressive systemic sclerosis. Br J Ind Med 1985;42(12):838–43.

21. Rodnan GP, Benedek TG, Medsger TA, et al. The association of progressive systemic sclerosis (Scleroderma) with Coal Miners' pneumoconiosis and other forms of silicosis. Ann Intern Med 1967;66(2):323–34.

22. Haustein UF, Ziegler V. Environmentally induced systemic sclerosis-like disorders. Int J Dermatol 1985;24(3):147–51.

23. Abbot S, Bossingham D, Proudman S, et al. Risk factors for the development of systemic sclerosis: a systematic review of the literature. Rheumatol Adv Pract 2018;2(2):rky041.

24. Englert H, Small-McMahon J, Davis K, et al. Male systemic sclerosis and occupational silica exposure-a population-based study. Aust N Z J Med 2000;30(2): 215–20.

25. Slimani S, Ben Ammar A, Ladjouze-Rezig A. Connective tissue diseases after heavy exposure to silica: a report of nine cases in stonemasons. Clin Rheumatol 2010;29(5):531–3.

26. Brown JM, Pfau JC, Holian A. Immunoglobulin and lymphocyte responses following silica exposure in New Zealand Mixed mice. Inhalation Toxicol 2004; 16(3):133–9.

27. Ferri C, Artoni E, Sighinolfi GL, et al. High serum levels of silica nanoparticles in systemic sclerosis patients with occupational exposure: Possible pathogenetic role in disease phenotypes. Semin Arthritis Rheum 2018;48(3):475–81.

28. Rocha LF, Luppino Assad AP, Marangoni RG, et al. Systemic sclerosis and silica exposure: a rare association in a large Brazilian cohort. Rheumatol Int 2016;36(5): 697–702.

29. Wong O. A critical assessment of the relationship between silicone breast implants and connective tissue diseases. Regul Toxicol Pharmacol 1996;23(1): 74–85.

30. Whorton D, Wong O. Scleroderma and silicone breast implants. West J Med 1997;167(3):159–65.

31. Janowsky EC, Kupper LL, Hulka BS. Meta-analyses of the relation between silicone breast implants and the risk of connective-tissue diseases. N Engl J Med 2000;342(11):781–90.

32. Aryal BK, Khuder SA, Schaub EA. Meta-analysis of systemic sclerosis and exposure to solvents. Am J Ind Med 2001;40(3):271–4.

33. Kettaneh A, Al Moufti O, Tiev KP, et al. Occupational exposure to solvents and gender-related risk of systemic sclerosis: a metaanalysis of case-control studies. J Rheumatol 2007;34(1):97–103.

34. Zhao JH, Duan Y, Wang YJ, et al. The influence of different solvents on systemic sclerosis: an updated meta-analysis of 14 case-control studies. J Clin Rheumatol 2016;22(5):253–9.

35. Griffin JM, Blossom SJ, Jackson SK, et al. Trichloroethylene accelerates an autoimmune response by Th1 T cell activation in MRL+/+ mice. Immunopharmacology 2000;46(2):123–37.

36. Yamakage A, Ishikawa H, Saito Y, et al. Occupational scleroderma-like disorder occurring in men engaged in the polymerization of epoxy resins. Dermatologica 1980;161(1):33–44.

37. Silman AJ, Jones S. What is the contribution of occupational environmental factors to the occurrence of scleroderma in men? Ann Rheum Dis 1992;51(12): 1322–4.

38. Marie I, Gehanno JF, Bubenheim M, et al. Prospective study to evaluate the association between systemic sclerosis and occupational exposure and review of the literature. Autoimmun Rev 2014;13(2):151–6.

39. Diot E, Lesire V, Guilmot JL, et al. Systemic sclerosis and occupational risk factors: a case-control study. Occup Environ Med 2002;59(8):545–9.

40. Diegel R, Black B, Pfau JC, et al. Case series: rheumatological manifestations attributed to exposure to Libby Asbestiform Amphiboles. J Toxicol Environ Health A 2018;81(15):734–47.

41. Noonan CW, Pfau JC, Larson TC, et al. Nested case-control study of autoimmune disease in an asbestos-exposed population. Environ Health Perspect 2006; 114(8):1243–7.

42. Gold LS, Ward MH, Dosemeci M, et al. Systemic autoimmune disease mortality and occupational exposures. Arthritis Rheum 2007;56(10):3189–201.

43. Marie I, Gehanno JF, Bubenheim M, et al. Systemic sclerosis and exposure to heavy metals: a case control study of 100 patients and 300 controls. Autoimmun Rev 2017;16(3):223–30.

44. Clark JG, Starcher BC, Uitto J. Bleomycin-induced synthesis of type I procollagen by human lung and skin fibroblasts in culture. Biochim Biophys Acta 1980;631(2): 359–70.

45. INAOKI M, KAWABATA C, NISHIJIMA C, et al. Case of bleomycin-induced sclero-derma. J Dermatol 2012;39(5):482–4.
46. Winkelmann RR, Yiannias JA, DiCaudo DJ, et al. Paclitaxel-induced diffuse cuta-neous sclerosis: a case with associated esophageal dysmotility, Raynaud's phe-nomenon, and myositis. Int J Dermatol 2016;55(1):97–100.
47. Cleveland MG, Ajaikumar BS, Reganti R. Cutaneous fibrosis induced by doce-taxel: a case report. Cancer 2000;88(5):1078–81.
48. Meridor K, Levy Y. Systemic sclerosis induced by CNS stimulants for ADHD: a case series and review of the literature. Autoimmun Rev 2020;19(1):102439.
49. Kerr LD, Spiera H. Scleroderma in association with the use of bleomycin: a report of 3 cases. J Rheumatol 1992;19(2):294–6.
50. Verhulst L, Noë E, Morren MA, et al. Scleroderma-like cutaneous lesions during treatment with paclitaxel and gemcitabine in a patient with pancreatic adenocar-cinoma. Review of literature. Int J Dermatol 2018;57(9):1075–9.
51. Alexandrescu DT, Bhagwati NS, Wiernik PH. Chemotherapy-induced sclero-derma: a pleiomorphic syndrome. Clin Exp Dermatol 2005;30(2):141–5.
52. Silver RM, Heyes MP, Maize JC, et al. Scleroderma, fasciitis, and eosinophilia associated with the ingestion of tryptophan. N Engl J Med 1990;322(13):874–81.
53. Sternberg EM, Van Woert MH, Young SN, et al. Development of a scleroderma-like illness during therapy with L-5-hydroxytryptophan and carbidopa. N Engl J Med 1980;303(14):782–7.
54. Pokhai G. Letrozole-induced very early systemic sclerosis in a patient with breast cancer: a case report. Arch Rheumatol 2014;29:126–9.
55. Tomlinson IW, Jayson MI. Systemic sclerosis after therapy with appetite suppres-sants. J Rheumatol 1984;11(2):254.
56. Palestine RF, Millns JL, Spigel GT, et al. Skin manifestations of pentazocine abuse. J Am Acad Dermatol 1980;2(1):47–55.
57. Kluger N, Girard C, Bessis D, et al. Methysergide-induced scleroderma-like changes of the legs. Br J Dermatol 2005;153(1):224–5.
58. Leshin B, Piette WW, Caplan RM. Morphea after bromocriptine therapy. Int J Der-matol 1989;28(3):177–9.
59. Terrier B, Humbert S, Preta LH, et al. Risk of scleroderma according to the type of immune checkpoint inhibitors. Autoimmun Rev 2020;19(8):102596.
60. Silva JL, Faria DS, Teixeira F, et al. Systemic sclerosis induced by interferon-alfa treatment of melanoma. Acta Reumatologica Portuguesa 2017;42(3):263–4.
61. Balbi GGM, Montes RA, Vilela VS, et al. Rapidly progressive diffuse systemic sclerosis after local vitamins A, D and E complex injections: literature review and report of two cases. Immunol Res 2017;65(1):285–92.
62. Pang BK, Munro V, Kossard S. Pseudoscleroderma secondary to phytomena-dione (vitamin K1) injections: Texier's disease. Australas J Dermatol 1996; 37(1):44–7.
63. Vera-Lastra O, Medina G, Cruz-Dominguez Mdel P, et al. Human adjuvant dis-ease induced by foreign substances: a new model of ASIA (Shoenfeld's syn-drome). Lupus 2012;21(2):128–35.
64. Ueda T, Niiyama S, Amoh Y, et al. Linear scleroderma after contusion and injec-tion of mepivacaine hydrochloride. Dermatol Online J 2010;16:11.
65. Magnavita N. Can scleroderma be induced by anesthetics? Case report. Med Pr 2016;6:557–60.
66. Rose T, Nothjunge J, Schlote W. Familial occurrence of dermatomyositis and pro-gressive scleroderma after injection of a local anaesthetic for dental treatment. Eur J Pediatr 1985;143(3):225–8.

67. Andreussi R, Silva LMB, da Silva HC, et al. Systemic sclerosis induced by the use of cocaine: is there an association? Rheumatol Int 2019;39(2):387–93.
68. Sternbæk L, Draborg AH, Østerlund MT, et al. Increased antibody levels to stage-specific Epstein-Barr virus antigens in systemic autoimmune diseases reveal a common pathology. Scand J Clin Lab Invest 2019;79(1–2):7–16.
69. Farina A, Peruzzi G, Lacconi V, et al. Epstein-Barr virus lytic infection promotes activation of Toll-like receptor 8 innate immune response in systemic sclerosis monocytes. Arthritis Res Ther 2017;19(1):39.
70. Ferri C, Cazzato M, Giuggioli D, et al. Systemic sclerosis following human cytomegalovirus infection. Ann Rheum Dis 2002;61(10):937–8.
71. Lunardi C, Bason C, Navone R, et al. Systemic sclerosis immunoglobulin G auto-antibodies bind the human cytomegalovirus late protein UL94 and induce apoptosis in human endothelial cells. Nat Med 2000;6(10):1183–6.
72. Caselli E, Soffritti I, D'Accolti M, et al. HHV-6A infection and systemic sclerosis: clues of a possible association. Microorganisms 2020;8(1):39.
73. Rizzo R, D'Accolti M, Bortolotti D, et al. Human Herpesvirus 6A and 6B inhibit in vitro angiogenesis by induction of Human Leukocyte Antigen G. Scientific Rep 2018;8(1):17683.
74. Soffritti I, D'Accolti M, Ravegnini G, et al. Modulation of microRNome by Human Cytomegalovirus and Human Herpesvirus 6 Infection in Human Dermal Fibroblasts: Possible Significance in the Induction of Fibrosis in Systemic Sclerosis. Cells 2021;10(5):1060.
75. Efthymiou G, Dardiotis E, Liaskos C, et al. A comprehensive analysis of antigen-specific antibody responses against human cytomegalovirus in patients with systemic sclerosis. Clin Immunol 2019;207:87–96.
76. Ferri C, Giuggioli D, Sebastiani M, et al. Parvovirus B19 infection of cultured skin fibroblasts from systemic sclerosis patients: comment on the article by Ray et al. Arthritis Rheum 2002;46(8):2262–3 [author reply: 2263-2264].
77. Zakrzewska K, Cortivo R, Tonello C, et al. Human parvovirus B19 experimental infection in human fibroblasts and endothelial cells cultures. Virus Res 2005; 114(1):1–5.
78. Ferri C, Zakrzewska K, Longombardo G, et al. Parvovirus B19 infection of bone marrow in systemic sclerosis patients. Clin Exp Rheumatol 1999;17(6):718–20.
79. Zakrzewska K, Arvia R, Torcia MG, et al. Effects of Parvovirus B19 In Vitro Infection on Monocytes from Patients with Systemic Sclerosis: Enhanced Inflammatory Pathways by Caspase-1 Activation and Cytokine Production. J Invest Dermatol 2019;139(10):2125–33.e2121.
80. Jimenez SA, Diaz A, Khalili K. Retroviruses and the Pathogenesis of Systemic Sclerosis. Int Rev Immunol 1995;12(2–4):159–75.
81. Query CC, Keene JD. A human autoimmune protein associated with U1 RNA contains a region of homology that is cross-reactive with retroviral p30gag antigen. Cell 1987;51(2):211–20.
82. Tiosano S, Cohen AD, Amital H. The association between hepatitis B, hepatitis C and systemic sclerosis: a cross-sectional study. Curr Opin Rheumatol 2019;31(5): 493–8.
83. Chen M-L, Huang J-Y, Hung Y-M, et al. Association of human papillomavirus and systemic sclerosis: a population based cohort study. Int J Clin Pract 2021;75(5): e13887.
84. Urano J, Kohno H, Watanabe T. Unusual case of progressive systemic sclerosis with onset in early childhood and following infectious mononucleosis. Eur J Pediatr 1981;136(3):285–9.

85. Longo F, Saletta S, Lepore L, et al. Localized scleroderma after infection with Epstein-Barr virus. Clin Exp Rheumatol 1993;11 6:681–3.
86. Jansen AFM, Raijmakers RPH, van Deuren M, et al. Chronic Q fever associated with systemic sclerosis. Eur J Clin Invest 2019;49(7):e13123.
87. Fineschi S. Case Report: Systemic Sclerosis After Covid-19 Infection. Front Immunol 2021;12:686699.
88. Yong WC, Upala S, Sanguankeo A. Helicobacter pylori infection in systemic sclerosis: a systematic review and meta-analysis of observational studies. Clin Exp Rheumatol 2018;36(Suppl 113):168–74.
89. Yasuda M, Amano H, Yamanaka M, et al. Coincidental association of mycosis fungoides and occupational systemic sclerosis? J Dermatol 2008;35(1):21–4.
90. Arnson Y, Amital H, Guiducci S, et al. The Role of Infections in the Immunopathogensis of Systemic Sclerosis–Evidence from Serological Studies. Ann N Y Acad Sci 2009;1173(1):627–32.
91. Arron ST, Dimon MT, Li Z, et al. High Rhodotorula sequences in skin transcriptome of patients with diffuse systemic sclerosis. J Invest Dermatol 2014;134(8):2138–45.
92. Kalabay L, Fekete B, Czirják L, et al. Helicobacter pylori Infection in Connective Tissue Disorders is Associated with High Levels of Antibodies to Mycobacterial hsp65 but not to Human hsp60. Helicobacter (Cambridge, Mass) 2002;7(4):250–6.
93. Boyanova L, Markovska R, Yordanov D, et al. High prevalence of virulent Helicobacter pylori strains in symptomatic Bulgarian patients. Diagn Microbiol Infect Dis 2009;64(4):374–80.
94. Gasbarrini A, Massari I, Serricchio M, et al. Helicobacter pylori eradication ameliorates primary Raynaud's phenomenon. Dig Dis Sci 1998;43(8):1641–5.
95. Volkmann ER, Chang Y-L, Barroso N, et al. Association of systemic sclerosis with a unique colonic microbial consortium. Arthritis Rheumatol 2016;68(6):1483–92.
96. Andréasson K, Alrawi Z, Persson A, et al. Intestinal dysbiosis is common in systemic sclerosis and associated with gastrointestinal and extraintestinal features of disease. Arthritis Res Ther 2016;18(1):278.
97. Patrone V, Puglisi E, Cardinali M, et al. Gut microbiota profile in systemic sclerosis patients with and without clinical evidence of gastrointestinal involvement. Sci Rep 2017;7(1):14874.
98. Johnson ME, Franks JM, Cai G, et al. Microbiome dysbiosis is associated with disease duration and increased inflammatory gene expression in systemic sclerosis skin. Arthritis Res Ther 2019;21(1):49.
99. Denton CP, Murray C. Cause or effect? Interpreting emerging evidence for dysbiosis in systemic sclerosis. Arthritis Res Ther 2019;21(1):81.

Environmental Risks for Inflammatory Myopathies

Weng Ian Che, MMSc[a,b], Ingrid E. Lundberg, MD, PhD[c,d,e,*],
Marie Holmqvist, MD, PhD[a,b,c,d]

KEYWORDS

- Idiopathic inflammatory myopathies • Myositis • Antisynthetase syndrome
- Environmental factors • Ultraviolet radiation • Smoking • Infectious agents
- Pollutants

KEY POINTS

- It has been suggested that the onset of idiopathic inflammatory myopathies (IIMs) requires environmental triggers besides underlying genetic susceptibility. Ultraviolet radiation, smoking, infectious agents, certain pollutants, medications, and vitamin D deficiency are potential environmental triggers for IIM.
- Many of the suggested environmental factors for IIM enter human body via lungs and are related to features of lung involvement in IIM, supporting lung as the initial onset site of autoimmunity for some subgroups of IIM.
- Some presented environmental factors are linked to specific IIM phenotypes and the presence of specific autoantibodies, such as anti-Mi2, anti-Jo1, and anti-3-hydroxy-3-methyl-glutaryl-coenzyme A reductase autoantibodies, indicating the relevance of different environmental factors in different autoantibody-defined subgroups of IIM.
- Future investigations should consider exploring the associations between environmental factors and subsets of IIM defined by autoantibody profile.

INTRODUCTION

Inflammatory myopathies are a group of heterogenous diseases. Some rare conditions in this group are associated with infections but the larger group, idiopathic inflammatory myopathies (IIMs), the focus of this review, does not have a causative agent. IIM is characterized by proximal muscle weakness accompanied by various extramuscular

[a] Department of Medicine, Solna, Eugeniahemmet, T2, Karolinska Universitetssjukhuset, Solna, Stockholm 171 76, Sweden; [b] Clinical Epidemiology Division, Department of Medicine, Solna, Karolinska Institutet, Stockholm, Sweden; [c] Rheumatology, Karolinska University Hospital, Anna Steckséns gata 30A, Stockholm 171 76, Sweden; [d] Division of Rheumatology, Department of Medicine, Solna, Karolinska Institutet, Stockholm, Sweden; [e] ME Gastro, Derm and Rheuma, Theme Inflammation and Aging, Karolinska University Hospital, Stockholm, Sweden
* Corresponding author. Rheumatology, Karolinska University Hospital, Anna Steckséns gata 30A, Stockholm 171 76, Sweden.
E-mail address: Ingrid.lundberg@ki.se

Rheum Dis Clin N Am 48 (2022) 861–874
https://doi.org/10.1016/j.rdc.2022.06.007   rheumatic.theclinics.com
0889-857X/22/© 2022 The Authors. Published by Elsevier Inc. This is an open access article under the CC BY license (http://creativecommons.org/licenses/by/4.0/).

manifestations, for example, in skin, lungs, joints, heart, and gastrointestinal tract.[1,2] The major subtypes of IIM classified based on clinical, serologic, and histologic features are dermatomyositis (DM), polymyositis (PM), inclusion body myositis (IBM), antisynthetase syndrome (ASSD), immune-mediated necrotizing myopathy (IMNM), and juvenile IIM.[1] More homogenous subsets can be identified by using myositis-specific and myositis-associated autoantibodies (MSAs and MAAs).[1]

The pathogenic mechanisms of IIM are complex and not fully understood but it has been suggested that the onset of IIM requires environmental triggers in genetically susceptible individuals.[3] The geospatial and seasonal pattern of IIM onset as well as exposure to different environmental factors before the diagnosis of IIM have been studied and findings suggest associations between various environmental factors and IIM[4–8] but only a few of them have been reproduced in large-scale studies with comparison to the general population.[9–12] In this review, we systemically review and discuss the external environmental factors with suggestive evidence mainly from cross-sectional, case-control, and cohort studies for adult-onset IIM (Table 1). We also highlight their potential implications in IIM development, identify current challenges, and provide insight into future investigation.

Ultraviolet Radiation

Ultraviolet (UV) radiation has long been considered a risk factor for IIM, in particular for DM. The supportive evidence include (1) photosensitivity being a common cutaneous manifestation associated with DM[2], (2) prevalence of DM showing a geographic gradient negatively correlated with latitude[13,14], and (3) prevalence of DM positively associated with UV radiation intensity.[15,16] The association between UV radiation and the development of DM is further supported by evidence from the study using MYOVISION registry data. Based on the self-reported data on sun exposure in 1,350 patients, patients with DM were more likely to experience 2 times or more of sunburn and high/moderate job-related sun exposure 12 months before disease diagnosis than patients with PM or IBM.[17] Moreover, sun exposure may not only confer the risk of DM development but also DM flare.[5]

The association between UV radiation and presence of some MSAs/MAAs has been examined, and a positive correlation between the prevalence of DM-specific anti-Mi2 autoantibodies and UV radiation has been suggested.[15,16] A systematic review analyzing prevalence data from 92 studies across 22 countries showed a significant trend of increasing prevalence of anti-Mi2 autoantibodies with lower latitudes, whereas the trend to increase in higher global solar UV index (UVI) was not significant.[4] Because UVI was estimated based on data in 2010 while data collection of the included studies spread over a much wider time period (up to 10 years), and because UV radiation was correlated with latitude, it was suggested that analyses of geographic gradient might provide more precise findings than UVI.[4] Interestingly, the review study also first reported positive associations with UVI for anti-Ro52, anti-PM-Scl, and anti-Ku autoantibodies and a negative association for anti-threonyl-tRNA synthetase autoantibodies,[4] suggesting that UV radiation may affect the development of other IIM phenotypes besides DM. Further investigation of these associations is warranted given the limitations, such as cross-sectional design and lack of measurement of personal exposure to UV radiation, of the included studies.[4,15,16]

It has also been suggested that associations between UV radiation and DM and anti-Mi2 autoantibodies differ across sex and ethnicity. The risk of having DM and anti-Mi2 autoantibodies associated with UV radiation and sunburn was solely significant in women, whereas the association between occupational sun exposure and DM was more apparent in men.[16,17] Moreover, UV radiation was more likely a risk factor of

Table 1
Environmental factors and their associations with idiopathic inflammatory myopathies and related features

Factors	Association	IIM Phenotypes	MSAs	Genetic Factors	Evidence from
UV radiation	Risk	DM	Anti-Mi2		4,15–17
Smoking	Risk	PM	Anti-Jo1	HLA-DRB1*03:01	19–21
	Protective		Anti-TIF1γ	HLA-DRB1*03:01	
Pollutants					
Silica	Risk	DMᵇ	Anti-Jo1[a]		9,23
Inorganic dust	Risk	IIM[b]			10
Dust, gas, fume	Risk	ASSD			24
World Trade Center dust	Risk	DM/PM[b]	Anti-Jo1[a]		26,27
Infectious agents	Risk	DM ASSD IMNM IBM PM	Anti-TIF1γ[c] Anti-MDA5[a]		11,12,34–38,42–44
Medications					
Statins	Risk	IMNM DM PM	Anti-HMGCR	HLA-DRB1*11:01	34,47,48,52,54,59,61
Immune checkpoint inhibitors	Risk	IIM			63–66
Vitamin D deficiency	Risk	IIM	Anti-Jo1 Anti-Mi2		68,69

Abbreviations: ASSD, antisynthetase syndrome; DM, dermatomyositis; HLA-DRB1, major histocompatibility complex, class II, DR beta 1; IBM, inclusion body myositis; IIM, idiopathic inflammatory myopathies; ILD, interstitial lung disease; IMNM, immune-mediated necrotizing myopathy; MDA5, melanoma differentiation-associated gene 5; MSAs, myositis-specific autoantibodies; PM, polymyositis; TIF1γ, transcriptional intermediary factor 1γ; UV, ultraviolet.

[a] Based on descriptive data.
[b] Evidence from combined analyses including other autoimmune diseases.
[c] Based on serologic data.

DM and anti-Mi2 autoantibodies in Caucasian populations than in non-Caucasian populations.[16] The absence of associations in men and in non-Caucasian populations could be due to small sample size because most patients included were women and Caucasians.[16,17]

It is not fully known how UV radiation may trigger the onset of DM but there are findings showing upregulation of the Mi2 protein but not the other subunits of the nucleosome remodeling and deacetylase complex in keratinocytes shortly after 30 minutes exposure to UV treatment.[18] In addition, upregulations of Mi2 protein after UV exposure were also noted in several cancer cell types. In addition, ionizing radiation that cause DNA damage could also result in rapid accumulation of Mi2 protein.[18] These findings combined suggest that UV radiation may contribute to the development of DM by causing DNA damage and by increasing antigen presentation in the affected cells.[18]

Smoking

Smoking has been found to confer an increased risk for anti-Jo1 autoantibodies in particular in genetically susceptible individuals with IIM. Anti-Jo1 positive patients were more likely to have a smoking history than anti-Jo1 negative patients.[6,19] Smokers with IIM carrying allele in the major histocompatibility complex, class II, DR beta 1 gene (*HLA-DRB1*03*) had the greatest risk of anti-Jo1 autoantibody positivity compared with other combinations of smoking history and positivity of anti-Jo1 autoantibodies among patients with IIM.[19] Consistent findings were noted in the analysis stratified by sex but women had a stronger association than men.[19] A follow-up study with higher resolution imputation data found an even stronger association between anti-Jo1 autoantibodies and smoking in *HLA-DRB1*03:01* positive patients.[20] Interactions on the multiplicative scale between *HLA-DRB1*03/*03:01* allele and smoking when modeling the risk of anti-Jo1 autoantibodies has been tested without significant interaction, potentially due to lack of power.[19,20] It has also been suggested that the association between smoking and anti-Jo1 autoantibodies could be independent of *HLA-DRB1*03:01*.[20] Together, these findings indicate that smoking is a risk factor of developing the anti-Jo1 autoantibodies and confers an additional risk in patients carrying *HLA-DRB1*03:01* allele.

There is a study analyzing smoking in pack-years and reporting that the likelihood was increased by 2% for PM and IIM-associated interstitial lung disease (ILD) and by 1% for anti-Jo1 autoantibodies but was decreased by 7% for anti-transcriptional intermediary factor 1 α/γ (TIF1α/γ) autoantibodies for every increased unit of pack-years.[21] However, the estimate for anti-Jo1 autoantibodies was not statistically significant.[21] Similar associations were observed in the analyses including only Caucasian patients while no significant associations were noted in African American patients, probably due to a smaller number of patients.[21] Importantly, this study also revealed that smoking had the strongest positive associations with PM, ILD, and anti-Jo1 autoantibodies, as well as a greatest inverse association with anti-TIF1α/γ autoantibodies in patients with *HLA-DRB1*03:01* allele.[21]

In summary, although lack of evidence from studies with longitudinal data raises uncertainty of a causal link between smoking and IIM, observational data support that smoking may have a role in the pathogenesis of anti-Jo1 positive IIM, potentially by triggering the development of anti-Jo1 autoantibodies in susceptible individuals carrying *HLA-DRB1*03:01* allele.

Pollutants

A wide range of environmental pollutants has been reported to potentially trigger the onset of IIM. Earlier case series found that some DM patients had long-term occupational exposure to silica or organic solvents before disease onset.[22,23] The association between silica and DM has been examined further in a Swedish cohort study including 241,077 men employed in the construction industry.[9] This study revealed that the risk of developing systemic lupus erythematosus, systemic sclerosis (SSc), or DM was almost doubled in workers exposed to silica dust compared with those unexposed office workers after controlling for age and smoking.[9] A recent study including 438,068 US discharge military veterans found that the odds of SSc, vasculitis, or IIM was significantly increased by 23% for those exposed to inorganic dust during services in Afghanistan or in Iraq than those unexposed after adjusting for age, sex, race, and smoking status, and the association became stronger as the length of service was increased.[10]

There is more evidence supporting a role of occupational pollutants in the pathogenesis of ASSD compared with other IIM phenotypes although findings are based on self-reported case-control data, and might therefore be subject to recall bias,[24] and some more descriptive data.[23,25–28] A case-control study observed a significantly higher frequency of lifetime occupational exposure to dust, gases, or fumes in 32 patients with ASSD (n = 25) or ILD (n = 7) than 32 IIM patients without ASSD (50% vs 22%).[24] Moreover, patients with ASSD with high occupational exposure (94%) were more likely to have ILD than those exposed to no or low occupational pollutants (75%).[24] Furthermore, a high likelihood of anti-Jo1 autoantibody positivity was observed in several studies investigating the association between environmental exposure and risk of autoimmune diseases. Both acute and chronic exposures to aerosolized World Trade Center dust after the 9/11 attack in firefighters were associated with increased risk of autoimmune diseases.[26] Among the identified autoimmune diseases, there were 8 cases of DM/PM and 2 of them were positive to anti-Jo1 autoantibodies.[26,27] In a study of 10 patients with ASSD, 6 had hypersensitivity pneumonitis preceding the onset of ASSD, 9 were exposed to significant levels of domiciliary exposures including mold, birds, pigeon and feather pillow, and 6 were anti-Jo1 positive.[28] One of the 3 patients with silica-associated DM was with the presence of anti-Jo1 autoantibodies.[23] These findings suggest a triggering role of environmental pollutants in onset of autoimmunity, perhaps in lungs, which may result in systemic onset of autoimmunity later affecting other tissues.

Infectious Agents

Seasonality of birth or IIM disease onset observed in several studies suggests a nonrandom disease development, which may be affected by environmental exposures with a seasonal pattern such as infectious agents.[29–32] For example, there are studies reporting aggregations of disease onset of patients with antimelanoma differentiation-associated gene 5 (MDA5) autoantibodies in winter where flu season coincided.[29,30,33] However, no causal inference could be drawn from these seasonal patterns.

The role of infectious agents in pathogenesis of IIM implicated by seasonality is further supported by the epidemiologic findings of preceding infections in patients with IIM. A nationwide cohort study in Denmark noted that the risk of DM/PM in individuals with history of hospital contact for viral, bacterial, and other infections was significantly increased and was 2-fold higher than those without hospital contact for infections after adjusting for calendar year, sex and its interaction with age, and comorbidities.[11] Furthermore, this association was strengthened when the number of hospitalizations increased and as the time since hospitalization with an infection to diagnosis of DM/PM decreased.[11] These findings are in line with the results of 2 case-control studies.[12,34] In one of the studies, the risk of reverse causality was minimized by excluding infections diagnosed in the year of IIM diagnosis.[12] Specifically, the types of infections associated with IIM were mainly respiratory and gastrointestinal infections.[12,34]

Serologic evidence suggests that the link between previous infection and IIM may be attributable to certain microbial agents, particularly viruses. Higher titers of antibodies against hepatitis C virus, Epstein-Barr virus (EBV), influenza A and B, parainfluenza, coxsackie virus, or cytomegalovirus (CMV) in patients with IIM than in controls were observed in several studies.[35–37] A recent case-control study also found that antibodies against viral families of Coronaviridae, Geminiviridae, Herpesviridae, Orthomyxoviridae, and Poxviridae in adult patients with anti-TIF1γ autoantibodies were enriched, whereas the enriched viral families in matched healthy controls were Picornaviridae, Caliciviridae, Orthomyxoviridae, Coronaviridae, and Retroviridae.[38] Specifically, a previous study found that, in comparison to matched healthy controls, patients with PM had higher levels of immunoglobulin M (IgM) and immunoglobulin G (IgG) against EBV, and IgM against CMV.[36] Interestingly, infiltrates of CD4+ CD28^{null} T cells in muscle biopsies of patients with DM has been found solely in patients with IgG against CMV and not in patients without.[39] Although no causality between these viral species and onset of IIM can be drawn from these serologic findings, they support the hypothesis for a role of acute (IgM) or latent (IgG) infection in the development of IIM.

Severe acute respiratory syndrome coronavirus 2 (SARS-CoV-2) has also been suggested as a trigger of IIM. The evidence supporting this assumption is weak, and includes the presence of DM-specific autoantibodies including anti-MDA5 and antinuclear matrix protein 2 autoantibodies in patients with coronavirus diseases 19 (COVID-19),[40] and a remarkable similarity of pathophysiological features between autoimmune anti-MDA5 syndrome and COVID-19[41] and onset of the DM subgroup presenting with anti-MDA5 autoantibodies.[42] However, acute-onset IIM related to COVID-19 could be a transient epiphenomenon.[42] Future studies with longer follow-up time are warranted to evaluate if COVID-19 is associated with chronic IIM evolved from acute IIM.

It is still unclear how microbes may trigger the onset of IIM but the abovementioned observations suggest a potential linkage to lung involvement in IIM.[12,34,41,43] The elevated risks of ASSD on exposure to pneumonia, of ILD in patients with IIM exposed to pneumonia, tuberculosis, or sarcoidosis observed, respectively, in 2 studies further support this hypothesis.[34,44] Molecular mimicry may be a mechanism involved in the onset of autoimmunity because shared epitope sequences have been observed between variola virus and tripartite motif-containing protein 3, which shared high sequence identity with TIF1γ,[38] and between 3 immunogenic linear epitopes derived from patients with DM and SARS-CoV-2 proteins.[45]

Medications

Statin

Statins are drugs widely used for reducing the risk of cardiovascular diseases by binding to 3-hydroxy-3-methyl-glutaryl-coenzyme A reductase (HMGCR) and thus interfering in the cholesterol biosynthesis. Discontinuation due to associated adverse events including muscle toxicity is common.[46] Statin-induced myopathy usually resolves after discontinuation but when the symptoms persist and require immunomodulatory treatment, statin-associated autoimmune IIM may have developed.[47–58]

Among all the IIM phenotypes, IMNM with anti-HMGCR autoantibodies is strongly related to statin exposure; up to 67% of patients from North America were exposed to statins before disease onset.[47,48] Moreover, compared with IMNM patients with anti-signal recognition particle autoantibodies, patients with anti-HMGCR autoantibodies were 33-fold more likely to have history of statin use.[59]

Unlike patients from North America, statin exposure in anti-HMGCR positive IMNM patients from eastern countries is much lower, ranging from 15% to 38%.[60,61] Because naturally occurring HMGCR inhibitors have been found in dietary products commonly used in eastern cuisine,[62,63] this discrepancy may suggest an association between natural sources of HMGCR inhibitors and anti-HMGCR positive IMNM. Indeed, this assumption has been supported by 2 cases of statin naïve anti-HMGCR positive patients with consumption of shiitake mushroom and red rice, respectively.[64,65] However, there is lack of supportive evidence from epidemiologic studies and the mechanisms of how these dietary compounds can inhibit the activity of HMGCR are unknown, similarly how they can lead to the production of anti-HMGCR autoantibodies.

Statins may also be a risk factor for other IIM phenotypes, although evidence show weaker associations to other subsets than to IMNM. In a study exclusively including patients with DM or PM but not IMNM, the odds of regular statin use 6 months before disease onset in these patients was 6 times higher than the age-matched and sex-matched controls.[52] This finding was reproduced in a case-control study comparing patients with biopsy confirmed IIM excluding IMNM to age-matched and sex-matched controls, although the association was weaker than that observed in anti-HMGCR-positive patients.[54,59] Another case-control study reported that patients with DM and patients with PM were 2 times more likely to be exposed to statin use a year before disease diagnosis than patients with IBM after adjusting for age, gender, race, and year of diagnosis.[34]

It has been suggested that statins contribute to the pathogenesis of IIM by upregulating HMGCR in regenerating muscle cells.[66] If self-tolerance is lost to HMGCR, production of anti-HMGCR autoantibodies will be initiated, contributing to autoimmunity attacking muscle tissue. Individuals carrying the genetic variant *HLA-DR11* may be more susceptible to this mechanism because this variant has been found to be strongly associated with statin-induced IMNM who are anti-HMGCR positive.[67] This evidence supports a role of the adaptive immune system in this subset of IIM. Other proinflammatory effects related to statins such as increased expression of major histocompatibility complex class I in myofibers may be involved in the disease development as well.[47,56]

Little is known what nongenetic factors are related to statin-associated autoimmune IIM. Characteristics such as older age, female sex, chronic statin exposure, and comorbidities including Type 2 diabetes, hypertension, and hyperlipidemia have frequently been reported in cases of statin-associated autoimmune IIM.[47–49,51,52,55,58,68] Interestingly, patients with prior exposure to simvastatin or pravastatin were at higher risk of having chronic muscular diseases including DM and PM than patients exposed to atorvastatin or fluvastatin but the associations were not statistically significant.[52] Significant interaction between statins and proton pump inhibitors was also found when estimating the odds ratio of statin-associated DM or PM.[52]

The association between statins and IMNM has led to a safety concern about statin use in patients with IIM for cardiovascular disease prevention. Although evidence is sparse, a study observed that 22 out of 23 patients with non-HMGCR IIM tolerated statins well.[57]

Immune checkpoint inhibitors

Immune checkpoint inhibitors (ICIs) are a group of medications that have revolutionized cancer treatment in recent years. Because they interfere with immune pathways, they have been associated with rheumatic immune-related adverse events, for example, myositis. Symptoms typically occur shortly after monotherapy or combination therapy with programmed death (PD)-1/PD-ligand 1 inhibitor or/and cytotoxic T lymphocyte antigen-4 inhibitor.[69–72] The pathogenesis of ICI-associated myositis is not well-understood but enhanced activation of T cells may partially explain the phenomenon because antigen-specific T cells play an important role in IIM development.[1,73] Importantly, even though lymphocytic infiltration is presented in muscle biopsy of patients with ICI-associated myositis,[69] characteristics such as concurrence with myasthenia gravis or myocarditis, infrequent positivity of MSAs/MAAs, high mortality, and resolution after steroid and intravenous immunoglobin treatments highlight a distinct pathologic mechanism different from that of IIM.[69,71,72]

Vitamin D Deficiency

Vitamin D deficiency has been suggested as a risk factor for adult IIM. Previous evidence has shown that vitamin D deficiency was not only more commonly seen in patients with newly diagnosed IIM than matched controls; it was also correlated with elevated muscle enzymes, increased number of proinflammatory cells, as well as anti-Jo1 and anti-Mi2 autoantibodies in newly diagnosed and untreated patients with IIM.[74,75] Heliotrope rash, gastrointestinal and liver involvements were also frequently seen in patients with IIM with extremely low levels of vitamin D at diagnosis.[74] Interestingly, vitamin D receptor polymorphisms associated with IIM have been suggested but these findings are inconsistent.[76,77] Given that only one time-point measurement of vitamin D was analyzed and that the observed low level at IIM diagnosis can be due to less outdoor activity because of muscle weakness, it remains unclear if vitamin D deficiency is causally associated with IIM.

SUMMARY

In this review, we have discussed several suggested environmental factors and their influence on clinically or serologically defined IIM phenotypes. This knowledge provides important clues to infer into the pathogenic mechanisms of IIM. Importantly, there is a growing body of evidence implicating lungs as the initial site of autoimmunity, which later may lead to the onset of some subsets of IIM in particular those with ILD.[78,79] As presented above, many of the external environmental factors suggested as risk factors for IIM, including smoking, occupational pollutants, and infectious agents, are associated with the subtype ASSD, IIM-associated ILD, or the presence of either anti-Jo1 or anti-MDA5 autoantibodies,[10,20,34,44,80] which are features of lung involvement in IIM. These observations further support that autoimmunity of IIM may first take place in lungs in response to environmental insults in susceptible individuals. Furthermore, the links to specific MSAs provide insight into the site of antigen presentation and production of autoantibodies, as seen in anti-Jo1, anti-Mi2, and anti-HMGCR autoantibodies.[18,66,81] The dose-dependent manners of correlations found in smoking, occupational dust, infections, and vitamin D deficiency suggest proportional correlations between accumulation of environmental exposure and IIM onset.[10,11,21,74] Besides pathogenic implications, information on environmental factors for IIM and IIM-related complications is useful for disease prevention and management.

FUTURE DIRECTIONS

Although several attempts have been made to identify potential environmental factors associated with IIM, no causal relationship has been established for a single factor.

Given the fact that IIM is a complex and rare disease, this is not surprising. Small sample size, lack of valid and longitudinal data on environmental exposure and potential confounders, as well as lack of proper control groups, confounding adjustment, and analysis by serologic profile are common limitations of many of the previously published studies, and these also reflect the challenges for future studies. It is impossible to overcome all these limitations in one study but establishing international collaborations to increase sample size and data diversity, and to enable standardized data collection and proper selection of controls is crucial to explore the role of environmental factors in the development of IIM. Moreover, although the pathogenesis of IIM is multifactorial, it is interesting that previous studies seldom considered interactions between environmental factors or between environmental and genetic factors. There is also a lack of mechanistic studies exploring the role of environmental factors for IIM at molecular level. Future epidemiologic and basic science studies should focus on answering these questions.

CLINICS CARE POINTS

- Little is currently known about the clinical relevance of avoiding the suggested environmental triggers in patients with idiopathic inflammatory myopathies (IIMs). However, in clinical practice, patients with dermatomyositis are recommended to protect skin from sun exposure.

- Although smoking cessation is recommended for general long-term health benefits, we suggest all providers counsel patients on smoking cessation after IIM diagnosis.

- Current evidence suggests that statin use as secondary cardiovascular prophylaxis is safe and tolerable for patients with non-3-hydroxy-3-methyl-glutaryl-coenzyme A reductase IIM.

ACKNOWLEDGMENTS

This article was supported by grants from The Swedish Research Council No 2020-01378, the Swedish Rheumatism Association, King Gustaf V 80 Year Foundation, Stockholm Regional Council (ALF), and Heart and Lung foundation.

DISCLOSURE

Dr I.E. Lundberg has received consulting fees from Corbus Pharmaceuticals, Inc and research grants from AstraZeneca and has been serving on the advisory board for Astra Zeneca, Bristol Myers Squibb, EMD Serono Research & Development Institute, Argenx, Octapharma, Kezaar, Orphazyme, Pfizer and Janssen and has stock shares in Roche and Novartis. The other authors declare no conflicts of interest.

REFERENCES

1. Lundberg IE, Fujimoto M, Vencovsky J, et al. Idiopathic inflammatory myopathies. Nat Rev Dis Primers 2021;7(1):86.
2. Aggarwal R, Oddis CV. Managing myositis: a practical guide. Switzerland: Springer International Publishing; 2019.
3. O'Hanlon TP, Rider LG, Gan L, et al. Gene expression profiles from discordant monozygotic twins suggest that molecular pathways are shared among multiple systemic autoimmune diseases. Arthritis Res Ther 2010;13(2):R69.

4. Aguilar-Vazquez A, Chavarria-Avila E, Pizano-Martinez O, et al. Geographical Latitude Remains as an Important Factor for the Prevalence of Some Myositis Autoantibodies: A Systematic Review. Front Immunol 2021;12:672008.

5. Mamyrova G, Rider LG, Ehrlich A, et al. Environmental factors associated with disease flare in juvenile and adult dermatomyositis. Rheumatology 2017;56(8): 1342–7.

6. Griger Z, Csige I, Vincze M, et al. Smoking and alcohol consumption may increase the development of anti-jo-1 antibodies in patients with idiopathic inflammatory myopathies. Ann Rheum Dis 2013;71.

7. Lyon MG, Bloch DA, Hollak B, et al. Predisposing factors in polymyositis-dermatomyositis: results of a nationwide survey. J Rheumatol 1989;16(9): 1218–24.

8. Sarkar K, Weinberg CR, Oddis CV, et al. Seasonal influence on the onset of idiopathic inflammatory myopathies in serologically defined groups. Arthritis Rheum 2005;52(8):2433–8.

9. Blanc PD, Järvholm B, Torén K. Prospective risk of rheumatologic disease associated with occupational exposure in a cohort of male construction workers. Am J Med 2015;128(10):1094–101.

10. Ying DV, Schmajuk G, Trupin L, et al. Inorganic Dust Exposure During Military Service as a Predictor of Rheumatoid Arthritis and Other Autoimmune Conditions. Acr Open Rheumatol 2021;3(7):466–74.

11. Nielsen PR, Kragstrup TW, Deleuran BW, et al. Infections as risk factor for autoimmune diseases - A nationwide study. J Autoimmun 2016;74:176–81.

12. Svensson J, Holmqvist M, Lundberg IE, et al. Infections and respiratory tract disease as risk factors for idiopathic inflammatory myopathies: a population-based case-control study. Ann Rheum Dis 2017;76(11):1803–8.

13. Dourmishev L, Meffert H, Piazena H. Dermatomyositis: comparative studies of cutaneous photosensitivity in lupus erythematosus and normal subjects. Photodermatol Photoimmunol Photomed 2004;20(5):230–4.

14. Hengstman GJ, van Venrooij WJ, Vencovsky J, et al. The relative prevalence of dermatomyositis and polymyositis in Europe exhibits a latitudinal gradient. Ann Rheum Dis 2000;59(2):141–2.

15. Okada S, Weatherhead E, Targoff IN, et al. Int Myositis Collab Study G. Global surface ultraviolet radiation intensity may modulate the clinical and immunologic expression of autoimmune muscle disease. Arthritis Rheum 2003;48(8):2285–93.

16. Love LA, Weinberg CR, McConnaughey DR, et al. Ultraviolet radiation intensity predicts the relative distribution of dermatomyositis and anti-Mi-2 autoantibodies in women. Arthritis Rheum 2009;60(8):2499–504.

17. Parks CG, Wilkerson J, Rose KM, et al. Association of Ultraviolet Radiation Exposure With Dermatomyositis in a National Myositis Patient Registry. Arthritis Care Res (Hoboken) 2020;72(11):1636–44.

18. Burd CJ, Kinyamu HK, Miller FW, et al. UV Radiation Regulates Mi-2 through Protein Translation and Stability. J Biol Chem 2008;283(50):34976–82.

19. Chinoy H, Adimulam S, Marriage F, et al. Interaction of HLA-DRB1*03 and smoking for the development of anti-Jo-1 antibodies in adult idiopathic inflammatory myopathies: a European-wide case study. Ann Rheum Dis 2012;71(6):961–5.

20. Pipis N, Rothwell S, Cooper R, et al. Gene-Environmental Interaction of HLA-DRB1*03:01 and Smoking for the Development of Anti-Jo-1 Autoantibodies in Idiopathic Inflammatory Myopathies: A UK Study. Arthritis Rheumatol 2016; 68(Suppl 10).

21. Schiffenbauer A, Faghihi-Kashani S, O'Hanlon TP, et al. The effect of cigarette smoking on the clinical and serological phenotypes of polymyositis and dermatomyositis. Semin Arthritis Rheum 2018;48(3):504–12.

22. Goldman JA. Connective tissue disease in people exposed to organic chemical solvents: systemic sclerosis (scleroderma) in dry cleaning plant and aircraft industry workers. J Clin Rheumatol 1996;2(4):185–90.

23. Koeger AC, Lang T, Alcaix D, et al. Silica-associated connective tissue disease. A study of 24 cases. Medicine (Baltimore) 1995;74(5):221–37.

24. Labirua-Iturburu A, Selva-O'Callaghan A, Zock JP, et al. Occupational exposure in patients with the antisynthetase syndrome. Clin Rheumatol 2014;33(2):221–5.

25. Campos G, Eisenreich MA, Lopes LM, et al. Antisynthetase syndrome after acute massive inhalation of wood and paint dust. Scand J Rheumatol 2016;45(5):425–6.

26. Webber MP, Moir W, Zeig-Owens R, et al. Nested Case-Control Study of Selected Systemic Autoimmune Diseases in World Trade Center Rescue/Recovery Workers. Arthritis Rheumatol 2015;67(5):1369–76.

27. Selva-O'Callaghan A, Labirua-Iturburu A, Pinal-Fernandez I. Antisynthetase antibodies in World Trade Center rescue and recovery workers with inflammatory myositis: comment on the article by Webber et al. Arthritis Rheumatol 2015;67(10):2791.

28. Kawassaki AM, Kairalla RA, Carvalho CR, et al. Hypersensitive pneumonitis: A trigger of autoimmunity in inflammatory myositis - A case series. Am J Respir Crit Care Med 2010;181(1).

29. So H, Shen Y, Wong TLV, et al. Seasonal variation in idiopathic inflammatory myopathies incidence and presentation: A retrospective study in Beijing and Hong Kong. Ann Rheum Dis 2020;79(SUPPL 1):1601–2.

30. Nishina N, Sato S, Masui K, et al. Seasonal and residential clustering at disease onset of anti-MDA5-associated interstitial lung disease. RMD Open 2020;6(2):e001202.

31. Toquet S, Granger B, Uzunhan Y, et al. The seasonality of Dermatomyositis associated with anti-MDA5 antibody: An argument for a respiratory viral trigger. Autoimmun Rev 2021;20(4):102788.

32. Woodman R, Hakendorf P, Limaye V. Seasonality of birth patterns in an Australian cohort of patients with biopsy-confirmed idiopathic inflammatory myopathy. Intern Med J 2016;46(5):619–21.

33. Rath B, Conrad T, Myles P, et al. Influenza and other respiratory viruses: standardizing disease severity in surveillance and clinical trials. Expert Rev Anti Infect Ther 2017;15(6):545–68.

34. Rider LG, Farhadi PN, Bayat N, et al. Infections and medications associated with onset of myositis in myovision, a national myositis patient registry. Arthritis Rheumatol 2017;69(Suppl 10).

35. Kalinova D, Todorova E, Kyurkchiev D, et al. AB0493 Association between antiviral IGM antibodies and myositis autoantibodies in patients with autoimmune myositis in Bulgarian population. Ann Rheum Dis 2013;72(Suppl 3):A939.

36. Barzilai O, Sherer Y, Ram M, et al. Epstein-Barr virus and cytomegalovirus in autoimmune diseases - Are they truly notorious? A preliminary report. Ann N Y Acad Sci 2007;1108:567–77. Shoenfeld Y, Gershwin ME, eds. Autoimmunity, Pt D: autoimmune disease, Annus Mirabilis.

37. Uruha A, Noguchi S, Hayashi YK, et al. Hepatitis C virus infection in inclusion body myositis: A case-control study. Neurology 2016;86(3):211–7.

38. Megremis S, Walker TDJ, He X, et al. Analysis of human total antibody repertoires in TIF1gamma autoantibody positive dermatomyositis. Commun Biol 2021; 4(1):419.
39. Fasth AE, Dastmalchi M, Rahbar A, et al. T cell infiltrates in the muscles of patients with dermatomyositis and polymyositis are dominated by CD28null T cells. J Immunol 2009;183(7):4792–9.
40. De Santis M, Isailovic N, Motta F, et al. Environmental triggers for connective tissue disease: the case of COVID-19 associated with dermatomyositis-specific autoantibodies. Curr Opin Rheumatol 2021;33(6):514–21.
41. Giannini M, Ohana M, Nespola B, et al. Similarities between COVID-19 and anti-MDA5 syndrome: what can we learn for better care? Eur Respir J 2020;56(3).
42. Gokhale Y, Patankar A, Holla U, et al. Dermatomyositis during COVID-19 Pandemic (A Case Series): Is there a Cause Effect Relationship? J Assoc Physicians India 2020;68(11):20–4.
43. Balseiro A, Oleaga A, Polledo L, et al. Clostridium sordellii in a Brown Bear (Ursus arctos) from Spain. J Wildl Dis 2013;49(4):1047–51.
44. Helmers SB, Jiang X, Pettersson D, et al. Inflammatory lung disease a potential risk factor for onset of idiopathic inflammatory myopathies: results from a pilot study. Rmd Open 2016;2(2):e000342.
45. Megremis S, Walker TDJ, He X, et al. Antibodies against immunogenic epitopes with high sequence identity to SARS-CoV-2 in patients with autoimmune dermatomyositis. Ann Rheum Dis 2020;79(10):1383–6.
46. Zhu Y, Chiang CW, Wang L, et al. A multistate transition model for statin-induced myopathy and statin discontinuation. CPT Pharmacometrics Syst Pharmacol 2021;10(10):1236–44.
47. Christopher-Stine L, Casciola-Rosen LA, Hong G, et al. A novel autoantibody recognizing 200-kd and 100-kd proteins is associated with an immune-mediated necrotizing myopathy. Arthritis Rheum 2010;62(9):2757–66.
48. Wu YF, Lach B, Provias JP, et al. Statin-associated Autoimmune Myopathies: A Pathophysiologic Spectrum. Can J Neurol Sci 2014;41(5):638–47.
49. Gonzales L, Ali M, Rodriguez-Cruz R, et al. Statin-induced necrotizing autoimmune myopathy: A novel diagnosis requiring a more widespread recognition. J Gen Intern Med 2016;31(2):S734–5.
50. Hinschberger O, Lohmann C, Lannes B, et al. [Immune-mediated necrotizing myopathy associated with antibodies to hydroxy-methyl-glutaryl-coenzyme A reductase]. Rev Med Interne 2014;35(8):546–9.
51. Borges IBP, Silva MG, Misse RG, et al. Lipid-lowering agent-triggered dermatomyositis and polymyositis: a case series and literature review. Rheumatol Int 2018;38(2):293–301.
52. Sailler L, Pereira C, Bagheri A, et al. Increased exposure to statins in patients developing chronic muscle diseases: a 2-year retrospective study. Ann Rheum Dis 2008;67(5):614–9.
53. Keithler A, Pomerantz B, Trang DN, et al. Statin-induced necrotizing autoimmune myopathy: A case of delayed onset following statin discontinuation. J Hosp Med 2018;13(4).
54. Caughey GE, Gabb GM, Ronson S, et al. Association of Statin Exposure With Histologically Confirmed Idiopathic Inflammatory Myositis in an Australian Population. JAMA Intern Med 2018;178(9):1224–9.
55. John SG, Thorn J, Sobonya R. Statins as a Potential Risk Factor for Autoimmune Diseases: A Case Report and Review. Am J Ther 2014;21(4):E94–6.

56. Kanth R, Shah MS, Flores RM. Statin-associated polymyositis following omeprazole treatment. Clin Med Res 2013;11(2):91–5.
57. Bae SS, Oganesian B, Golub I, et al. Statin use in patients with non-HMGCR idiopathic inflammatory myopathies: A retrospective study. Clin Cardiol 2020;43(7): 732–42.
58. Machado H, Andre A, Félix A, et al. Immune-mediated necrotizing myopathy associated with statin exposure: A rare side effect of a commonly used medication. Eur J Neurol 2021;28(SUPPL 1):642.
59. Tiniakou E, Pinal-Fernandez I, Lloyd TE, et al. More severe disease and slower recovery in younger patients with anti-3-hydroxy-3-methylglutaryl-coenzyme A reductase-associated autoimmune myopathy. Rheumatology (Oxford) 2017; 56(5):787–94.
60. Watanabe Y, Suzuki S, Nishimura H, et al. Statins and myotoxic effects associated with anti-3-hydroxy-3-methylglutaryl-coenzyme A reductase autoantibodies: an observational study in Japan. Medicine (Baltimore) 2015;94(4):e416.
61. Ge Y, Lu X, Peng Q, et al. Clinical Characteristics of Anti-3-Hydroxy-3-Methylglutaryl Coenzyme A Reductase Antibodies in Chinese Patients with Idiopathic Inflammatory Myopathies. PLoS One 2015;10(10):e0141616.
62. Wang TH, Lin TF. Monascus rice products. Adv Food Nutr Res 2007;53:123–59.
63. Lee J-W, Lee S-M, Gwak K-S, et al. Screening of edible mushrooms for the production of lovastatin and its HMG-CoA reductase inhibitory activity. Korean J Microbiol 2006;42(2):83–8.
64. Yoshida T, Chikazawa H, Kumon Y, et al. Did Shiitake Mushrooms Induce Immune-Mediated Necrotizing Myopathy? Rheumatologist 2019.
65. Barbacki A, Fallavollita SA, Karamchandani J, et al. Immune-Mediated Necrotizing Myopathy and Dietary Sources of Statins. Ann Intern Med 2018;168(12): 893–904.
66. Mammen AL, Chung T, Christopher-Stine L, et al. Autoantibodies Against 3-Hydroxy-3-Methylglutaryl-Coenzyme A Reductase in Patients With Statin-Associated Autoimmune Myopathy. Arthritis Rheum 2011;63(3):713–21.
67. Limaye V, Bundell C, Hollingsworth P, et al. Clinical and genetic associations of autoantibodies to 3-hydroxy-3-methyl-glutaryl-coenzyme a reductase in patients with immune-mediated myositis and necrotizing myopathy. Muscle Nerve 2015; 52(2):196–203.
68. Close RM, Close LM, Galdun P, et al. Potential implications of six American Indian patients with myopathy, statin exposure and anti-HMGCR antibodies. Rheumatology 2021;60(2):692–8.
69. Aldrich J, Pundole X, Tummala S, et al. Inflammatory Myositis in Cancer Patients Receiving Immune Checkpoint Inhibitors. Arthritis Rheumatol 2021;73(5):866–74.
70. Xu M, Nie Y, Yang Y, et al. Risk of Neurological Toxicities Following the Use of Different Immune Checkpoint Inhibitor Regimens in Solid Tumors: A Systematic Review and Meta-analysis. Neurologist 2019;24(3):75–83.
71. Moreira A, Loquai C, Pföhler C, et al. Myositis and neuromuscular side-effects induced by immune checkpoint inhibitors. Eur J Cancer 2019;106:12–23.
72. Anquetil C, Salem JE, Lebrun-Vignes B, et al. Immune Checkpoint Inhibitor-Associated Myositis: Expanding the Spectrum of Cardiac Complications of the Immunotherapy Revolution. Circulation 2018;138(7):743–5.
73. Okiyama N, Ichimura Y, Shobo M, et al. Immune response to dermatomyositis-specific autoantigen, transcriptional intermediary factor 1gamma can result in experimental myositis. Ann Rheum Dis 2021;80(9):1201–8.

74. Yu Z, Cheng H, Liang Y, et al. Decreased Serum 25-(OH)-D Level Associated With Muscle Enzyme and Myositis Specific Autoantibodies in Patients With Idiopathic Inflammatory Myopathy. Front Immunol 2021;12:642070.

75. Azali P, Helmers SB, Kockum I, et al. Low serum levels of vitamin D in idiopathic inflammatory myopathies. Ann Rheum Dis 2013;72(4):512–6.

76. Dzhebir G, Kamenarska Z, Hristova M, et al. Association of vitamin D receptor gene BsmI B/b and FokI F/f polymorphisms with adult dermatomyositis and systemic lupus erythematosus. Int J Dermatol 2016;55(8):e465–8.

77. Bodoki L, Chen JQ, Zeher M, et al. Vitamin D receptor gene polymorphisms and haplotypes in Hungarian patients with idiopathic inflammatory myopathy. Biomed Res Int 2015;2015:809895.

78. Notarnicola A, Preger C, Lundström S, et al. Longitudinal assessment of reactivity and affinity profile of anti-Jo1 autoantibodies to distinct HisRS domains and a splice variant in a cohort of patients with myositis and anti-synthetase syndrome. Arthritis Res Ther 2022;24(1):62.

79. Galindo-Feria AS, Albrecht I, Fernandes-Cerqueira C, et al. Proinflammatory Histidyl-Transfer RNA Synthetase-Specific CD4+ T Cells in the Blood and Lungs of Patients With Idiopathic Inflammatory Myopathies. Arthritis Rheumatol 2020; 72(1):179–91.

80. Chen HH, Yong YM, Lin CH, et al. Air pollutants and development of interstitial lung disease in patients with connective tissue disease: a population-based case-control study in Taiwan. Bmj Open 2020;10(12):e041405.

81. Levine SM, Raben N, Xie D, et al. Novel conformation of histidyl-transfer RNA synthetase in the lung: the target tissue in Jo-1 autoantibody-associated myositis. Arthritis Rheum 2007;56(8):2729–39.

Environmental Triggers for Vasculitis

Guy Katz, MD[a], Zachary S. Wallace, MD, MSc[b],*

KEYWORDS

- Vasculitis • Environmental • Infection • Exposure • ANCA • Kawasaki • Arteritis

KEY POINTS

- Environmental exposures are hypothesized to be a triggering event in genetically susceptible individuals with certain vasculitis syndromes.
- Many infections have been hypothesized or observed to trigger various types of vasculitis.
- Seasonal and geographic variation in incidence suggests a potential role for environmental factors in the onset of multiple vasculitis syndromes.
- Airborne and occupational exposures have been identified as risk factors for certain
vasculitides.
- The literature on this topic continues to evolve, and it is likely that specific triggers of
vasculitis may vary according to the type of vasculitis and the individual patient.

INTRODUCTION

Systemic vasculitis is a group of heterogenous immune-mediated inflammatory diseases characterized by vascular inflammation. Vasculitides are frequently categorized
according to the size of blood vessels involved: small (eg, antineutrophil cytoplasmic
antibody [ANCA]-associated vasculitis [AAV], immunoglobulin A [IgA] vasculitis), medium (eg, polyarteritis nodosa [PAN], Kawasaki disease [KD]), large (eg, giant cell
arteritis [GCA], Takayasu arteritis [TAK]), or variable (eg, Behçet disease, Cogan syndrome).[1] Each syndrome is associated with different epidemiologic characteristics,[2]
symptoms, patterns of vascular involvement, and extravascular manifestations
(**Table 1**).

As vasculitides are relatively rare diseases, much remains unknown about their
pathogenesis, but an expanding body of literature suggests that exposure to environmental triggers in genetically susceptible individuals may contribute to vasculitis onset

[a] Rheumatology Unit, Division of Rheumatology, Allergy, and Immunology, Massachusetts
General Hospital, Bulfinch 165, 55 Fruit Street, Boston, MA 02114, USA; [b] Clinical Epidemiology
Program, Rheumatology Unit, Division of Rheumatology, Allergy, and Immunology, Mongan
Institute, Massachusetts General Hospital, Harvard Medical School, 100 Cambridge Street,
Boston, MA 02114, USA
* Corresponding author.
E-mail address: zswallace@mgh.harvard.edu

Rheum Dis Clin N Am 48 (2022) 875–890
https://doi.org/10.1016/j.rdc.2022.06.008
0889-857X/22/© 2022 Elsevier Inc. All rights reserved.

Table 1
Blood vessels involved and common clinical manifestations of selected systemic vasculitides

Vessels Involved	Diseases	Common Manifestations	
Large: • Aorta • Arch vessels • Subclavian arteries • Axillaries • External carotid artery branches • Renal arteries • Pulmonary arteries • Iliac arteries	Giant cell arteritis Takayasu arteritis	• Headache • Jaw claudication • Scalp tenderness • Temporal artery tenderness • Diplopia • Monocular vision loss • Limb claudication • Polymyalgia rheumatic • Limb claudication • Carotidynia • Angina • Hypertension • Blood pressure discrepancy between limbs • Reduced peripheral pulses • Vascular bruits, aneurysms, or stenosis • Arthritis	
Medium (ie, parenchymal vessels within organs): • Coronary arteries • Branches of renal arteries • Mesenteric vasculature • Cutaneous arteries and arterioles • Vasa nervorum • Skeletal muscle vasculature	Polyarteritis nodosa Kawasaki disease	• Abdominal pain • Hematochezia • Flank pain • Testicular pain • Myalgias • Arthralgias • Mononeuritis multiplex • Hypertension • Skin nodules • Livedo reticularis • Conjunctivitis • Pharyngitis • Dry, cracked lips • Strawberry tongue • Cervical lymphadenopathy • Edema of the hands and feet • Arthritis • Rash • Myocarditis • Coronary artery aneurysms	
Small (ie, capillary beds, arteries, and venules within organs): • Kidneys • Lungs • Skin • Upper respiratory tract • Peripheral nerves	ANCA-associated vasculitis	MPA, GPA, and EGPA: • Inflammatory eye disease • Alveolar hemorrhage • Glomerulonephritis • Purpura • Mononeuritis multiplex MPA • Interstitial lung disease	GPA and EGPA: • Orbital inflammation • Lung nodules • Sinonasal disease EGPA: • Asthma • Atopy • Eosinophilic organ inflammation

(**Table 2**). This is of particular interest as some may represent "modifiable" risk factors for what are rare but often highly morbid diseases. Several consistent themes characterize the literature on this topic, particularly the search for infectious causes of

Table 2
Known or suspected environmental triggers in giant cell arteritis, Kawasaki disease, and antineutrophil cytoplasmic antibody-associated vasculitis

Environmental Exposure/ Association	Giant Cell Arteritis	Takayasu Arteritis	Polyarteritis Nodosa	Kawasaki Disease	ANCA-Associated Vasculitis
Infection	✔		✔	✔	✔
Seasonality	✔			✔	✔
Latitude	✔				✔
Rurality/farming					✔
Wind patterns				✔	
Smoking				✔	✔
Air pollution				✗	✔
Ozone				✔	
Silica					✔
Solvents					✔
Heavy metals					✔
Earthquakes					✔

Notes: Blank cells indicate insufficient data to determine the presence or absence of associations. "X" indicates current evidence suggests no association is present.

vasculitis given the observed temporal and geographic variations in the incidence of many vasculitides (**Table 3**). Here, we review the known and suspected environmental triggers for vasculitis, with a particular focus on GCA, TAK, PAN, KD, and AAV.

Giant Cell Arteritis

GCA is a large-vessel vasculitis that almost exclusively affects individuals above the age of 50 and presents as headache, scalp tenderness, jaw claudication, vision-threatening ischemic optic neuropathy, and inflammation of the aorta and its branches (see **Table 1**).[3,4] Although GCA has a well-described genetic predisposition, particularly with the major histocompatability complex (MHC) class II allele human leukocyte antigen-DRB (HLA-DRB)1*04, its pathophysiology suggests an antigen-driven etiology, which has long been suspected to represent an infectious or other environmental trigger.[5–8]

Geographic and temporal variations in giant cell arteritis incidence

Indirect evidence of an environmental trigger for GCA includes the varied incidence of GCA around the world. Indeed, a recent meta-analysis reported a strong association between incidence and latitude, with the highest incidence observed in Scandinavian countries.[9] Although higher latitude has also been shown to be associated with an increased frequency of the HLA-DRB1*04 susceptibility allele, analyses suggested that the associations between latitude and GCA incidence persist after adjusting for differences in this HLA frequency.[7] There have been conflicting studies regarding whether incidence varies across rural and urban locations.[10–12]

In addition to geographic variations in GCA incidence, there have been several studies evaluating temporal variations in GCA incidence, but these have yielded conflicting results. Some studies have found associations between GCA incidence and different seasons (eg, spring vs winter), whereas others have found no such

Table 3
Seasonality and potential infectious triggers in giant cell arteritis, Kawasaki disease, and antineutrophil cytoplasmic antibody-associated vasculitis

Disease	Seasonality	Potential Infectious Triggers
Giant cell arteritis	Conflicting results: • Winter or spring predominance in some studies • No seasonality in some studies	• Varicella zoster virus
Takayasu arteritis	• Unknown	• Unknown
Polyarteritis nodosa	• Unknown	• Hepatitis B virus • Human immunodeficiency virus • Parvovirus B19 • Cytomegalovirus
Kawasaki disease	• Winter predominance	• Enteroviruses • Adenovirus • Rhinovirus • Human metapneumovirus • Coronaviruses, including SARS-CoV-2 • *M pneumonia* • Bocavirus
ANCA-associated vasculitis	• Winter predominance in most studies that show seasonality • Many studies show no seasonality	• *S aureus* • Changes in nasal microbiome

Abbreviation: SARS-CoV-2, severe acute respiratory syndrome coronavirus 2.

associations.[13–17] Similarly, some studies have suggested differences in incidence year to year, whereas others have not.[13–16,18–20]

Reports of associations between geography, season, and calendar time with GCA incidence suggest a yet-to-be identified environmental trigger that varies because of climate such as an infection (eg, virus) or other climate-related factor.[19]

Infection

Infections have been intensely investigated as a potential trigger of GCA. One study demonstrated a correlation between peaks in GCA incidence in Denmark and epidemics of *Mycoplasma pneumonia*, parvovirus B19, and *Chlamydia pneumonia*, but subsequent studies have failed to replicate these findings or identify genetic material from these pathogens in temporal artery (TA) biopsies from patients with GCA.[20–26]

More recently, there has been interest in the role of varicella zoster virus (VZV) in the pathogenesis of GCA because of observations regarding the temporal association between VZV and GCA onset (reviewed in Ref.[27]). Although early studies demonstrated more frequent VZV antigen in TA biopsies from patients with GCA than controls, the staining methods used may have resulted in false positives and follow-up studies have failed to consistently reproduce these results or otherwise demonstrate a direct pathogenic role for the virus in GCA.[24,27–29]

At this time, the pathogenic antigen in GCA remains unknown, but additional studies investigating potential infectious and noninfectious environmental triggers are needed, recognizing that the infectious or noninfectious causes contributing to GCA may vary around the world and over time.

Takayasu Arteritis

TAK is a granulomatous large-vessel vasculitis that tends to affect women under the age of 40 and frequently manifests with constitutional symptoms, vascular aneurysms and stenoses, and limb claudication (see **Table 1**).[30] There is a well-established genetic predisposition to TAK, particularly with the HLA-B*52:01 allele[31]; however, like GCA, our current understanding of the pathogenesis of TAK supports an antigen-dependent immune response, suggesting the possibility of an environmental trigger.[32] A recent systematic review and meta-analysis showed a significant variation in reported incidence across various populations, implying a genetic or environmental effect on the development of the disease.[33] Indeed, some of this geographic variation in incidence may be explained by differences in HLA-B*52:01 allele frequency, but additional studies are needed to evaluate the potential role of environmental triggers in TAK.[31]

Polyarteritis Nodosa

PAN is a rare, heterogenous medium-vessel necrotizing vasculitis that frequently affects the skin, joints, muscles, nervous system, and abdominal vasculature but spares the lungs (see **Table 1**).[34] Our understanding of PAN has evolved considerably in recent decades. Since the 1970s, a strong association between PAN and hepatitis B virus (HBV) infection has been known.[35–37] Reported incidences varied, but in the 1970s and 1980s, HBV likely accounted for over 30% of cases of PAN.[38] In contrast, two recent cohorts demonstrated that HBV-associated PAN accounted for 3% and 11% of PAN cases, and many of these were in patients who were born before the implementation of broad population-level vaccination efforts.[39,40] Nevertheless, most of the US adults have not been fully vaccinated against HBV, and in some regions, the incidence of HBV has increased in recent years due to an increase in the use of injection drugs.[41] These trends emphasize the need for ongoing public health measures to prevent HBV transmission and by extension, HBV-associated PAN.

Although the incidence of HBV-associated PAN has decreased substantially, there remain non-HBV-associated cases of PAN (eg, classic PAN).[37,42,40] A portion of these cases have now been attributed to a monogenic cause—deficiency of adenosine deaminase-2 —and others have been reclassified as microscopic polyangiitis (MPA) with the expanding availability of ANCA testing.[43] Additional studies of otherwise classic PAN are needed to determine whether these patients can also be better reclassified or if they represent a unique vasculitis syndrome.

The evolving classification of PAN and other medium vessel vasculitides makes it difficult to interpret some of the studies on PAN pathogenesis. Although the association with HBV is well established, there have been reported associations between PAN and other viral infections, including human immunodeficiency virus, parvovirus B19, and cytomegalovirus.[44–47] In addition, one study showed a higher prevalence of PAN in an urban study population than a historical rural control group.[48] Such a difference in prevalence based on proximity to urban centers could potentially suggest an environmental trigger for the disease, but this result has not been replicated to date, and the study's conclusions are limited by the use of historical controls and potential for referral bias. Ultimately, a consistent viral or other environmental trigger for the development of classic, non-HBV-related PAN has yet to be established.

Kawasaki Disease

KD is a medium-vessel vasculitis that almost exclusively affects children under the age of 5.[49] KD typically manifests as fever, lymphadenopathy, and mucocutaneous disease (see **Table 1**). If left untreated, it can lead to coronary arteritis with resulting coronary aneurysms.[49] Although its complete etiopathogenesis remains unknown, it is largely suspected that an infectious or other environmental exposure in a genetically susceptible host is central to the disease process.[50,51]

Infection

Unlike most other systemic vasculitides, which typically present as chronic inflammatory syndromes, KD is usually a monophasic, acute, febrile illness.[49] Also, unlike most other primary systemic vasculitides, it affects almost exclusively young children.[49] These features, as well as the overwhelming overlap in clinical manifestations between KD and certain pediatric infections, has led to a long-standing hypothesis that infection is an important trigger. This hypothesis has been supported by the observed "epidemic" variations in KD incidence and clustering of cases in short periods of time, especially during winter.[52–56] Indeed, recent observations regarding the similarities between KD and multisystem inflammatory syndrome in children recovered from COVID-19 has renewed interest in these potential associations.[57,58]

Interestingly, siblings between ages 0 and 4 years of patients with KD have a 10-fold higher risk for developing KD, and when the siblings develop KD, they do so within 10 days of each other in over half of instances.[59] Although this familial clustering highlights a likely genetic predisposition to developing KD, the temporal association between cases also suggests that an environmental exposure is central in the pathogenesis of KD.[49,50] Furthermore, bronchial epithelial tissue from patients with KD has been found to have intracytoplasmic inclusion bodies containing ribonucleic acid (RNA), but not deoxyribonucleaic acid (DNA), an observation that would be supportive of a recent viral infection as a potential contributing factor.[60,61] Indeed, there have been reports potentially linking KD with various infectious agents, suggesting the possibility that KD is an aberrant immune response that can be triggered by a variety of infections.[50,57,62–65]

Airborne exposures

In addition to potential infectious data, some studies also point to potential noninfectious factors contributing to KD onset. Several studies have found associations between KD incidence and pollen spikes and global wind patterns,[52,66,67] suggesting that an airborne exposure may contribute to the etiopathogenesis of KD. For instance, one study observed that up to 38% of the variance in KD incidence rates in Santiago, Chile, could be explained by weather patterns; they found that that northerly winds from the Atacama Desert correlated with incidence of disease.[67] Similarly, incidence of KD cases in Japan has been correlated with wind traveling from northeastern China to Japan with an incubation period of less than 1 day after exposure and rapid spread of cases geographically after exposure.[68] Not only do these results suggest that an airborne etiologic agent is carried from one location to the site of disease incidence, but also the short incubation period and rapid spread noted in the latter study suggest that this may be a noninfectious agent or a preformed microbial toxin. Other studies of potential environmental exposures have not consistently identified clear associations between air pollutants and KD incidence, but one study found an association between ozone exposure and KD hospitalization.[68–72]

In contrast to other vasculitis syndromes which predominantly affect adults at the later part of the age spectrum, KD tends to affect children, prompting interest in the association of maternal risk factors or prenatal exposures. There has been a study suggesting an association between maternal smoking exposure and KD hospitalization.[73] In addition, a prospective longitudinal study in Japan found that prenatal exposure to air pollutants was associated with an increased risk of KD hospitalization in early childhood.[74] This observation notably contrasts with the previously discussed studies suggesting associations between acute changes in tropospheric wind patterns with KD incidence.[52,67,68] A challenge to this research is that linked prenatal and postnatal data are not typically available in many data sources used to conduct this type of research. Additional studies are needed to better describe the role of airborne exposures in the development of KD and the biological basis for these findings.

Antineutrophil Cytoplasmic Antibody-Associated Vasculitis

Three conditions with similar manifestations caused by a small-to-medium-vessel vasculitis are classified as AAV but defined by unique clinical features: MPA, granulomatosis with polyangiitis (GPA), and eosinophilic GPA (EGPA) (see **Table 1**).[75] AAV is associated with ANCAs, which are classically autoantibodies to proteinase-3 (PR3) or myeloperoxidase (MPO), at various frequencies depending on disease.[75] Like the other types of vasculitis discussed thus far, the pathogenesis of AAV is also thought to be triggered by antigenic exposure in a genetically susceptible, aging individual which leads to loss of tolerance to PR3 or MPO and ultimately activation of neutrophils (in MPA and GPA) or eosinophils (in EGPA) in addition to other effector cells that lead to tissue destruction.[75,76] Although AAV is well-known to be caused by specific drug exposures in certain cases, there are likely environmental exposures contributing to AAV as well.

Geographic and temporal variations in antineutrophil cytoplasmic antibody-associated vasculitis incidence

Similar to GCA, several studies have demonstrated variation in the prevalence of AAV by latitude, with most studies showing that GPA and EGPA tend to have higher incidence further from the equator, whereas MPA incidence tends to be higher close to the equator.[77–80] These observed differences have led some to hypothesize that ultraviolet radiation may have a protective effect in GPA and EGPA.[80] Observations regarding the striking differences in the incidence of GPA (or PR3-ANCA + AAV) and MPA (or MPO-ANCA + AAV) in people of Northern European (where PR3-ANCA+ and MPO-ANCA + AAV are observed) versus East Asian ancestry (where AAV is almost exclusively due to MPO-ANCA + AAV) have been hypothesized to result from differences in genetic predisposition but also raise the possible role of an environmental exposure.[75]

Data on the seasonality of AAV incidence have yielded conflicting results. Many studies have suggested a winter predominance,[81–84] whereas one showed an increase in frequency of GPA in the summer,[85] one showed discordance in seasonality between GPA and MPA,[86] and some showed no seasonal variation.[87–92] Much of this variation is likely attributable to differing study designs and the challenge of clearly defining the onset of disease. Similarly, some studies have shown periodicity or annual fluctuations in AAV diagnoses,[82,90,93,94] whereas other studies have not.[81,91,95] The conflicting data on the temporal fluctuations in AAV diagnoses suggest that there are potentially many different environmental exposures underlying AAV pathogenesis.

Infection

As with other systemic vasculitides, there are data to support an infectious trigger in the pathogenesis of AAV. Some animal models have demonstrated molecular mimicry between bacterial adhesion molecule *FimH* and lysosomal-associated membrane protein-2, one of the targets of ANCAs[96,97]; further, autoreactive B cells from AAV patients have been found to produce ANCA in response to bacterial motifs that activate B cell toll-like receptors, establishing a potential link between bacteria exposure and this autoimmune disease.[97–99] In contrast to other vasculitides, there has not been much data suggesting the role of other infections as AAV triggers.[87]

Importantly, although bacteria may play a role in AAV pathogenesis, this is not necessarily in the context of an infection. Indeed, there have been extensive data in the past supporting an association between nasal carriage of *Staphylococcus aureus* and risk of relapse in GPA,[100–102] and more recent research has demonstrated other alterations in the nasal microbiome that may distinguish patients with GPA.[103,104] These observations are supported by clinical studies demonstrating that patients with GPA who are treated with the combination antibiotic trimethoprim–sulfamethoxazole may have a lower risk of relapse[105,106], although the mechanism underlying this effect is not known, it may relate to the antibiotic's effect on respiratory microbiome.[107]

Airborne and occupational exposures

Epidemiologic studies have suggested a role for different potential environmental exposures in the pathogenesis of AAV. The incidence and severity of AAV have been found to be higher following earthquakes in China and Japan,[84,108,109] suggesting an association between airborne release of a natural element and AAV pathogenesis. However, a similar finding was not observed after a 2011 earthquake in New Zealand, possibly reflecting geographic differences in elements released during earthquakes.[110] Studies have also shown an association between AAV and farming, as well as rural residence, further supporting a potential role for elements in the soil or earth driving risk in these individuals, although this could also be explained by inhaled toxins from agricultural products used for farming.[48,92,111–115] One study that suggested an increased frequency of AAV in urban, rather than rural, populations may have been skewed by referral bias.[11]

There has been a long-documented apparent association between silica exposure and AAV, and this was strongly supported in a recent capture–recapture and geospatial analysis in France that demonstrated an association between AAV and proximity to quarries.[112,115–117] Other potential exposures associated with AAV in the literature have included carbon monoxide,[84] organic solvents,[111,112,115,118] and heavy metal exposure,[111,113,115,118,119] though the studies on these topics have yielded conflicting results.

Smoking

Data on the influence of smoking on the development of AAV have been mixed. Although some studies have shown statistically insignificant trends, no association, or a protective effect of smoking on risk of AAV, these studies have largely focused on GPA or PR3-ANCA + AAV, had limited sample sizes, or used general population controls that may not have been adequately representative of their study population.[111,112,120–122] In contrast, a recent, large case-control study found that patients with AAV were more likely to be current or former smokers and that this association was largely driven by MPO-ANCA + AAV.[123] Moreover, in a multicenter Japanese cohort, there was a dose-dependent relationship between smoking and risk of relapse of MPA.[124] These results suggest that smoking may have a different role in the different AAV syndromes and may increase the risk of MPA diagnosis and relapse.

DISCUSSION

Despite the variations in epidemiology, pathogenesis, and clinical features across vasculitis syndromes, there are several similarities in the suspected environmental triggers driving many of them. The expanding literature on this topic has highlighted the potential role of infections, seasonal and geographic factors, airborne exposures, and occupational exposures (see **Tables 2** and **3**). In recent decades, there have been advances in our understanding of the pathophysiology, improved vasculitis subtype classification, and development of cohorts that will enable robust studies evaluating environmental triggers of vasculitis, including reassessment of those previously associated with vasculitis risk. Advances in immunology will enable parallel work closely linking potential environmental triggers with the immunologic events underlying the pathogenesis of these syndromes. This approach is likely to advance our understanding of disease mechanisms, enable identification of potential pathogenic antigens, and guide management strategies specific to different vasculitis types.

SUMMARY

Systemic vasculitides are rare autoimmune conditions that result from a complex interaction between antigen exposures and genetically susceptible hosts' immune systems. Environmental exposures likely have a central role in the pathogenesis of most vasculitides. The variation in data on environmental triggers both between different vasculitis syndromes and within each disease emphasizes the heterogenous nature of these conditions and their pathophysiology. Further research is needed to better characterize the mechanisms by which environmental exposures lead to the development of systemic vasculitis.

CLINICS CARE POINTS

- In some forms of systemic vasculitis, infections may be a trigger.
- In most cases, infection-induced vasculitis represents immune dysregulation triggered by infection rather than active infection causing the vasculitis.
- Modifiable environmental risk factors for certain vasculitides include smoking and occupational exposures.

FUNDING

Z.S. Wallace is funded by the National Institutes of Health and the National Institute of Arthritis and Musculoskeletal and Skin Diseases [K23AR073334 and R03AR078938].

DISCLOSURE

The authors declare no conflicts of interest pertinent to the content of this article.

REFERENCES

1. Jennette JC, Falk RJ, Bacon PA, et al. 2012 revised international chapel hill consensus conference nomenclature of vasculitides. Arthritis Rheum 2013; 65:1–11.
2. Watts RA, Hatemi G, Burns JC, et al. Global epidemiology of vasculitis. Nat Rev Rheumatol 2022;18:22–34.

3. van der Geest KSM, Sandovici M, Brouwer E, et al. Diagnostic Accuracy of Symptoms, Physical Signs, and Laboratory Tests for Giant Cell Arteritis: A Systematic Review and Meta-analysis. JAMA Intern Med 2020;180:1295–304.

4. Koster MJ, Matteson EL, Warrington KJ. Large-vessel giant cell arteritis: diagnosis, monitoring and management. Rheumatology (Oxford) 2018;57:ii32–42.

5. Carmona FD, González-Gay MA, Martín J. Genetic component of giant cell arteritis. Rheumatology (Oxford) 2014;53:6–18.

6. Liozon E, Ouattara B, Rhaiem K, et al. Familial aggregation in giant cell arteritis and polymyalgia rheumatica: a comprehensive literature review including 4 new families. Clin Exp Rheumatol 2009;27:S89–94.

7. Mackie SL, Taylor JC, Haroon-Rashid L, et al. Association of HLA-DRB1 amino acid residues with giant cell arteritis: genetic association study, meta-analysis and geo-epidemiological investigation. Arthritis Res Ther 2015;17:195.

8. Borchers AT, Gershwin ME. Giant cell arteritis: a review of classification, pathophysiology, geoepidemiology and treatment. Autoimmun Rev 2012;11:A544–54.

9. Li KJ, Semenov D, Turk M, et al. A meta-analysis of the epidemiology of giant cell arteritis across time and space. Arthritis Res Ther 2021;23:82.

10. Reinhold-Keller E, Zeidler A, Gutfleisch J, et al. Giant cell arteritis is more prevalent in urban than in rural populations: results of an epidemiological study of primary systemic vasculitides in Germany. Rheumatology (Oxford) 2000;39:1396–402.

11. Herlyn K, Buckert F, Gross WL, et al. Doubled prevalence rates of ANCA-associated vasculitides and giant cell arteritis between 1994 and 2006 in northern Germany. Rheumatology (Oxford) 2014;53:882–9.

12. Schmidt D, Schulte-Mönting J. Giant cell arteritis is more prevalent in urban than in rural populations. Rheumatology (Oxford) 2001;40:1193.

13. Bas-Lando M, Breuer GS, Berkun Y, et al. The incidence of giant cell arteritis in Jerusalem over a 25-year period: annual and seasonal fluctuations. Clin Exp Rheumatol 2007;25:S15–7.

14. Petursdottir V, Johansson H, Nordborg E, et al. The epidemiology of biopsy-positive giant cell arteritis: special reference to cyclic fluctuations. Rheumatology (Oxford) 1999;38:1208–12.

15. González-Gay MA, Garcia-Porrua C, Rivas MJ, et al. Epidemiology of biopsy proven giant cell arteritis in northwestern Spain: trend over an 18 year period. Ann Rheum Dis 2001;60:367–71.

16. Gonzalez-Gay MA, Miranda-Filloy JA, Lopez-Diaz MJ, et al. Giant cell arteritis in northwestern Spain: a 25-year epidemiologic study. Medicine (Baltimore) 2007;86:61–8.

17. De Smit E, Clarke L, Sanfilippo PG, et al. Geo-epidemiology of temporal artery biopsy-positive giant cell arteritis in Australia and New Zealand: is there a seasonal influence? RMD Open 2017;3:e000531.

18. Brekke LK, Fevang B-T, Myklebust G. Increased Incidence of Giant Cell Arteritis in Urban Areas? J Rheumatol 2019;46:327–8.

19. Wing S, Rider LG, Johnson JR, et al. Do solar cycles influence giant cell arteritis and rheumatoid arthritis incidence? BMJ Open 2015;5:e006636.

20. Elling P, Olsson AT, Elling H. Synchronous variations of the incidence of temporal arteritis and polymyalgia rheumatica in different regions of Denmark; association with epidemics of Mycoplasma pneumoniae infection. J Rheumatol 1996;23:112–9.

21. Njau F, Ness T, Wittkop U, et al. No correlation between giant cell arteritis and Chlamydia pneumoniae infection: investigation of 189 patients by standard and improved PCR methods. J Clin Microbiol 2009;47:1899–901.
22. Regan MJ, Wood BJ, Hsieh Y-H, et al. Temporal arteritis and Chlamydia pneumoniae: failure to detect the organism by polymerase chain reaction in ninety cases and ninety controls. Arthritis Rheum 2002;46:1056–60.
23. Haugeberg G, Bie R, Nordbø SA. Chlamydia pneumoniae not detected in temporal artery biopsies from patients with temporal arteritis. Scand J Rheumatol 2000;29:127–8.
24. Rodriguez-Pla A, Bosch-Gil JA, Echevarria-Mayo JE, et al. No detection of parvovirus B19 or herpesvirus DNA in giant cell arteritis. J Clin Virol 2004; 31:11–5.
25. Cooper RJ, D'Arcy S, Kirby M, et al. Infection and temporal arteritis: a PCR-based study to detect pathogens in temporal artery biopsy specimens. J Med Virol 2008;80:501–5.
26. Helweg-Larsen J, Tarp B, Obel N, et al. No evidence of parvovirus B19, Chlamydia pneumoniae or human herpes virus infection in temporal artery biopsies in patients with giant cell arteritis. Rheumatology (Oxford) 2002;41:445–9.
27. Ostrowski RA, Metgud S, Tehrani R, et al. Varicella Zoster Virus in Giant Cell Arteritis: A Review of Current Medical Literature. Neuroophthalmology 2019; 43:159–70.
28. Verdijk RM, Ouwendijk WJD, Kuijpers RWAM, et al. No Evidence of Varicella-Zoster Virus Infection in Temporal Artery Biopsies of Anterior Ischemic Optic Neuropathy Patients With and Without Giant Cell Arteritis. J Infect Dis 2021; 223:109–12.
29. Abendroth A, Slobedman B. Varicella-Zoster Virus and Giant Cell Arteritis. J Infect Dis 2021;223:4–6.
30. Seyahi E. Takayasu arteritis: an update. Curr Opin Rheumatol 2017;29:51–6.
31. Terao C. Revisited HLA and non-HLA genetics of Takayasu arteritis—where are we? J Hum Genet 2016;61:27–32.
32. Zaldivar Villon MLF, de la Rocha JAL, Espinoza LR. Takayasu Arteritis: Recent Developments. Curr Rheumatol Rep 2019;21:45.
33. Rutter M, Bowley J, Lanyon PC, et al. A systematic review and meta-analysis of the incidence rate of Takayasu arteritis. Rheumatology (Oxford) 2021;60: 4982–90.
34. Hernández-Rodríguez J, Alba MA, Prieto-González S, et al. Diagnosis and classification of polyarteritis nodosa. J Autoimmun 2014;48–49:84–9.
35. Trepo C, Thivolet J. Hepatitis associated antigen and periarteritis nodosa (PAN). Vox Sang 1970;19:410–1.
36. Gocke DJ, Hsu K, Morgan C, et al. Association between polyarteritis and Australia antigen. Lancet 1970;2:1149–53.
37. Wang C-R, Tsai H-W. Human hepatitis viruses-associated cutaneous and systemic vasculitis. World J Gastroenterol 2021;27:19–36.
38. Guillevin L, Lhote F, Cohen P, et al. Polyarteritis nodosa related to hepatitis B virus. A prospective study with long-term observation of 41 patients. Medicine (Baltimore) 1995;74:238–53.
39. Karadag O, Erden A, Bilginer Y, et al. A retrospective study comparing the phenotype and outcomes of patients with polyarteritis nodosa between UK and Turkish cohorts. Rheumatol Int 2018;38:1833–40.
40. Sönmez HE, Armağan B, Ayan G, et al. Polyarteritis nodosa: lessons from 25 years of experience. Clin Exp Rheumatol 2019;37(Suppl 117):52–6.

41. Haber P, Schillie S. Hepatitis B. In: Epidemiology and prevention of vaccine-preventable diseases. Washington, D.C: Public Health Foundation; 2021.

42. Guillevin L, Mahr A, Callard P, et al. Hepatitis B virus-associated polyarteritis nodosa: clinical characteristics, outcome, and impact of treatment in 115 patients. Medicine (Baltimore) 2005;84:313–22.

43. Ozen S. The changing face of polyarteritis nodosa and necrotizing vasculitis. Nat Rev Rheumatol 2017;13:381–6.

44. Font C, Miró O, Pedrol E, et al. Polyarteritis nodosa in human immunodeficiency virus infection: report of four cases and review of the literature. Br J Rheumatol 1996;35:796–9.

45. Corman LC, Dolson DJ. Polyarteritis nodosa and parvovirus B19 infection. Lancet 1992;339:491.

46. Kouchi M, Sato S, Kamono M, et al. A case of polyarteritis nodosa associated with cytomegalovirus infection. Case Rep Rheumatol 2014;2014:604874.

47. Fernandes SR, Bértolo MB, Rossi CL, et al. Polyarteritis nodosa and cytomegalovirus: diagnosis by polymerase chain reaction. Clin Rheumatol 1999;18:501–3.

48. Mahr A, Guillevin L, Poissonnet M, et al. Prevalences of polyarteritis nodosa, microscopic polyangiitis, Wegener's granulomatosis, and Churg-Strauss syndrome in a French urban multiethnic population in 2000: a capture-recapture estimate. Arthritis Rheum 2004;51:92–9.

49. Sundel RP. Kawasaki disease. Rheum Dis Clin North Am 2015;41:63–73 viii.

50. Agarwal S, Agrawal DK. Kawasaki disease: etiopathogenesis and novel treatment strategies. Expert Rev Clin Immunol 2017;13:247–58.

51. Rodó X, Ballester J, Curcoll R, et al. Revisiting the role of environmental and climate factors on the epidemiology of Kawasaki disease. Ann N Y Acad Sci 2016;1382:84–98.

52. Rodó X, Ballester J, Cayan D, et al. Association of Kawasaki disease with tropospheric wind patterns. Sci Rep 2011;1:152.

53. Rypdal M, Rypdal V, Burney JA, et al. Clustering and climate associations of Kawasaki Disease in San Diego County suggest environmental triggers. Sci Rep 2018;8:16140.

54. Burney JA, DeHaan LL, Shimizu C, et al. Temporal clustering of Kawasaki disease cases around the world. Sci Rep 2021;11:22584.

55. Nagao Y, Urabe C, Nakamura H, et al. Predicting the characteristics of the aetiological agent for Kawasaki disease from other paediatric infectious diseases in Japan. Epidemiol Infect 2016;144:478–92.

56. Burns JC, Herzog L, Fabri O, et al. Seasonality of Kawasaki disease: a global perspective. PLoS One 2013;8:e74529.

57. Ravelli A, Martini A. Kawasaki disease or Kawasaki syndrome? Ann Rheum Dis 2020;79:993–5.

58. Bautista-Rodriguez C, Sanchez-de-Toledo J, Clark BC, et al. Multisystem Inflammatory Syndrome in Children: An International Survey. Pediatrics 2021;147.

59. Fujita Y, Nakamura Y, Sakata K, et al. Kawasaki disease in families. Pediatrics 1989;84:666–9.

60. Rowley AH, Baker SC, Shulman ST, et al. Cytoplasmic inclusion bodies are detected by synthetic antibody in ciliated bronchial epithelium during acute Kawasaki disease. J Infect Dis 2005;192:1757–66.

61. Rowley AH, Baker SC, Shulman ST, et al. RNA-containing cytoplasmic inclusion bodies in ciliated bronchial epithelium months to years after acute Kawasaki disease. PLoS One 2008;3:e1582.

62. Lee MN, Cha JH, Ahn HM, et al. Mycoplasma pneumoniae infection in patients with Kawasaki disease. Korean J Pediatr 2011;54:123–7.

63. Chang L-Y, Lu C-Y, Shao P-L, et al. Viral infections associated with Kawasaki disease. J Formos Med Assoc 2014;113:148–54.

64. Bajolle F, Meritet J-F, Rozenberg F, et al. Markers of a recent bocavirus infection in children with Kawasaki disease: "a year prospective study. Pathol Biol (Paris) 2014;62:365–8.

65. Patra PK, Das RR, Banday AZ, et al. Non-SARS, non-MERS human coronavirus infections and risk of Kawasaki disease: a meta-analysis. Future Virol 2021. https://doi.org/10.2217/fvl-2021-0176.

66. Awaya A, Sahashi N. The etiology of Kawasaki disease: does intense release of pollen induce pollinosis in constitutionally allergic adults, while constitutionally allergic infants develop Kawasaki disease? Biomed Pharmacother 2004;58: 136–40.

67. Jorquera H, Borzutzky A, Hoyos-Bachiloglu R, et al. Association of Kawasaki disease with tropospheric winds in Central Chile: is wind-borne desert dust a risk factor? Environ Int 2015;78:32–8.

68. Rodó X, Curcoll R, Robinson M, et al. Tropospheric winds from northeastern China carry the etiologic agent of Kawasaki disease from its source to Japan. Proc Natl Acad Sci U S A 2014;111:7952–7.

69. Oh J, Lee JH, Kim E, et al. Is short-term exposure to PM2.5 relevant to childhood kawasaki disease? Int J Environ Res Public Health 2021;18:924.

70. Zeft AS, Burns JC, Yeung RS, et al. Kawasaki disease and exposure to fine particulate air pollution. J Pediatr 2016;177:179–83.e1.

71. Lin Z, Meng X, Chen R, et al. Ambient air pollution, temperature and kawasaki disease in Shanghai, China. Chemosphere 2017;186:817–22.

72. Jung C-R, Chen W-T, Lin Y-T, et al. Ambient air pollutant exposures and hospitalization for kawasaki disease in taiwan: a case-crossover study (2000-2010). Environ Health Perspect 2017;125:670–6.

73. Yorifuji T, Tsukahara H, Doi H. Early childhood exposure to maternal smoking and kawasaki disease: a longitudinal survey in Japan. Sci Total Environ 2019; 655:141–6.

74. Yorifuji T, Tsukahara H, Kashima S, et al. Intrauterine and early postnatal exposure to particulate air pollution and kawasaki disease: a nationwide longitudinal survey in japan. J Pediatr 2018;193:147–54.e2.

75. Kitching AR, Anders H-J, Basu N, et al. ANCA-associated vasculitis. Nat Rev Dis Primers 2020;6:71.

76. Gapud EJ, Seo P, Antiochos B. ANCA-associated vasculitis pathogenesis: a commentary. Curr Rheumatol Rep 2017;19:15.

77. Watts RA, Lane SE, Scott DG, et al. Epidemiology of vasculitis in Europe. Ann Rheum Dis 2001;60:1156–7.

78. Watts RA, Gonzalez-Gay MA, Lane SE, et al. Geoepidemiology of systemic vasculitis: comparison of the incidence in two regions of Europe. Ann Rheum Dis 2001;60:170–2.

79. O'Donnell JL, Stevanovic VR, Frampton C, et al. Wegener's granulomatosis in New Zealand: evidence for a latitude-dependent incidence gradient. Intern Med J 2007;37:242–6.

80. Gatenby PA, Lucas RM, Engelsen O, et al. Antineutrophil cytoplasmic antibody-associated vasculitides: could geographic patterns be explained by ambient ultraviolet radiation? Arthritis Rheum 2009;61:1417–24.

81. Carruthers DM, Watts RA, Symmons DPM, et al. Wegener's granulomatosis—increased incidence or increased recognition? Rheumatology 1996;35:142–5.
82. Draibe J, Rodó X, Fulladosa X, et al. Seasonal variations in the onset of positive and negative renal ANCA-associated vasculitis in Spain. Clin Kidney J 2018;11:468–73.
83. Falk RJ. Clinical course of anti-neutrophil cytoplasmic autoantibody-associated glomerulonephritis and systemic vasculitis. Ann Intern Med 1990;113:656.
84. Li J, Cui Z, Long J-Y, et al. The frequency of ANCA-associated vasculitis in a national database of hospitalized patients in China. Arthritis Res Ther 2018;20:226.
85. Mahr A, Artigues N, Coste J, et al. Seasonal variations in onset of Wegener's granulomatosis: increased in summer? J Rheumatol 2006;33:1615–22.
86. Pavone L, Grasselli C, Chierici E, et al. Outcome and prognostic factors during the course of primary small-vessel vasculitides. J Rheumatol 2006;33:1299–306.
87. Scott J, Hartnett J, Mockler D, et al. Environmental risk factors associated with ANCA associated vasculitis: a systematic mapping review. Autoimmun Rev 2020;19:102660.
88. Aries PM, Herlyn K, Reinhold-Keller E, et al. No seasonal variation in the onset of symptoms of 445 patients with Wegener's granulomatosis. Arthritis Rheum 2008;59:904.
89. Cotch MF, Hoffman GS, Yerg DE, et al. The epidemiology of Wegener's granulomatosis. Estimates of the five-year period prevalence, annual mortality, and geographic disease distribution from population-based data sources. Arthritis Rheum 1996;39:87–92.
90. Tidman M, Olander R, Svalander C, et al. Patients hospitalized because of small vessel vasculitides with renal involvement in the period 1975-95: organ involvement, anti-neutrophil cytoplasmic antibodies patterns, seasonal attack rates and fluctuation of annual frequencies. J Intern Med 1998;244:133–41.
91. Lane SE, Watts RA, Scott DGI. Seasonal variations in onset of Wegener's granulomatosis: increased in summer? J Rheumatol 2007;34:889–90 ; author reply 890.
92. Aiyegbusi O, Frleta-Gilchrist M, Traynor JP, et al. ANCA-associated renal vasculitis is associated with rurality but not seasonality or deprivation in a complete national cohort study. RMD Open 2021;7:e001555.
93. Watts RA, Mooney J, Skinner J, et al. The contrasting epidemiology of granulomatosis with polyangiitis (Wegener's) and microscopic polyangiitis. Rheumatology 2012;51:926–31.
94. Koldingsnes W, Nossent H. Epidemiology of Wegener's granulomatosis in Northern Norway. Arthritis Rheum 2000;43:2481–7.
95. Reinhold-Keller E. No difference in the incidences of vasculitides between north and south Germany: first results of the German vasculitis register. Rheumatology 2002;41:540–9.
96. Kain R, Exner M, Brandes R, et al. Molecular mimicry in pauci-immune focal necrotizing glomerulonephritis. Nat Med 2008;14:1088–96.
97. Berti A, Dejaco C. Update on the epidemiology, risk factors, and outcomes of systemic vasculitides. Best Pract Res Clin Rheumatol 2018;32:271–94.
98. Tadema H, Abdulahad WH, Lepse N, et al. Bacterial DNA motifs trigger ANCA production in ANCA-associated vasculitis in remission. Rheumatology (Oxford) 2011;50:689–96.
99. Lepse N, Land J, Rutgers A, et al. Toll-like receptor 9 activation enhances B cell activating factor and interleukin-21 induced anti-proteinase 3 autoantibody production in vitro. Rheumatology (Oxford) 2016;55:162–72.

100. Stegeman CA, Tervaert JW, Sluiter WJ, et al. Association of chronic nasal car-riage of Staphylococcus aureus and higher relapse rates in Wegener granulo-matosis. Ann Intern Med 1994;120:12–7.
101. Laudien M, Gadola SD, Podschun R, et al. Nasal carriage of Staphylococcus aureus and endonasal activity in Wegener s granulomatosis as compared to rheumatoid arthritis and chronic Rhinosinusitis with nasal polyps. Clin Exp Rheu-matol 2010;28:51–5.
102. Salmela A, Rasmussen N, Tervaert JWC, et al. Chronic nasal Staphylococcus aureus carriage identifies a subset of newly diagnosed granulomatosis with pol-yangiitis patients with high relapse rate. Rheumatology (Oxford) 2017;56: 965–72.
103. Rhee RL, Sreih AG, Najem CE, et al. Characterisation of the nasal microbiota in granulomatosis with polyangiitis. Ann Rheum Dis 2018;77:1448–53.
104. Rhee RL, Lu J, Bittinger K, et al. Dynamic changes in the nasal microbiome associated with disease activity in patients with granulomatosis with polyangiitis. Arthritis Rheumatol 2021;73:1703–12.
105. Stegeman CA, Tervaert JW, de Jong PE, et al. Trimethoprim-sulfamethoxazole (co-trimoxazole) for the prevention of relapses of Wegener's granulomatosis. Dutch Co-Trimoxazole Wegener Study Group. N Engl J Med 1996;335:16–20.
106. Zycinska K, Wardyn KA, Zielonka TM, et al. Co-trimoxazole and prevention of relapses of PR3-ANCA positive vasculitis with pulmonary involvement. Eur J Med Res 2009;14(Suppl 4):265–7.
107. Cohen Tervaert JW. Trimethoprim-sulfamethoxazole and antineutrophil cyto-plasmic antibodies-associated vasculitis. Curr Opin Rheumatol 2018;30: 388–94.
108. Takeuchi Y, Saito A, Ojima Y, et al. The influence of the Great East Japan earth-quake on microscopic polyangiitis: A retrospective observational study. PLoS One 2017;12:e0177482.
109. Yashiro M, Muso E, Itoh-Ihara T, et al. Significantly high regional morbidity of MPO-ANCA-related angitis and/or nephritis with respiratory tract involvement af-ter the 1995 great earthquake in Kobe (Japan). Am J Kidney Dis 2000;35: 889–95.
110. Farquhar HJ, McGettigan B, Chapman PT, et al. Incidence of anti-neutrophil cytoplasmic antibody-associated vasculitis before and after the February 2011 Christchurch Earthquake. Intern Med J 2017;47:57–61.
111. Lane SE, Watts RA, Bentham G, et al. Are environmental factors important in pri-mary systemic vasculitis? A case-control study. Arthritis Rheum 2003;48: 814–23.
112. Maritati F, Peyronel F, Fenaroli P, et al. Occupational Exposures and Smoking in Eosinophilic Granulomatosis With Polyangiitis: A Case-Control Study. Arthritis Rheumatol 2021;73:1694–702.
113. Stamp LK, Chapman PT, Francis J, et al. Association between environmental ex-posures and granulomatosis with polyangiitis in Canterbury, New Zealand. Arthritis Res Ther 2015;17:333.
114. Canney M, Induruwage D, McCandless LC, et al. Disease-specific incident glomerulonephritis displays geographic clustering in under-serviced rural areas of British Columbia, Canada. Kidney Int 2019;96:421–8.
115. Chung EY, Risi D, Holt JL, et al. A retrospective study on the epidemiology of ANCA-associated vasculitis in two Australian health districts. Intern Med J 2020. https://doi.org/10.1111/imj.15098.

116. Gómez-Puerta JA, Gedmintas L, Costenbader KH. The association between silica exposure and development of ANCA-associated vasculitis: systematic review and meta-analysis. Autoimmun Rev 2013;12:1129–35.

117. Giorgiutti S, Dieudonne Y, Hinschberger O, et al. Prevalence of Antineutrophil Cytoplasmic Antibody-Associated Vasculitis and Spatial Association With Quarries in a Region of Northeastern France: A Capture-Recapture and Geospatial Analysis. Arthritis Rheumatol 2021;73:2078–85.

118. Stratta P, Messuerotti A, Canavese C, et al. The role of metals in autoimmune vasculitis: epidemiological and pathogenic study. Sci Total Environ 2001;270: 179–90.

119. Albert D, Clarkin C, Komoroski J, et al. Wegener's granulomatosis: Possible role of environmental agents in its pathogenesis. Arthritis Rheum 2004;51:656–64.

120. Khabbazi A, Alinejati B, Hajialilo M, et al. Cigarette smoking and risk of primary systemic vasculitis: a propensity score matching analysis. Sarcoidosis Vasc Diffuse Lung Dis 2019;36:243–50.

121. Haubitz M, Woywodt A, de Groot K, et al. Smoking habits in patients diagnosed with ANCA associated small vessel vasculitis. Ann Rheum Dis 2005;64:1500–2.

122. Hogan SL, Satterly KK, Dooley MA, et al. Silica exposure in anti-neutrophil cytoplasmic autoantibody-associated glomerulonephritis and lupus nephritis. J Am Soc Nephrol 2001;12:134–42.

123. McDermott G, Fu X, Stone JH, et al. Association of cigarette smoking with antineutrophil cytoplasmic antibody-associated vasculitis. JAMA Intern Med 2020; 180:870–6.

124. Yamaguchi M, Ando M, Katsuno T, et al. Smoking is a risk factor for relapse of antimyeloperoxidase antibodies-associated vasculitis. J Clin Rheumatol 2018; 24:361–7.

Environmental Triggers of Hyperuricemia and Gout

Lindsay N. Helget, MD[a,b,*], Ted R. Mikuls, MD, MSPH[a,b]

KEYWORDS

- Gout • Hyperuricemia • Environmental exposures • Diet • Epidemiology

KEY POINTS

- Hyperuricemia results as an imbalance between purine intake, endogenous uric acid synthesis, and its excretion via the kidneys or gastrointestinal tract; an imbalance that may relate to several different environmental exposures.
- Increased purine consumption from meat, alcohol, and high fructose corn syrup contributes to both hyperuricemia leading to gout, as well as the risk of flare.
- Medications such as cyclosporine, low-dose aspirin, diuretics, and other select treatments contribute to hyperuricemia, whereas calcium channel blockers, losartan, and sodium/glucose transporter-2 inhibitors demonstrate urate-lowering effects.
- Environmental exposures to lead, air pollution, and ambient temperature increases may also act as triggers for gout flares.

Gout, characterized by hyperuricemia and recurrent episodes of an acute painful inflammatory arthritis separated by asymptomatic intercritical periods, is the most common type of inflammatory arthritis. Gout incidence has increased in recent decades, an increase that seems to be due in part to changes in several environmental factors including dietary patterns, medication use, and other select environmental toxins and exposures.

Historically, the first documented evidence of gout appeared in ancient Egypt. Egyptians are credited with the first use of the word "podagra" for descriptions of gout flares of the first metatarsophalangeal joint in 2640 BC.[1] In addition to the documentation of the term podagra on papyrus, there has been archeological evidence of

Funding: T.R. Mikuls is supported by grants from the VA (BX004600), U.S. Department of Defense (PR200793) and grants from the National Institutes of Health (U54GM115458 and R25AA020818).
Conflicts of Interest: T.R. Mikuls has served as a consultant for Horizon Therapeutics, Pfizer, Gilead, and Sanofi.

[a] Veterans Affairs Nebraska-Western Iowa Health Care System, 4101 Woolworth Avenue, Omaha, NE 68105, USA; [b] Department of Internal Medicine, University of Nebraska Medical Center, 986270 Nebraska Medical Center, Omaha, NE 68198-6270, USA
* Corresponding author. 986270 Nebraska Medical Center, Omaha, NE 68198-6270.
E-mail address: lindsay.helget@unmc.edu

Rheum Dis Clin N Am 48 (2022) 891–906
https://doi.org/10.1016/j.rdc.2022.06.009
0889-857X/22/Published by Elsevier Inc.
rheumatic.theclinics.com

urate crystals in joints of Egyptian mummies. Although today we understand that gout can affect people of all racial and socioeconomic backgrounds, the disease was historically associated with an "indulgent" lifestyle of the upper class. Hippocrates was among the first to make this observation, describing gout as "arthritis of the rich."[2]

Throughout history, there have been several gout "epidemics," each providing insight into environmental factors predisposing individuals to gout. A historical survey noted that more than two-thirds of all Roman Emperors from 30 to 220 AD suffered from gout.[3] Heavy consumption of port wines, a preferred beverage of the Roman ruling class, was typically produced in lead-lined pots or kettles. Nriagu estimates that the daily consumption of lead for the average Roman Emperor approached 150 μg, far exceeding thresholds deemed to be safe by contemporary standards. Chronic lead intoxication, in turn, led to the development of debilitating gout and neurologic disturbances in many, possibly contributing to the downfall of the Roman Empire.[3] These epidemics continued into the Renaissance period, most notably with King Henry VIII whose overindulgent nature supported the commonly used term for gout, "the disease of kings." It has been speculated that Michelangelo suffered from gout, possibly related to chronic exposure to lead-based paints used in his masterpieces such as the Sistine Chapel.[4] More recently, the popularity of moonshine in the southeastern United States, made in part by running alcohol through a lead-lined car radiator, led to another gout epidemic related to lead toxicity and plumbism.[5]

This review will examine modern environmental risk factors in the development of hyperuricemia and gout, some of which have persisted since historical times. We will first focus on triggers for the development of hyperuricemia such as diet, alcohol use, medications, and lead exposure. Additionally, we will review environmental factors associated with the occurrence of flares that in some cases may act independently of serum urate concentrations such as physiologic stress, trauma, temperature changes, and air pollution.

TRIGGERS FOR HYPERURICEMIA LEADING TO GOUT

Considered a "necessary but insufficient" risk factor for gout, hyperuricemia results as an imbalance between dietary intake of purines that serve as building blocks of uric acid or endogenous uric acid synthesis (produced during cell turnover) and its excretion via the kidneys or gastrointestinal tract. Defined by serum concentrations exceeding its solubility threshold (>6.8 mg/dL or 400 μmol/L), hyperuricemia may result from environmental exposures that tip the balance, particularly those related to increased purine consumption (eg, diet, alcohol) or factors leading to diminished urate excretion (eg, lead intoxication, medications; **Fig. 1**).

Diet

Several foods are linked to the development of hyperuricemia and gout based on high purine content (**Table 1**). Red meat (a staple of the Western diet) is often implicated in the development of hyperuricemia, although most cuts of beef contain only moderate quantities of purine (~ 100 mg purine/100g).[6] Veal, chicken breast with skin, and lamb have higher purine contents (~ 170–180 mg purine/100g) with organ meats such as heart, liver, kidney, thymus demonstrating the highest purine content of any foods, with calf thymus yielding ~ 1260 mg of purines/100g.[6]

Fish and seafood consumption may also precipitate hyperuricemia, again due to elevated purine content. Similar to different meats, not all fish and seafoods have equal purine content. Anchovies, trout, mackerel, herring, tuna, salmon, sardines,

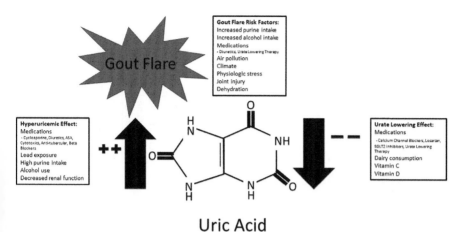

Uric Acid

Fig. 1. Environmental factors associated with hyperuricemia, serum urate lowering, and gout flare risk. Hyperuricemia results as an imbalance between uric acid its excretion via the kidneys or gastrointestinal tract and may result from environmental exposures that tip the balance, particularly those related to increased purine consumption (eg, diet, alcohol) or factors leading to diminished urate excretion (eg, lead intoxication, medications).

and shellfish have substantially higher purine content. In general, processed, dried, and canned fish have a higher purine content than fresh fish, with dried anchovies containing ∼1100 mg of purines/100g.[6] Given potential cardiovascular protection and reduction in gout flare frequency observed with omega-3 fatty acid consumption, the choice of fish/seafood may be important to optimize overall health benefits.[7] Fish with lower purine content such as cod, haddock, perch, pike, and sole contain only ∼110 to 130 mg of purines/100g.

Using the National Health and Nutrition Examination Survey (NHANES), the link between increased dietary consumption of purines and increased serum urate has been shown. Individuals consuming less than 1 meat serving/d demonstrate serum urate concentrations approximately 0.5 mg/dL lower than in those consuming greater than 2 meat servings/d.[8] Similarly, daily fish consumption of greater than 2 servings corresponds to modest serum urate elevations, 0.16 mg/dL higher compared with individuals consuming less than 1 fish serving/d.[8]

Although there are several vegetables containing high quantities of purine (eg, asparagus, mushrooms, spinach, green peas, and cauliflower), there is little data to suggest that these purine-rich foods contribute to hyperuricemia or gout risk. Two prospective studies found that vegetarians had the overall lowest risk of developing gout when compared with both vegans and nonvegetarians.[9] These findings were echoed in a 12-year prospective cohort study demonstrating no increased risk of gout with 1 or more servings of high-purine vegetables per day.[8] An additional meta-analysis of 19 studies found no associations between consumption of high-purine vegetables and hyperuricemia.[10] The combination of this data indicates that purine content alone may not fully explain the association between diet and hyperuricemia. These studies would suggest that health-care providers should avoid "blanket" recommendations of a low-purine diet in gout, and rather suggest one lower in foods such as high-purine meats or seafood that have been more strongly implicated to raise serum urate concentrations.

Table 1
Selected studies examining associations of high-purine content food intake with hyperuricemia and gout

First Author, Publication Year	Study Design, Population Source	Dietary Exposure	Sample Size	Results
Choi et al,[78] 2004	Prospective cohort, American Health Professionals Follow-up Study	Meat, seafood, purine-rich vegetables, daily products	47,150	RR of gout when comparing highest and lowest quintiles of meat and seafood consumption were 1.41 and 1.51, respectively
Choi et al,[8] 2005	Prospective cohort, NHANES	Meat, seafood, dairy	14,809	Uric acid difference when comparing highest and lowest quintiles of meat and seafood consumption was 0.48 and 0.16 mg/dL, respectively
Villegas et al,[79] 2012	Cross-sectional, Shanghai Men's Health Study	Rice, poultry, red meat, fish, eggs, vegetables, soy, fruits	3978	OR of hyperuricemia when comparing highest and lowest quintiles of seafood consumption was 1.56, no association with meat or vegetable consumption
Schmidt et al,[80] 2013	Cross-sectional, European Prospective Investigation into Cancer and Nutrition Oxford Cohort	Meat, fish, dairy, eggs, alcohol, coffee, tea, fructose-rich drinks	1693	Vegans had the highest concentrations of uric acid followed by meat eaters; vegetarians and fish (but not meat) eaters had the lowest concentrations of uric acid
Teng et al,[81] 2015	Prospective cohort, Singapore Chinese Health Study	Rice/noodles, meats, vegetables, fruits, soy, nonsoy legumes, nuts/seeds, dairy, beverages, condiments, preserved food	51,114	HRs of gout when comparing highest and lowest quartiles of protein, poultry, and fish consumption were 1.27, 1.27, and 1.16, respectively

Study	Study type	Dietary factors	Sample size	Findings
Rai et al,[82] 2017	Prospective cohort, American Health Professional Follow-up Study	Fruits, vegetables, nuts/legumes, dairy, whole grains, sodium, sweetened beverages, red and processed meats	44,444	RR of gout when comparing highest adherent DASH diet to lowest adherent DASH diet was 0.68. RR of gout when comparing highest adherent Western diet to lowest adherence Western diet was 1.42
Aihemaitijiang et al,[83] 2020	Cross-sectional, China Health and Nutrition Survey	Red meat, poultry, seafood, legumes, vegetables, fungi	6813	RRs of hyperuricemia when comparing each 10g increase of meat and legumes were 1.024 and 1.10, respectively
Yokose et al,[84] 2022	Prospective cohort, US Nurses' Health Study	DASH, Alternate Mediterranean Diet Score, AHEI, Prudent diet, Western diet	80,039 women	HRs of gout when comparing highest and lowest adherence quintiles to a particular diet included: DASH (0.68), Alternate Mediterranean Diet Score (0.88), AHEI (0.79), Prudent (0.75), and Western (1.49) diet; High adherence to DASH diet with normal BMI compared with low adherence to DASH diet and abnormal BMI lead to HR of 0.32 for the development of gout

Abbreviations: AHEI, alternative healthy eating index; BMI, body mass index; DASH, dietary approaches to stop hypertension; HR, hazards ratio; NHANES, National Health and Nutrition Examination Survey; OR, odds ratio; RR, relative risk.

In addition to meat, another staple of the Western diet includes high-fructose corn syrup, an artificial sweetener introduced in 1967. This product is used in many heavily processed foods and beverages, most notably soft drinks. Increased consumption of high-fructose corn syrup has correlated with the increased prevalence of gout.[11] Mechanistically, fructose intake leads to uric acid production by increasing adenosine triphosphate degradation to adenosine monophosphate, a precursor to uric acid. Indeed, intravenous fructose infusions significantly increased serum urate concentrations one small study.[12] A systematic review and meta-analysis subsequently supported the existence of a dose-dependent relationship between the consumption of high-fructose corn syrup and serum urate levels, with "high consumers" ($\geq$2 servings/d) demonstrating a 62% higher rate of incident gout compared with "low consumers" (<1 serving/d).[11] Interestingly, fructose occurring in its natural form (eg, fruit) does not seem to confer the same risk as artificially manufactured fructose in the form of corn syrup. In fact, a study of male runners found that fruit consumption ($\geq$2 servings/d) was associated with a 27% lower risk of incident gout compared with those with lower amounts of intake.[13]

There are several foods available that seem to decrease serum urate, subsequently lowering gout risk. Consumption of 1 or more daily servings of dairy products (ie, milk/yogurt), for example, has been associated with significant, although modest decreases in serum urate approaching 0.25 mg/dL.[8] Low in overall purine content, dairy products contain casein and lactalbumin, which have uricosuric properties.[8] Along this same line, patients with Vitamin D insufficiency and deficiency have significantly higher serum urate levels (0.33 and 0.45 mg/dL, respectively) based on a meta-analysis of 7 cross-sectional studies that specifically included studies which compared serum urate acid values between Vitamin D replete and Vitamin D insufficiency groups.[14] This data suggests (but does not prove) that supplementation with this vitamin could portend urate-lowering effects. A meta-analysis of 32 studies, which had less strict inclusion criteria than the prior study and included any studies that examined an association between serum urate and Vitamin D levels, reported a pooled odds ratio of 1.5 between Vitamin D deficiency and hyperuricemia.[15] Given the potential of bias in these observational studies, future randomized controlled trials (RCTs) are needed to adequately assess the potential utility of vitamin D supplementation in gout. One small randomized control trial has shown a small reduction in serum urate concentration in prediabetic patients with hyperuricemia.[16]

In contrast to the more limited evidence for Vitamin D, several RCTs have shown that serum urate levels are reduced with Vitamin C supplementation[17–19] with a meta-analysis of 13 RCTs equating Vitamin C doses of 500 mg/d to serum urate reductions approaching 0.35 mg/dL.[20] Although cherry juice and/or extract are well-advertised as gout remedies, evidence supporting their use is mixed. A meta-analysis of 6 studies (including RCTs and observational studies) found that cherry consumption yields only modest urate-lowering effects.[21] More recently, Stamp and colleagues found no significant decrease in serum urate with varying amounts of cherry concentrate.[22] With reports of decreased rates of gout flares with cherry consumption, this effect may more likely be due to anti-inflammatory pathways rather than urate-lowering properties.[23,24]

The consumption of coffee, another staple of the Western diet, may also lead to decreased serum urate. A meta-analysis of 9 observational studies by Park and colleagues showed a dose-dependent relationship with the highest decrease in serum urate (0.36 mg/dL) attributable to the consumption of 4 to 6 cups of coffee daily compared with those with no consumption.[25] In addition to coffee consumption, tea may also exert a urate-lowering effect. In a mouse model, both green and black teas were shown to have a hypouricemic effect,[26] findings, however, that have not been consistently replicated in human subjects.[27–30] Although coffee and green tea contain many compounds including caffeine, it is speculated that polyphenols (which can inhibit xanthine oxidase) explain any urate-lowering effects.[31–33]

Alcohol

Increased alcohol consumption may also contribute to elevated serum urate levels, an effect that likely relates to purine content in some alcohol products as well as reduced secretion of uric acid induced by lactate, a metabolic byproduct of alcohol.[34] Using NHANES, investigators have shown that compared with individuals reporting no alcohol intake, those consuming 1 or more daily servings of beer (0.46 mg/dL higher) or liquor (0.29 mg/dL higher) have higher serum urate concentrations, an association not seen with wine.[35] The potential for a differential impact of different forms of alcohol may relate to the highly variable purine content across products. A study leveraging high-performance liquid chromatography demonstrated that 1 beer serving contains up to 1000 µg/L of purines, whereas whiskey, brandy, and wine each contain less than 100 µg/L.[36]

Lead

As noted above, historical gout epidemics may be at least partially explained by increased exposures to lead, leading to saturnine gout. Increased blood lead levels cause tubulointerstitial nephritis, subsequent decreases in the renal secretion of uric acid coupled with increased reabsorption, that together contribute to the development of hyperuricemia.[37] In addition to this mechanism, it is also proposed that increased blood lead levels cause glomerular disruption, albuminuria, chronic kidney disease and decreased renal urate filtration,[37] all of which conspire to further exacerbate hyperuricemia.[38–42]

A 2010 Nigerian study demonstrated a dose-dependent relationship between occupational exposures to lead and serum urate concentration.[43] Although current studies suggest that exposures resulting in blood lead levels less than 5 to 10 µg/dL are considered "safe,"[44] an NHANES study noted a dose-dependent relationship between blood lead concentrations considered "safe" and the risk of both gout and hyperuricemia.[45] Even after accounting for confounders, those in the highest quartile of blood lead concentration (concentrations deemed safe based on US standards) had a 3.6-fold higher risk of gout and 1.9-fold higher risk of hyperuricemia when compared with those in the lowest quartile.[45] Additionally, a study done on US adolescents aged 12 to 19 years showed a positive linear relationship with blood lead levels and serum urate, suggesting that no level of lead is likely "safe" and without adverse physiologic effects.[46]

Medications

Several different medications may contribute to hyperuricemia and gout risk (**Table 2**). The calcineurin inhibitor cyclosporine gained popularity as a posttransplant immunosuppressant in the 1980s and has been correlated with both increased rates of hyperuricemia and an increased risk of gout.[47] More recently, there has been increased use of tacrolimus over cyclosporine for long-term immunosuppression in the setting of transplant. A 2020 study found that nearly 20% of patients on cyclosporine had a diagnosis of gout, whereas patients on tacrolimus had approximately half the rate of gout and this was similar to rates observed in the absence of immunosuppressant therapy.[48]

Table 2
Nongout medications with documented effects on serum urate concentrations

Increased serum urate	Proposed Mechanism
Antitubercular • Pyrazinamide • Ethambutol	Reduces renal excretion of uric acid[85]
Aspirin (low-dose)	Inhibits tubular secretion, decrease GFR[86,87]
Beta blockers (eg, metoprolol)	Increases intracellular glucose, increasing serum urate by the pentose phosphate pathway[51]
Cyclosporine	Decreases GFR, reduces uric acid secretion in proximal tubule[88,89]
Cytotoxins (eg, chemotherapies)	Increases cell turnover leading to increased purine burden
Diuretics	Decreases fractional excretion of urate[90]
Nicotinic acid (Niacin)	Interacts with URAT1 and OAT2 transporters in the nephron leading to decrease urinary excretion of uric acid[91,92]

Decreased Serum Urate	Proposed Mechanism
Aspirin (high-dose)	Inhibits tubular reabsorption of uric acid[93]
Calcium channel blocker, dihydropiridines (eg, amlodipine)	Dilates afferent arterioles and increases GFR and subsequent uric acid filtration; vasodilates blood vessels causing hemodilution effect[52]
Losartan	Inhibits uptake of uric acid by URAT1 transporter in nephron[94]
Sodium/glucose transporter-2 inhibitor (eg, empagliflozin)	Increases glycosuria stimulates uric acid excretion and inhibits reabsorption[95]

Abbreviations: GFR, glomerular filtration rate; OAT2, Organic Anion Transporter 2; URAT1, Urate Transporter 1.

Other medications implicated in hyperuricemia and gout include diuretics, select antihypertensives, low-dose aspirin, antitubercular drugs (ie, pyrazinamide, etham-butol), cytotoxins in the context of chemotherapy and resulting cell turnover, testosterone replacement, and nicotinic acid.[49] Of these, diuretics may pose the most meaningful impact given frequent use and potent effects on serum urate levels. In a study of nearly 6000 hypertensive patients, the use of loop and thiazide diuretics were associated with a 2.3-fold and 1.4-fold increased risk, respectively, with gout risk.[50] Metoprolol, another commonly prescribed medication for hypertension and heart disease and used commonly in combination with diuretics has also been shown to increase serum urate, particularly among black or African American patients.[51] A study examining dihydropyridine calcium channel blockers (eg, amlodipine) reported a serum urate-lowering effect for these agents, an association that was particularly strong when blood pressure was well controlled.[52] These findings were supported by results of the Antihypertensive and Lipid-Lowering Treatment to Prevent Heart Attack Trial (ALLHAT), which found that amlodipine administration lowered gout risk by 37%.[53] A urate-lowering effect has previously been well attributed to the angiotensin II receptor blocker (ARB) losartan,[54] an effect that does not seem to be shared by other ARBs or ACE inhibitors.[53,55] Together, these data suggest that for patients with hyperuricemia or at high risk for gout, careful selection of antihypertensives could yield benefit.

The management of diabetes mellitus type II (DMT2), another common comorbidity in gout, has evolved during the past 10 years with several novel therapies available. In addition to glucose-lowering effects, sodium/glucose transporter-2 inhibitors (SGLT2) also reduce cardiovascular risk.[56] In addition, SGLT2 inhibitors seem to reduce gout risk compared with glucagon-like-peptide-1 receptor agonists or dipeptidyl peptidase inhibitors in the treatment of DMT2,[57,58] a protective effect that may result from urate-lowering. A meta-analysis of 62 studies found that various SGLT2 inhibitors lowered serum urate by a mean of 0.6 mg/dL with empagliflozin yielding the greatest effect with mean reductions approaching 0.8 mg/dL.[59]

TRIGGERS FOR GOUT FLARES
Diet

In addition to contributing to hyperuricemia and increased risk for gout development, a select number of environmental exposures have also been examined as potential triggers of gout flare, an effect that in select circumstances may be attributable to resulting fluctuations in serum urate concentration. Using questionnaire data from more than 500 patients with gout, investigators found that more than one-third of patients reported at least 1 such trigger for gout flare with the most frequent triggers including red meat or seafood consumption, alcohol use, dehydration, injury or excess activity, or ambient temperature/weather.[60] In addition to associations with increased serum urate concentrations in large epidemiologic studies, the consumption of foods with high-purine content has been linked with the risk of experiencing recurrent gout flare in other observational studies. Using a novel Internet-based case-crossover study design, investigators found that increasing purine intake (>3 g during a 2-day span vs those consuming <1g over the same time period) increased the odds of experiencing a gout flare by almost 5-fold.[61]

Alcohol

Alcohol consumption may also act as a potential trigger for acute gout flares in addition to adversely affecting serum urate concentrations.[62] Again, using an Internet-based case-crossover study, Neogi and colleagues observed a dose-dependent relationship between alcohol consumption over the preceding 24 hours and flare risk.[63] Compared with those reporting no alcohol consumption, there was a 36% (95% confidence interval [CI] 1.00–1.88) increased risk of flare with more than 1 to 2 servings of any type of alcohol (beer, liquor, wine) and a 51% (95% CI 1.09–2.09) increased risk of flare with more than 2 to 4 servings, respectively.[63] Of note, this risk seemed to be independent of alcohol type, suggesting that the increased flare risk posed by alcohol intake may related to factors other than purine content.

Medications

In addition to affecting long-term changes in serum urate, the use of select medications that acutely raise or lower serum urate have been implicated as precipitants of gout flare. This has perhaps been best detailed with the initiation of gout treatments such as allopurinol or febuxostat where flares are considered to be a "physiologic" consequence of urate-lowering and serve as the basis for recommendations supporting anti-inflammatory prophylaxis.[64,65] Similarly, acute urate increases accompanying therapies such as diuretics may also increase flare risk.[66] Adjusting for alcohol consumption and purine intake, investigators found that diuretic use during the previous 2-day period increased the risk of flare by 3.6-fold (95% CI 1.4–9.7) with a similar magnitude of risk between loop and thiazide diuretics.[67]

Climate

In addition to the aforementioned, climate could also affect the natural course of gout, specifically the occurrence of flares. A study examining the frequency of Google searches for "gout" found that this search term was used most frequently during spring and early summer months,[68] suggesting a seasonal or weather-based influence on gout-related symptoms. Cooler temperatures promote uric acid crystallization, a fact that might explain the predominance of gout in cooler body regions such as the first metatarsophalangeal joint. A meta-analysis by Park and colleagues found that gout flares were most likely to accompany extreme variations (particularly increases) in day-to-day temperatures, which are most common during spring months.[69] Besides ambient temperature, humidity may also play a role in flare occurrence, with one study showing that most flares occur under conditions of both high temperature and low humidity.[70] Although the precise association and potential mechanisms linking weather and ambient temperatures to flare risk remain unknown, current trends in global warming could significantly effect the burden posed by gout.

Air Pollution

Ambient air pollution has also recently been associated with an increased risk of gout flares. A 2021 study found that for every 1 mg/m^3 increase in carbon monoxide concentration, the rate of gout hospitalizations increased by almost 4%.[71] Another study reported that exposures to ozone and particulate matter increased the risk of gout-related emergency department visits by 7% and 2%, respectively.[72] An additional study found that particulate matter levels greater than 100 $\mu g/m^3$ showed a positive linear relationship with number of gout flares.[73] Although mechanisms underpinning the associations of air pollution with flare risk are not well understood, there is speculation that inhalant particulate matter could potentiate activation of the NLR family pyrin domain containing 3 (NLRP3) inflammasome, which in turn facilitates interleukin-1β production and acts as a key inflammatory mediator in flares.[74] NLRP3 inflammasome activation has been shown, for example, to be increased following quartz dust inhalation in iron workers.[75] Of note, these studies did not adequately adjust for socioeconomic status, which may confound study findings.

Physiologic Stress

Physiologic stress (and its downstream consequences) also seems to act as a trigger of gout flares. For example, postsurgical gout flares are common in the inpatient setting. In a study of 70 gout patients undergoing surgery, nearly half experienced a flare with mean occurrence on day 4 postoperatively.[76] Flares in this study most often accompanied large serum urate fluctuations (preoperatively to postoperatively) as well as in patients not receiving urate-lowering therapy, suggesting prior control of gout and continuation of urate-lowering therapy during the perioperative period are most important factors in preventing flare in this setting. Although empiric data is limited, joint trauma is anecdotally reported to precede flare in many. Dehydration may also be tied to flare risk. A study of primary care patients found that nearly 5% reported dehydration before a gout flare.[60] Neogi and colleagues reported nearly a 50% reduction in gout flare risk in individuals consuming greater than 8 glasses of water/day versus those drinking only 0 to 1 glasses of water.[77]

SUMMARY

In summary, there are several environmental factors that promote hyperuricemia, increase gout risk, and predispose patients to recurrent flares. In this review, we have summarized dietary patterns, medication use, and other select environmental exposures that have been implicated in the pathogenesis of gout. In general, the influence of individual environmental exposures on serum urate concentration or gout risk often cluster and thus is difficult to tease apart. Moreover, the effect of individual factors seems to be modest, suggesting that interventions targeting these exposures may be best suited as part of a holistic approach to disease prevention or as adjuvant therapies among patients with established gout.

CLINICS CARE POINTS

- High-purine content foods in the form of meat, alcohol, and high-fructose corn syrup contribute to hyperuricemia, gout, and gout flare risk, whereas high purine content vegetables and fruits do not seem to contribute to this risk.

- Medications such as amlodipine, losartan, and sodium/glucose transporter-2 inhibitors have shown serum urate and gout risk lowering effects, whereas diuretics and β-blockers contribute to these risks.

- Lead exposure may serve as a relevant environmental risk factor for hyperuricemia and gout, even at levels that are typically considered safe by regulatory bodies.

REFERENCES

1. Nuki G, Simkin PA. A concise history of gout and hyperuricemia and their treatment. Arthritis Res Ther 2006;8(Suppl 1):S1.
2. Pasero G, Marson P. Hippocrates and rheumatology. Clin Exp Rheumatol 2004; 22(6):687–9.
3. Nriagu JO. Saturnine gout among Roman aristocrats. Did lead poisoning contribute to the fall of the Empire? N Engl J Med 1983;308(11):660–3.
4. Pinals RS, Schlesinger N. Did Michelangelo Have Gout? J Clin Rheumatol 2015; 21(7):364–7.
5. Dalvi SR, Pillinger MH. Saturnine gout, redux: a review. Am J Med 2013;126(5): 450.e1-8.
6. A Complete List of Purine Content In Foods. Available at: https://healthtopquestions.com/a-complete-list-of-purine-content-in-foods/#:~:text=Purine%20Content%20in%20Various%20Foods%20%20%20Content,%20%20%20%2059%20more%20rows%20. Accessed January 21, 2022.
7. Zhang M, Zhang Y, Terkeltaub R, et al. Effect of Dietary and Supplemental Omega-3 Polyunsaturated Fatty Acids on Risk of Recurrent Gout Flares. Arthritis Rheumatol 2019;71(9):1580–6.
8. Choi HK, Liu S, Curhan G. Intake of purine-rich foods, protein, and dairy products and relationship to serum levels of uric acid: the Third National Health and Nutrition Examination Survey. Arthritis Rheum 2005;52(1):283–9.
9. Jakše B, Jakše B, Pajek M, et al. Uric Acid and Plant-Based Nutrition. Nutrients 2019;11(8):1736.
10. Li R, Yu K, Li C. Dietary factors and risk of gout and hyperuricemia: a meta-analysis and systematic review. Asia Pac J Clin Nutr 2018;27(6):1344–56.
11. Jamnik J, Rehman S, Blanco Mejia S, et al. Fructose intake and risk of gout and hyperuricemia: a systematic review and meta-analysis of prospective cohort studies. BMJ Open 2016;6(10):e013191.

12. Raivio KO, Becker A, Meyer LJ, et al. Stimulation of human purine synthesis de novo by fructose infusion. Metabolism 1975;24(7):861–9.
13. Williams PT. Effects of diet, physical activity and performance, and body weight on incident gout in ostensibly healthy, vigorously active men. Am J Clin Nutr 2008; 87(5):1480–7.
14. Charoenngam N, Ponvilawan B, Ungprasert P. Vitamin D insufficiency and deficiency are associated with a higher level of serum uric acid: A systematic review and meta-analysis. Mod Rheumatol 2020;30(2):385–90.
15. Isnuwardana R, Bijukchhe S, Thadanipon K, et al. Association Between Vitamin D and Uric Acid in Adults: A Systematic Review and Meta-Analysis. Horm Metab Res 2020;52(10):732–41.
16. Nimitphong H, Saetung S, Chailurkit LO, et al. Vitamin D supplementation is associated with serum uric acid concentration in patients with prediabetes and hyperuricemia. J Clin Transl Endocrinol 2021;24:100255.
17. Biniaz V, Tayebi A, Ebadi A, et al. Effect of vitamin C supplementation on serum uric acid in patients undergoing hemodialysis: a randomized controlled trial. Iran J Kidney Dis 2014;8(5):401–7.
18. Huang HY, Appel LJ, Choi MJ, et al. The effects of vitamin C supplementation on serum concentrations of uric acid: results of a randomized controlled trial. Arthritis Rheum 2005;52(6):1843–7.
19. Kyllästinen MJ, Elfving SM, Gref CG, et al. Dietary vitamin c supplementation and common laboratory values in the elderly. Arch Gerontol Geriatr 1990;10(3): 297–301.
20. Juraschek SP, Miller ER 3rd, Gelber AC. Effect of oral vitamin C supplementation on serum uric acid: a meta-analysis of randomized controlled trials. Arthritis Care Res (Hoboken) 2011;63(9):1295–306.
21. Chen PE, Liu CY, Chien WH, et al. Effectiveness of Cherries in Reducing Uric Acid and Gout: A Systematic Review. Evid Based Complement Alternat Med 2019; 2019:9896757.
22. Stamp LK, Chapman P, Frampton C, et al. Lack of effect of tart cherry concentrate dose on serum urate in people with gout. Rheumatology (Oxford) 2020;59(9): 2374–80.
23. Zhang Y, Neogi T, Chen C, et al. Cherry consumption and decreased risk of recurrent gout attacks. Arthritis Rheum 2012;64(12):4004–11.
24. Schlesinger N, Schlesinger M. Previously reported prior studies of cherry juice concentrate for gout flare prophylaxis: comment on the article by Zhang et al. Arthritis Rheum 2013;65(4):1135–6.
25. Park KY, Kim HJ, Ahn HS, et al. Effects of coffee consumption on serum uric acid: systematic review and meta-analysis. Semin Arthritis Rheum 2016;45(5):580–6.
26. Zhu C, Tai LL, Wan XC, et al. Comparative effects of green and black tea extracts on lowering serum uric acid in hyperuricemic mice. Pharm Biol 2017;55(1): 2123–8.
27. Jatuworapruk K, Srichairatanakool S, Ounjaijean S, et al. Effects of green tea extract on serum uric acid and urate clearance in healthy individuals. J Clin Rheumatol 2014;20(6):310–3.
28. Zhang Y, Cui Y, Li XA, et al. Is tea consumption associated with the serum uric acid level, hyperuricemia or the risk of gout? A systematic review and meta-analysis. BMC Musculoskelet Disord 2017;18(1):95.
29. Choi HK, Curhan G. Coffee, tea, and caffeine consumption and serum uric acid level: the third national health and nutrition examination survey. Arthritis Rheum 2007;57(5):816–21.

30. Peluso I, Teichner A, Manafikhi H, et al. Camellia sinensis in asymptomatic hyperuricemia: A meta-analysis of tea or tea extract effects on uric acid levels. Crit Rev Food Sci Nutr 2017;57(2):391–8.

31. Zhao M, Zhu D, Sun-Waterhouse D, et al. In Vitro and In Vivo Studies on Adlay-Derived Seed Extracts: Phenolic Profiles, Antioxidant Activities, Serum Uric Acid Suppression, and Xanthine Oxidase Inhibitory Effects. J Agric Food Chem 2014;62(31):7771–8.

32. Huang XF, Li HQ, Shi L, et al. Synthesis of resveratrol analogues, and evaluation of their cytotoxic and xanthine oxidase inhibitory activities. Chem Biodivers 2008; 5(4):636–42.

33. Yahfoufi N, Alsadi N, Jambi M, et al. The Immunomodulatory and Anti-Inflammatory Role of Polyphenols. Nutrients 2018;10(11):1618.

34. Newcombe DS. Ethanol metabolism and uric acid. Metabolism 1972;21(12): 1193–203.

35. Choi HK, Curhan G. Beer, liquor, and wine consumption and serum uric acid level: the Third National Health and Nutrition Examination Survey. Arthritis Rheum 2004;51(6):1023–9.

36. Kaneko K, Yamanobe T, Fujimori S. Determination of purine contents of alcoholic beverages using high performance liquid chromatography. Biomed Chromatogr 2009;23(8):858–64.

37. Rastogi SK. Renal effects of environmental and occupational lead exposure. Indian J Occup Environ Med 2008;12(3):103–6.

38. Jing J, Kielstein JT, Schultheiss UT, et al. Prevalence and correlates of gout in a large cohort of patients with chronic kidney disease: the German Chronic Kidney Disease (GCKD) study. Nephrol Dial Transpl 2015;30(4):613–21.

39. Johnson RJ, Nakagawa T, Jalal D, et al. Uric acid and chronic kidney disease: which is chasing which? Nephrol Dial Transpl 2013;28(9):2221–8.

40. Lipkowitz MS. Regulation of uric acid excretion by the kidney. Curr Rheumatol Rep 2012;14(2):179–88.

41. Obermayr RP, Temml C, Gutjahr G, et al. Elevated uric acid increases the risk for kidney disease. J Am Soc Nephrol 2008;19(12):2407–13.

42. Roughley MJ, Belcher J, Mallen CD, et al. Gout and risk of chronic kidney disease and nephrolithiasis: meta-analysis of observational studies. Arthritis Res Ther 2015;17(1):90.

43. Alasia DD, Emem-Chioma PC, Wokoma FS. Association of lead exposure, serum uric acid and parameters of renal function in Nigerian lead-exposed workers. Int J Occup Environ Med 2010;1(4):182–90.

44. Adult Blood Lead Epidemiology and Surveillance (ABLES). Available at: https://www.cdc.gov/niosh/topics/ables/ReferenceBloodLevelsforAdults.html. Accessed January 21, 2022.

45. Krishnan E, Lingala B, Bhalla V. Low-level lead exposure and the prevalence of gout: an observational study. Ann Intern Med 2012;157(4):233–41.

46. Hu G, Jia G, Tang S, et al. Association of low-level blood lead with serum uric acid in U.S. adolescents: a cross-sectional study. Environ Health 2019;18(1):86.

47. Gores PF, Fryd DS, Sutherland DE, et al. Hyperuricemia after renal transplantation. Am J Surg 1988;156(5):397–400.

48. Brigham MD, Milgroom A, Lenco MO, et al. Immunosuppressant Use and Gout in the Prevalent Solid Organ Transplantation Population. Prog Transplant 2020; 30(2):103–10.

49. Ben Salem C, Slim R, Fathallah N, et al. Drug-induced hyperuricaemia and gout. Rheumatology (Oxford) 2017;56(5):679–88.

50. McAdams DeMarco MA, Maynard JW, Baer AN, et al. Diuretic use, increased serum urate levels, and risk of incident gout in a population-based study of adults with hypertension: the Atherosclerosis Risk in Communities cohort study. Arthritis Rheum 2012;64(1):121–9.
51. Juraschek SP, Appel LJ, Miller ER 3rd. Metoprolol Increases Uric Acid and Risk of Gout in African Americans With Chronic Kidney Disease Attributed to Hypertension. Am J Hypertens 2017;30(9):871–5.
52. Zhang D, Huang QF, Sheng CS, et al. Serum uric acid change in relation to antihypertensive therapy with the dihydropyridine calcium channel blockers. Blood Press 2021;30(6):395–402.
53. Juraschek SP, Simpson LM, Davis BR, et al. The effects of antihypertensive class on gout in older adults: secondary analysis of the Antihypertensive and Lipid-Lowering Treatment to Prevent Heart Attack Trial. J Hypertens 2020;38(5): 954–60.
54. Sutton Burke EM, Kelly TC, Shoales LA, et al. Angiotensin Receptor Blockers Effect on Serum Uric Acid-A Class Effect? J Pharm Pract 2020;33(6):874–81.
55. Schmidt A, Gruber U, Böhmig G, et al. The effect of ACE inhibitor and angiotensin II receptor antagonist therapy on serum uric acid levels and potassium homeostasis in hypertensive renal transplant recipients treated with CsA. Nephrol Dial Transpl 2001;16(5):1034–7.
56. Dave CV, Kim SC, Goldfine AB, et al. Risk of Cardiovascular Outcomes in Patients With Type 2 Diabetes After Addition of SGLT2 Inhibitors Versus Sulfonylureas to Baseline GLP-1RA Therapy. Circulation 2021;143(8):770–9.
57. Fralick M, Chen SK, Patorno E, et al. Assessing the Risk for Gout With Sodium-Glucose Cotransporter-2 Inhibitors in Patients With Type 2 Diabetes: A Population-Based Cohort Study. Ann Intern Med 2020;172(3):186–94.
58. Chung MC, Hung PH, Hsiao PJ, et al. Association of Sodium-Glucose Transport Protein 2 Inhibitor Use for Type 2 Diabetes and Incidence of Gout in Taiwan. JAMA Netw Open 2021;4(11):e2135353.
59. Zhao Y, Xu L, Tian D, et al. Effects of sodium-glucose co-transporter 2 (SGLT2) inhibitors on serum uric acid level: A meta-analysis of randomized controlled trials. Diabetes Obes Metab 2018;20(2):458–62.
60. Abhishek A, Valdes AM, Jenkins W, et al. Triggers of acute attacks of gout, does age of gout onset matter? A primary care based cross-sectional study. PLoS One 2017;12(10):e0186096.
61. Zhang Y, Chen C, Choi H, et al. Purine-rich foods intake and recurrent gout attacks. Ann Rheum Dis 2012;71(9):1448–53.
62. Zhang Y, Woods R, Chaisson CE, et al. Alcohol Consumption as a Trigger of Recurrent Gout Attacks. Am J Med 2006;119(9):800.e1-6.
63. Neogi T, Chen C, Niu J, et al. Alcohol quantity and type on risk of recurrent gout attacks: an internet-based case-crossover study. Am J Med 2014;127(4):311–8.
64. Hollingworth P, Reardon JA, Scott JT. Acute gout during hypouricaemic therapy: prophylaxis with colchicine. Ann Rheum Dis 1980;39(5):529.
65. FitzGerald JD, Dalbeth N, Mikuls T, et al. 2020 American College of Rheumatology Guideline for the Management of Gout. Arthritis Care Res (Hoboken) 2020;72(6):744–60.
66. Jeong S, Tan IJ. Characteristics of Acute Gout Flare in Patients Initiated on Intravenous Bumetanide for Acute Heart Failure Exacerbation. Cureus 2020;12(6): e8605.

67. Hunter DJ, York M, Chaisson CE, et al. Recent diuretic use and the risk of recurrent gout attacks: the online case-crossover gout study. J Rheumatol 2006;33(7): 1341–5.

68. Kardeş S. Seasonal variation in the internet searches for gout: an ecological study. Clin Rheumatol 2019;38(3):769–75.

69. Park KY, Kim HJ, Ahn HS, et al. Association between acute gouty arthritis and meteorological factors: An ecological study using a systematic review and meta-analysis. Semin Arthritis Rheum 2017;47(3):369–75.

70. Neogi T, Chen C, Niu J, et al. Relation of temperature and humidity to the risk of recurrent gout attacks. Am J Epidemiol 2014;180(4):372–7.

71. He YS, Wang GH, Wu Q, et al. The Relationship Between Ambient Air Pollution and Hospitalizations for Gout in a Humid Subtropical Region of China. J Inflamm Res 2021;14:5827–35.

72. Ryu H, Seo M, Choi H, et al. THU0427 Ambient air pollution and risk of acute gout flares; a time-series study. Ann Rheum Dis 2017;76(Suppl 2):369.

73. Ryu HJ, Seo MR, Choi HJ, et al. Particulate matter (PM(10)) as a newly identified environmental risk factor for acute gout flares: A time-series study. Joint Bone Spine 2021;88(2):105108.

74. Martinon F, Glimcher LH. Gout: new insights into an old disease. J Clin Invest 2006;116(8):2073–5.

75. Hedbrant A, Andersson L, Bryngelsson I-L, et al. Quartz dust exposure affects NLRP3 Inflammasome activation and plasma levels of IL-18 and IL-1Ra in iron foundry workers. Mediators Inflamm 2020;2020:8490908.

76. Jeong H, Jeon CH. Clinical characteristics and risk factors for gout flare during the postsurgical period. Adv Rheumatol 2019;59(1):31.

77. Neogi T, Chen C, Chaisson C, Hunter D, Zhang Y: Drinking water can reduce the risk of recurrent gout attacks. In: ACR Annual Scientific Meeting: 2009; 2009: 16-21. October 21, 2009, Pennsylvania Convention Center.

78. Choi HK, Atkinson K, Karlson EW, et al. Purine-Rich Foods, Dairy and Protein Intake, and the Risk of Gout in Men. New Engl J Med 2004;350(11):1093–103.

79. Villegas R, Xiang YB, Elasy T, et al. Purine-rich foods, protein intake, and the prevalence of hyperuricemia: the Shanghai Men's Health Study. Nutr Metab Cardiovasc Dis 2012;22(5):409–16.

80. Schmidt JA, Crowe FL, Appleby PN, et al. Serum uric acid concentrations in meat eaters, fish eaters, vegetarians and vegans: a cross-sectional analysis in the EPIC-Oxford cohort. PLoS One 2013;8(2):e56339.

81. Teng GG, Pan A, Yuan JM, et al. Food Sources of Protein and Risk of Incident Gout in the Singapore Chinese Health Study. Arthritis Rheumatol 2015;67(7): 1933–42.

82. Rai SK, Fung TT, Lu N, et al. The Dietary Approaches to Stop Hypertension (DASH) diet, Western diet, and risk of gout in men: prospective cohort study. BMJ 2017;357:j1794.

83. Aihemaitijiang S, Zhang Y, Zhang L, et al. The Association between Purine-Rich Food Intake and Hyperuricemia: A Cross-Sectional Study in Chinese Adult Residents. Nutrients 2020;12(12):3835.

84. Yokose C, McCormick N, Lu N, et al. Adherence to 2020 to 2025 Dietary Guidelines for Americans and the Risk of New-Onset Female Gout. JAMA Intern Med 2022;182(3):254–64.

85. Pham AQ, Doan A, Andersen M. Pyrazinamide-induced hyperuricemia. P t 2014; 39(10):695–715.

86. Kimberly RP, Plotz PH. Aspirin-induced depression of renal function. N Engl J Med 1977;296(8):418–24.
87. Yu TF, Gutman AB. Study of the paradoxical effects of salicylate in low, intermediate and high dosage on the renal mechanisms for excretion of urate in man. J Clin Invest 1959;38(8):1298–315.
88. Zürcher RM, Bock HA, Thiel G. Hyperuricaemia in cyclosporin-treated patients: GFR-related effect. Nephrol Dial Transpl 1996;11(1):153–8.
89. Laine J, Holmberg C. Mechanisms of hyperuricemia in cyclosporine-treated renal transplanted children. Nephron 1996;74(2):318–23.
90. Keenan RT, Nowatzky J, Pillinger MH. 94 - Etiology and Pathogenesis of Hyperuricemia and Gout. In: Firestein GS, Budd RC, Gabriel SE, et al, editors. Kelley's Textbook of Rheumatology. 9th edition. Philadelphia: W.B. Saunders; 2013. p. 1533–53.e5.
91. Enomoto A, Kimura H, Chairoungdua A, et al. Molecular identification of a renal urate anion exchanger that regulates blood urate levels. Nature 2002; 417(6887):447–52.
92. Bahn A, Hagos Y, Reuter S, et al. Identification of a new urate and high affinity nicotinate transporter, hOAT10 (SLC22A13). J Biol Chem 2008;283(24): 16332–41.
93. Caspi D, Lubart E, Graff E, et al. The effect of mini-dose aspirin on renal function and uric acid handling in elderly patients. Arthritis Rheum 2000;43(1):103–8.
94. Iwanaga T, Sato M, Maeda T, et al. Concentration-dependent mode of interaction of angiotensin II receptor blockers with uric acid transporter. J Pharmacol Exp Ther 2007;320(1):211–7.
95. Chino Y, Samukawa Y, Sakai S, et al. SGLT2 inhibitor lowers serum uric acid through alteration of uric acid transport activity in renal tubule by increased glycosuria. Biopharm Drug Dispos 2014;35(7):391–404.

Environmental Risk Factors for Osteoarthritis: The Impact on Individuals with Knee Joint Injury

David M. Werner, PT, DPT, OCS, CSCS[a,b,*],
Yvonne M. Golightly, PT, PhD[c], Matthew Tao, MD[b,d],
Austin Post, BS[e], Elizabeth Wellsandt, PT, DPT, PhD, OCS[b,d]

KEYWORDS

- Anterior cruciate ligament • Knee • Knee injury • Prevention • Disease management

KEY POINTS

- An interdisciplinary team is required to address all potential risk factors for osteoarthritis development and progression.
- An anterior cruciate ligament injury is associated with osteoarthritis development and progression, and individuals with these injuries require appropriate care and monitoring.
- Non-modifiable risk factors for osteoarthritis include previous joint injury and sociodemographic characteristics.
- Modifiable risk factors for osteoarthritis include body mass, physical activity, muscle strength, movement patterns, psychological factors, comorbidities, occupational demands, and anatomic alignment.

INTRODUCTION

Osteoarthritis (OA) is a chronic condition involving joint degeneration that impacts over 300 million people in the global population.[1] In the United States alone, 32.5 million individuals are diagnosed with OA.[2] Radiographic OA is often characterized by

[a] Office of Graduate Studies, Medical Sciences Interdepartmental Area, University of Nebraska Medical Center, 987815 Nebraska Medical Center, Omaha, NE 68198-7815, USA; [b] Division of Physical Therapy Education, College of Allied Health Professions, University of Nebraska Medical Center, 984420 Nebraska Medical Center, Omaha, NE 68198-4420, USA; [c] College of Allied Health Professions, University of Nebraska Medical Center, 984035 Nebraska Medical Center Omaha, NE 68198-4035, USA; [d] Department of Orthopedic Surgery and Rehabilitation, University of Nebraska Medical Center, 984420 Nebraska Medical Center, Omaha, NE 68198-4420, USA; [e] College of Medicine, University of Nebraska Medical Center, 984420 Nebraska Medical Center, Omaha, NE 68198-4420, USA
* Corresponding author.
E-mail address: dwerner@unmc.edu

Rheum Dis Clin N Am 48 (2022) 907–930
https://doi.org/10.1016/j.rdc.2022.06.010
0889-857X/22/© 2022 Elsevier Inc. All rights reserved.
rheumatic.theclinics.com

osteophyte formation, narrowing of the joint space, and altered shape of the bone end.[3] Individuals may or may not report joint-specific symptoms that correspond to imaging signs of OA. Symptomatic OA involves the presence of stiffness, pain, and/ or swelling. Symptomatic OA accounts for almost 10 additional health care visits per individual per year[4] and an estimated $140 to $185 billion in health care costs each year in the United States.[5,6] Individuals with symptomatic OA miss an average of three additional work days per year leading to an approximate $10 billion in absenteeism costs.[7,8] In addition, people with OA are less productive at work, regardless of the occupation's physical demands, resulting in an annual loss of up to $7100 per individual.[9]

OA most often impacts the hand, hip, and knee joints,[10] with knee OA occurring at twice the rate of hand and hip OA.[10] Approximately, 14 million adults in the United States suffer from symptomatic knee OA.[11] Major risk factors for knee OA include older age,[12] obesity,[13] and intra-articular injury,[13] and those with knee OA have reduced the quality of life[14,15] and impaired physical function, such as difficulty with walking, climbing stairs, or lifting.[1,16] The primary surgical treatment of end-stage knee OA is a total knee arthroplasty (TKA). It is estimated from 2005 to 2030, there will be a 673% increase in the number of TKA procedures performed in the United States, resulting in almost 3.5 million TKA procedures completed annually by 2030.[17] Of the 14 million adults that suffer from knee OA, almost 2 million cases are in individuals under the age of 45, largely driven by prior joint injury.[11,18] The onset of knee OA at a younger age has contributed to an increase in TKA in younger individuals,[19] which is particularly concerning because a younger age (50–54 years) at the time of initial TKA increases lifetime risk of revision up to 35%.[20] Accordingly, the demand for TKA revision is expected to increase 600% between 2005 and 2030 due to the increase in younger adults with knee OA, the overall aging of the population, and the obesity epidemic.[17]

Traumatic knee joint injuries that involve fractures, ligamentous, cartilage, or meniscal damage are a common cause for the development of knee OA early in adulthood. This type of OA is sometimes referred to as post-traumatic OA or early onset OA. Up to 12% of lower extremity OA is related to previous injury, translating to over 5.5 million people within the United States.[21] Injury to the anterior cruciate ligament (ACL) of the knee commonly leads to the development of early knee OA.[22,23] Within the first 5 years after ACL injury, 12% of individuals may progress to knee OA,[22] and over 50% may have knee OA by 15 years.[23] With an estimated 250,000 ACL injuries occurring annually in the United States,[24] this translates to potentially over 125,000 new individuals each year developing early knee OA.

The purpose of this review is to discuss non-modifiable and modifiable environmental risk factors for developing knee OA, with a focus on early knee OA after ACL injury. Although factors such as family history and genetics play a role in the risk of early knee OA development,[25–29] this review focuses on risk factors that are environmental in nature. We provide clinically applicable knowledge of early knee OA risk factors and current evidence-based recommendations for interventions to reduce the risk of knee OA after ACL injury.

DISCUSSION

Risk factors for the development and progression of early knee OA can be broken into two categories: non-modifiable and modifiable (**Table 1**). Non-modifiable risk factors are characteristics that can impact the risk for OA development but have no potential to be changed with interventions. Modifiable risk factors can be altered

Table 1
Modifiable and non-modifiable environmental risk factors for osteoarthritis development after anterior cruciate ligament injury

Modifiable	Non-Modifiable
Body mass index/weight	Previous joint injury
Physical activity	Sociodemographic characteristics
Muscle strength	
Movement patterns	
Psychological factors	
Comorbidities	
Occupational demands	
Anatomic alignment	

by interventions, both nonoperative and surgical, aimed at mitigating early knee OA development.

Non-Modifiable Risk Factors

Previous joint injury

Joint injury can be considered both a potentially modifiable and non-modifiable risk factor for OA. Evidence-based injury prevention programs exist, which reduce the risk of initial injury for a variety of joints with correct implementation.[30–32] Further, many modifiable risk factors described below can be targeted in interventions after joint injury to change the trajectory of OA development. However, the occurrence of joint injury cannot be reversed (ie, non-modifiable) and results in greater OA risk despite current secondary prevention strategies. Previous joint injury is strongly associated with OA and significantly accelerates progression to OA at various joint sites. After a distal radius fracture, up to 37% of individuals will develop OA within 31 months.[33] OA development in the hip joint increases drastically after acetabular fracture, with up to 48% of individuals presenting with radiographic OA within 2 years injury.[34,35] Almost 80% of individuals who have end-stage ankle OA had a previous injury to that ankle joint.[36]

Specific to the knee, previous injury was associated with a 4.2 higher odds of OA compared with individuals with no history of knee injury.[37] An estimated 10% of all knee OA diagnoses are related to a previous knee injury.[21] The type of injury sustained seems to impact OA development and progression as well. According to a meta-analysis of 24 observational studies, an injury to a ligament, tendon, meniscus, or fracture at the knee was strongly associated with knee OA (odds ratio [OR] 6.0; 95% confidence interval [CI] 4.6, 7.8).[37] Additional data from that meta-analysis found that a meniscus injury leads to a 6.9 higher odds of developing knee OA compared with uninjured knee (OR 6.9, 95% CI 4.6, 10.5).[37] Pernin and colleagues has also reported the high risk of developing knee OA after meniscal and chondral injuries.[38] Meniscal damage resulting in meniscectomy at time of ACL reconstruction leads to a 30% increase in the prevalence of radiographic knee OA at 22 years after surgery[39] and to almost 70% prevalence of radiographic OA at 24.5 years after surgery.[38] Eighty percent of individuals with chondral injuries present at the time of ACL reconstruction will have radiographic knee OA by 24.5 years after surgery.[38] Even before signs of OA are present on standing radiographs, and OA features on magnetic resonance imaging (MRI) can be detected. Patterson and colleagues reported that at only 1 year after ACL reconstruction in a cohort of 111 patients, 45%, 29%, and 26% had at least partial-thickness cartilage lesions in the patellofemoral, medial tibiofemoral, and lateral tibiofemoral compartments, respectively.[40] Bone marrow lesions, another defining feature of OA, were present 23% of the time in the patellofemoral compartment, 16% in the medial tibiofemoral compartment, and 20% in the lateral tibiofemoral compartment.[40] ACL graft ruptures and revision ACL reconstruction further increases the risk for early knee OA. Svantesson and colleagues found that 23% of patients undergoing ACL revision had cartilage defects that were not present at time of primary ACL reconstruction.[41]

Recommendation after ACL Injury: Clinicians need a thorough understanding of a patient's joint injury history to help understand the risk for OA development. One of the primary goals after ACL injury may be to return to pre-injury activity levels. Clinicians should use the best available evidence to mitigate modifiable OA risk factors and ensure that patients are safe to return to activity to minimize the risk for additional knee injuries.[42,43]

Sociodemographic characteristics

Sociodemographic characteristics have been shown to alter the progression of knee OA. A meta-analysis comparing OA prevalence between men and women found that when including all body regions together, there was no difference in the prevalence of OA across sex.[44] However, when only considering the knee and hand joints, men had a significantly lower prevalence of OA (risk ratios for knee OA: 0.63 [95% CI 0.53,0.75]; hand OA: 0.81 [95% CI 0.73–0.90]).[44] Regardless of sex, the prevalence of OA increases with age, peaking during the age range of 60 to 64 years.[1] Meanwhile, conflicting data exist regarding the association between education and income levels with OA. Globally, using a sociodemographic scoring system that includes income, education, and fertility, countries that were rated higher in sociodemographic status (eg, countries from North America, Southern Latin America, North Africa and Middle East, South Asia, and Oceania]) had more years lived with disability with OA compared with those with lower scores (eg, countries from Sub-Saharan Africa).[1] However, other studies have found no link between OA and income,[45] and even that lower levels of education and income are linked with a higher prevalence of OA in both the United States[46,47] and Portugal.[48]

With respect to individuals with ACL injury, current evidence suggests that sociodemographic characteristics may also impact the risk for the early development of knee OA. A recent systematic review found that those with lower income and public health insurance had longer times between ACL injury and treatment, increased rates of concomitant meniscal and chondral injury, and worse knee range of motion outcomes, and had a higher risk of requiring acute medical care within 30 days following ACL reconstruction.[49] As mentioned previously, any additional injury to the knee, including ACL re-rupture or meniscal or chondral injury increases the risk of early onset OA development.[37–39] However, sociodemographic characteristics can impact the injury–OA relationship as well. With regard to race and ethnicity, White race is a risk factor for second surgery (eg, revision ACL reconstruction, subsequent contralateral reconstruction).[49] Compared with White patients, Black and Hispanic patients have longer time from injury until they see a health care provider, higher rates of hospital admissions after ACL reconstruction,[50,51] and shorter postoperative follow-up length with their health care providers.[52–56]

Recommendation after ACL Injury: Advancing clinicians' understanding of the association between sociodemographic factors and early knee OA is needed to identify those at the greatest risk of early knee OA and drive policy change to narrow the gaps in patient outcomes after ACL injury. Clinicians and patients can learn more about OA prevention and management strategies through resources such as the Osteoarthritis Action Alliance to inform clinician–patient interactions and develop action plans to minimize OA risk.[57]

Clinical relevance of non-modifiable risk factors
Although non-modifiable risk factors inherently do not provide a target for change, they do provide vital information for health care providers who work with individuals after ACL injury. These characteristics allow for a better understanding of the risk for early OA development and progression and can accordingly help patients understand their individual risk profile. In addition, these non-modifiable characteristics allow for potential future work investigating OA treatments for specific subgroups that may benefit most from targeted interventions.

Modifiable Risk Factors

Body mass index/weight
There is a large body of literature exploring the role of body mass and the development and progression of knee OA. Obese individuals have been shown to have more consistent loading of their knee without relaxation of the load.[58] This inability to offload likely limits tissue perfusion and reduces cartilage health overall.[58] Early data from the Osteoarthritis Initiative (OAI) demonstrated that body mass index (BMI) over 30 was associated with the progression of knee OA.[59] Over a 4-year span, individuals in the OAI who had a 5% increase in BMI had an 11.3 higher odds of worse cartilage health as quantified on MRI compared with those who did not gain weight (OR 11.3, 95% CI 3.5,51.4).[60] BMI is more strongly associated with the incidence of radiographic knee OA than location of adipose tissue or waist to hip ratio.[61] Individuals with OA who are classified as obese (BMI >30 kg/m^2) are on more medications, report higher levels of disability, and have lower gait speeds.[62] In addition, it has been shown that in obese individuals with knee OA who lose weight, more weight loss leads to greater improvements in pain, function, mobility, and knee compressive forces.[63] In the intensive diet and exercise randomized controlled trial, exercise, diet, and the exercise + diet improved weight in overweight and obese patients with knee OA.[64] There was also 7.5% less knee joint loading in those that lost weight with the diet program[64] compared with exercise alone, but there was no change in radiographic findings.[65] Data over an 8-year period from over 4000 participants in the OAI suggest that for every 1% of weight loss, the risk of knee replacement is reduced by 2% and the risk of hip OA in those with painful hips is reduced by 3%, regardless of baseline BMI.[66] The relationship between a variety of diets and OA symptoms has been investigated. The Mediterranean diet seems to provide some benefit, with individuals with radiographic knee OA who adhere to it having lower risks of worsening pain (relative risk: 0.96, 95% CI 0.91, 0.999), but no impact of radiographic changes over 4 years.[67] However, other diets that focus on supervised caloric restriction reduce body weight and improve function.[64,68] There is also consistent improvement in knee OA-related symptoms after bariatric surgery,[69–71] further suggesting the important role of bodyweight in the disease course and patient experience of OA.

After ACL injuries, changes in body mass and composition occur in both the immediate time frame after injury and reconstruction, as well as years later. In the first decade after a knee joint injury, individuals are 3.75 times more likely to be obese compared with individuals without a previous knee injury.[72] This increased body mass is accompanied by a body fat percentage increase of 1.5% in the first year after injury.[73] If an ACL reconstruction is performed, individuals have an average increase in BMI of 3 to 5 points within the first year.[73,74] This increase in body mass after ACL reconstruction has a negative impact on patient-reported activity levels and physical function[75–77] and leads to a 3.1 increase in odds of developing patellofemoral OA (OR 3.1, 95% CI 1.22–7.89).[78]

Recommendation after ACL Injury: The European Alliance of Associations for Rheumatology and the American College of Rheumatology (ACR) recommends individualized care with education on weight loss for individuals who are at risk for progressive OA.[79,80] Patient education early after ACL injury should include weight management strategies from point-of-care clinicians including surgeons, physical therapists, and athletic trainers because of the impact of bodyweight on the development and progression of knee OA. Monitoring weight gain throughout recovery after ACL injury and reconstruction should be completed, with consultation and referral to nutritionists and mental health specialists as needed, both in the short-term when physical activity (PA) will be restricted for recovery and in the long-term if return to pre-injury activity levels is not achieved.

Physical activity

Although the benefits of PA have been established in all age groups, consistent data demonstrate that American adults with OA do not reach the recommended levels of PA.[81–84] Although multiple studies have shown that PA is not directly correlated with radiographic OA development,[85,86] a cohort from the OAI showed inactivity was associated with up to a 72% increased risk of developing functional limitations related to OA.[87] In addition, in a study of 4,179 participants from the OAI, individuals with symptomatic OA were almost nine times more likely to have dramatically reduced gait speed (2.75% decrease annually) over a 4-year span compared with individuals without symptomatic OA (OR 8.9, 95% CI 3.1, 25.5).[88] In those with OA, current evidence shows that PA is important because replacing 10 minutes of very light walking with moderately intense walking reduces the 5-year risk of TKA by 35%.[89] Large cohort studies demonstrate the benefits of improvements from PA. Results from 1,788 participants in the Multicenter Osteoarthritis Study (MOST) demonstrated every 1000 step/day increase in activity was associated with a 16% to 18% reduced risk of functional limitations over a 2-year period.[90] In a study with 3656 participants from both the MOST and OAI cohorts, replacing 20 min/d of sedentary time with moderate to vigorous PA reduced the risk of slowing gait speed over a 2-year span by almost 50%.[91] In a group of 1,873 participants from the OAI, replacing 60 min/d of sedentary time with 60 min/d of light activity was associated with a 17% reduction in risk for gait speed decline within 2 years.[92] Interventions that successfully improve PA also improve physical function and quality of life[93] and are recommended by several rheumatological organizations, including the European Alliance of Associations for Rheumatology,[79] the Osteoarthritis Research Society International,[94] the ACR,[80] and the Arthritis Foundation.[80] Last, forms of PA other than walking can also be performed to improve joint and general health. The incidence of knee OA is almost 7% lower in individuals who participate in moderate levels of running compared with sedentary individuals,[95] but strong longitudinal evidence does not exist.[96] Aquatic exercises also can improve pain, function, and quality of life.[97]

After ACL reconstruction, individuals regularly participate in less PA than their uninjured peers.[98–100] Individuals six to 36 months after ACL reconstruction record 1500 to 3000 less steps per day than their uninjured peers,[98,99] with almost 15 min/d less spent in moderate to vigorous PA.[98] In addition, women who have undergone an ACL reconstruction are 2.5 times more likely to not reach recommended PA guidelines than their uninjured peers.[100] Early evidence suggests PA levels are related to cartilage health after ACL injury, as altered objectively measured PA within 1 month after ACL injury is related to cartilage T2 relaxation time on MRI.[101] In addition to overall daily PA levels, participation in sports activities also declines after ACL injury and reconstruction despite most athletes expecting and planning to return initially after injury.[102] Up to 37% of individuals at all sports levels[103] and 27% of elite level athletes[104] do not return to their prior level of competition. Although further longitudinal study is needed, current evidence suggests that returning to sports that involve frequent pivoting does not increase the risk for worsening of OA features on MRI, radiographic knee OA, or knee symptoms and function.[105,106]

Recommendation after ACL Injury: Patient education and monitoring of PA should be completed with patients after ACL injury and reconstruction. PA may need to be objectively assessed to understand PA levels,[107] because self-reported PA levels are not consistent with objectively quantified PA using accelerometers in this population.[108] To successfully achieve increases in patient PA levels, personalized PA education considering factors such as baseline PA levels, patient preferences regarding modes of exercise and delivery mode of content, and other health conditions such as co-morbidities is recommended.[79,109] Although specific recommendations for levels of PA early after ACL reconstruction to promote knee joint health are unknown, the 2018 Physical Activity Guidelines for Americans[110] provide reasonable targets for children, adolescents and adults to achieve after completing ACL rehabilitation.

Return to sport: Current evidence does not support the avoidance of sport to decrease the risk for the development of early knee OA.[105,106] Properly incorporating a return-to-sport testing battery and systematic progression back to full sport participation and competition is recommended to allow for safe return to sport to decrease re-injury risk.[111] Return-to-sport test batteries should include assessments of strength, power, and both objective and self-reported function.[42,43] Timing of return to sport after ACL reconstruction should also be considered. For example, the risk of additional knee injury is reduced by 51% for each month return to sport is delayed up until nine months after ACL reconstruction.[42]

Muscle strength

Inadequate muscle strength is associated with both the development and progression of knee OA. Loss of knee extensor, or quadriceps, muscle strength is associated with an increase in the radiographic presence of OA[112] and reduced function[113,114] and increases the risk to develop OA by almost 1.65 compared with those who do not have weakness (OR 1.65, 95% CI 1.23, 2.21).[86] Men and women with low quadriceps strength have a 2.41 higher risk of radiographic knee OA compared with those with high quadriceps strength (OR 2.41, 95% CI 1.05, 7.31).[115] Addressing strength deficits is a common component of exercise programs in patients with hip and knee OA. Several large studies have investigated exercise interventions with strengthening components in patients with hip and knee OA. The Good Life with osteoArthritis in Denmark (GLA:D) is an exercise and education program that consists of 6 weeks of supervised treatment that includes patient education and neuromuscular exercise training.[116] A large analysis of the GLA:D program database of over 32,000 individuals with OA spanning three countries found that a structured exercise program was able to improve common OA-related signs and symptoms including joint pain, walking speed, and self-reported quality of life.[117] A large randomized clinical trial investigating high and low intensity strength training compared with group-based education, demonstrated no difference in pain between groups, but also no worsening of joint health with either form of strength training.[118]

Restoration of quadriceps strength is one of the primary goals after ACL injury and reconstruction[119] because of its reported associations with self-reported knee function,[120] movement patterns,[121] and re-injury risk.[42,43] Despite this, nearly 60% of young adults do not achieve 90% quadriceps strength compared with the uninjured limb despite already being cleared to return to sport.[122] Reduced quadriceps strength is related to the development of early symptomatic knee OA[123] and worse patient-reported physical function after ACL reconstruction.[124] Patients with quadriceps strength less than 85% of the uninjured limb at time of return to sport have worse cartilage T2 relaxation times, an MRI-based marker of cartilage structure and health, when compared with patients with at least 90% strength.[125] At 2 years after ACL reconstruction, quadriceps strength is associated with tibiofemoral joint cartilage volumes.[126] This emerging evidence in ACL-injured populations suggests quadriceps strength is likely a strong contributor to the development of early knee OA as it is in middle- and old-aged adult populations. In addition, quadriceps strength is an important factor for safely returning to sport.[42,43]

Recommendation after ACL Injury: Formal rehabilitation that includes muscle strengthening is recommended for individuals with OA[117] and after ACL injury and reconstruction[127] by guidelines from multiple professional organizations such as the Multicenter Orthopeadic Outcomes Network,[128] American Physical Therapy Association,[129] Dutch Orthopaedic Association,[130] and Royal Dutch Society for Physical Therapy.[131] Quadriceps strength should begin immediately after ACL injury and reconstruction, and current clinical guidelines recommend at least 90% quadriceps strength before progressing back to sports activities.[119]

Movement patterns

Gait, or walking, biomechanics have been regularly identified as an important risk factor for knee OA progression. A recent systematic review and meta-analysis found that individuals with knee OA have altered frontal plane mechanics during gait compared with healthy controls.[132] Frontal plane mechanics provide information about how joint loads are distributed across the medial and lateral compartments of the tibiofemoral joint. A greater knee adduction moment, a measurement of frontal plane mechanics, is frequently present in patients with knee OA, particularly in the presence of varus malalignment.[133] In addition, altered frontal plane knee loading during gait has been prospectively linked to future OA development in individuals with and without a history of knee injury.[134] In patients with knee OA, gait alterations designed to reduce the forces placed through the knee joint such as shifting load to the hip or leaning the trunk are evident.[135] Slower gait speed is another common altered movement pattern in individuals with knee OA.[136] Not only does slower walking speed result in impaired physical functioning, but also walking 0.2 m per second slower is associated with a 23% higher mortality risk in patients over 60 year old with radiographic knee OA.[137]

After ACL injury and reconstruction, altered movement patterns are ubiquitous and persist even after completion of rehabilitation.[138,139] Gait patterns after ACL injury are characterized by a stiffened knee pattern where knee loading and knee flexion motion are reduced. Biomechanical risk factors for knee OA differ between patients with a history of knee joint injury compared with nontraumatic mechanisms.[140] For example, although a greater knee adduction moment is associated with nontraumatic knee OA development,[133] the reduced frontal plane loading during walking has been associated with immediate worsening of cartilage T2 relaxation time on MRI[101] and radiographic OA development 5 years later.[141] However, other studies have shown different relationships between frontal plane loading and quantitative markers of cartilage health.[142,143] Sagittal plane gait biomechanics are also impacted by reduced knee flexion angles and moments present up to 40 months after ACL reconstruction, which may also be related to early knee OA development.[144] In addition, walking with varus thrust after ACL reconstruction is associated with long-term joint space narrowing in both men and women.[132,145] Walking speed, a factor in knee OA for patients without a history of knee injury,[136] may also influence early OA development after ACL reconstruction. Capin and colleagues and Pfeiffer and colleagues reported that slower walking speed was associated with worse cartilage quantitative MRI markers in the cartilage of the femoral trochlea and medial femoral condyle.[146,147]

Recommendation after ACL Injury: Improving movement patterns after ACL injury is both important and difficult. In clinical trials to improve gait mechanics after ACL reconstruction, additional perturbation training did not improve gait symmetry in men or women.[146,148] However, gait symmetry was noted to improve with perturbation versus strength training.[149] Using a metronome to force faster than self-selected gait speed also improved hip and knee joint angles during gait.[150] With regard to landing, neuromuscular training with an external focus on control improved landing movement patterns in a small sample after ACL reconstruction.[151] It is recommended that formal rehabilitation after ACL injury and reconstruction include progressive training to improve typical movement patterns.[152] A poor quality of movement should be addressed before clearance to sports activities. However, further research is needed to identify effective interventions to improve and maintain optimal movement patterns after ACL injury.

Psychological factors

Psychological well-being is often impacted in people with OA. Twenty percent of all individuals with OA report symptoms of depression,[153] as compared with estimates of close to 10% for the general population.[154] Individuals with OA and depressive symptoms report a lower quality of life,[155,156] take more medications,[156] experience higher levels of pain,[156] and have more contacts with medical providers[155,156] than individuals with OA who do not have depressive symptoms. In addition, the progression of knee OA is associated with onset of depression over time.[157] After TKA, pain catastrophizing scores explain over 50% of the variance in patient-reported outcomes.[158] There is evidence that interventions can improve psychological factors in individuals with OA. Learning pain coping skills,[159] participating in strength or multiple types of exercise,[160,161] and participating in cognitive behavioral therapy[160] have positive impacts on psychological factors in individuals with OA.

There has been increasing attention paid to the psychological wellness of individuals after ACL reconstruction. After injury and subsequent surgery, individuals often feel fear, frustration, anxiety, and lack of confidence.[162] Psychological wellness is a contributing factor to patient decisions whether to return to pre-injury activity levels and to self-perceived quality of life. A recent systematic review by Nwachukwu and colleagues reported that of the 36.6% of patients who did not return to sport after ACL reconstructions, nearly two-thirds of them cited a psychological reason for not returning.[163] Fear of re-injury was the most common psychological reason not to return, but other factors such as lack of knee confidence, depression, and lack of interest or motivation also prevented return to play. There is limited evidence on the role of psychological factors on early knee OA development after ACL injury. Filbay and colleagues have reported that radiographic knee OA 5 to 20 years after ACL reconstruction is associated with worse knee-related quality of life in symptomatic compared with asymptomatic individuals.[164] Although improving psychological wellness may not directly reduce early OA development and progression after ACL injury, it influences other OA risk factors such as participation in physical activity. For example, in individuals 28 ± 33 months after ACL reconstruction with symptoms consistent with early knee OA, greater self-reported knee quality of life is associated with greater participation in moderate to vigorous physical activity.[165]

Recommendation after ACL Injury: Tools to measure psychological factors after ACL injury and reconstruction should be serially used to identify potential barriers to recovery and patient goals, such as the Tampa Scale for Kinesiophobia,[166] Hospital Anxiety and Depression Scale,[167] ACL-Return to Sport after Injury scale,[168] and Knee Self-Efficacy Scale.[169] These outcome measures can also help clinicians identify mental health disorders where an appropriate referral to a mental health specialist is needed. Although evidence is limited, targeted strategies such as cognitive-behavioral-based treatments and advanced training programs that incorporate fear-evoking activities may facilitate participation in regular physical activity and decrease OA risks such as sedentary lifestyles and obesity.[170,171]

Comorbidities

Individuals with OA commonly have several other health conditions.[172] Diabetes mellitus is a common comorbidity in individuals with OA. However, a recent systematic review and meta-analysis of 31 studies, by Khor and colleagues, found no increased risk of developing OA in individuals who had preexisting diabetes mellitus.[173] Khor and colleagues note that obesity is one of the larger risk factors for both OA and diabetes mellitus and likely confounds the relationship between the two.[173] Cardiovascular disease is also frequently present in individuals with OA.[174] A systematic review and meta-analysis of 15 studies found that individuals with OA are three times as likely to have heart failure and twice as likely to have ischemic heart disease.[174] In a study of 4093 participants with OA, those with cardiovascular disease had a higher hazard of developing knee OA-related symptoms than people without cardiovascular disease (adjusted hazard ratio 1.5, 95% CI 1.1, 2.1).[175] Continued research is needed to fully quantify the relationship between OA and cardiovascular disease.

After ACL reconstruction, individuals who also have diabetes mellitus have a 2.6 higher odds to be rehospitalized within 90 days compared with those without diabetes (OR 2.6, 95% CI 1.9, 3.5).[176] The high risk for rehospitalization may be explained by the 18.8 increased odds of infection in individuals with diabetes mellitus who undergo ACL reconstruction compared with individuals without diabetes mellitus (OR 18.8, 95% CI 3.8, 94.0).[177] Current evidence linking ACL reconstruction and cardiovascular disease is scarce. Meehan and colleagues reported a 50% higher risk of myocardial infarction in former professional football players in the United States who sustained an ACL injury while playing compared with uninjured peers.[178] However, it is unknown if individuals with ACL injury who possess additional comorbidities have altered risk for early knee OA development.

Recommendation after ACL Injury: Given the known negative impact that ACL injury has on body mass,[72–74] physical activity,[98–100] and psychological factors, long-term monitoring for the development of metabolic or cardiovascular disease is worthy of further consideration. Although the development of metabolic or cardiovascular disease may not directly result in rapid knee OA development, the factors that contributed to the development of those diseases (eg, obesity, physical inactivity) may significantly impact the risk for early knee OA development and progression.

Occupational demands

The tasks that are required in one's job may impact the development, progression, and aggravation of OA symptoms. One in ten cases of OA is related to work.[179] Multiple systematic reviews and meta-analyses have found that lifting, kneeling, heavy lifting, and squatting as part of an individual's job requirements increase the odds of developing OA up to 7.3-fold.[180–183] Stair or ladder climbing also increases the odds for OA development up to 2.7-fold.[180,181,184] The associations between occupational demands and OA are stronger in men than women, and light work may be associated with a decreased risk of OA disease progression.[183]

After ACL reconstruction, some individuals will need to return to manual occupations that increase risk of OA development. In addition, a recent systematic review of 22 studies found that similar activities (kneeling, squatting, climbing stairs, and lifting) increase the risk of meniscal lesions.[185] This is significant because additional meniscal injury after ACL reconstruction further increases the risk of early knee OA development.[37–39]

Recommendation after ACL Injury: For patients returning to heavy manual occupations, patient education should be provided regarding the additional job-related risks for knee OA in addition to the existing risk from ACL injury. Clinicians can also make individualized recommendations to reduce specific knee stresses that an individual may be required to do as part of their employment. There have been efforts that show adding automation[186] and changing safety equipment[187] may reduce the stresses linked to OA pain and progression.

Anatomic and Surgical Considerations

Most evidence regarding the relationship between anatomic alignment and the development and progression of OA has focused on the knee joint. In the general population, varus alignment increases the odds of knee OA development up to 11.0 (OR 11.0, 95% CI 3.10, 37.8) compared with neutral or valgus alignment.[188] However, when combined with ACL injury, valgus alignment is also related to early knee OA development.[189] In addition, performing an ACL reconstruction to improve passive stability does not result in a reduced risk of OA development compared with nonsurgical management.[190] When injury to the meniscus is present, meniscus repair may reduce the risk of radiographic OA development.[191,192]

Recommendation after ACL Injury: Operative bony osteotomy can alter anatomical alignment. Recent systematic reviews have found that a high tibial osteotomy can lead to favorable outcomes in young, active patients in the absence of ACL or other injuries.[193,194] However, the combination of a high tibial osteotomy with ACL reconstruction is considered a salvage procedure and may not prevent or slow the progression of already established OA.[195] In addition, the use of high tibial osteotomy in the presence of significant posterior tibial slope or varus alignment may be completed with revision ACL reconstruction, but whether it results in superior outcomes to revision ACL reconstruction alone is unknown.[196] Because ACL reconstruction does not alter the risk for knee OA development, nonsurgical and surgical treatment options should be discussed. When concomitant meniscus injury is present, meniscal repair with ACL reconstruction may slow the progression of OA.[191,192]

SUMMARY

There are a variety of both modifiable and non-modifiable risk factors for developing OA, including early knee OA after ACL injury. Given the wide breath of knowledge required to adequately address all these factors, an interdisciplinary care team is recommended for each patient. There is an interconnectedness to the modifiable risk factors (**Fig. 1**) that demonstrate the need to address all factors to adequately reduce risk. A multifaceted, comprehensive care plan consisting of formal rehabilitation and/or

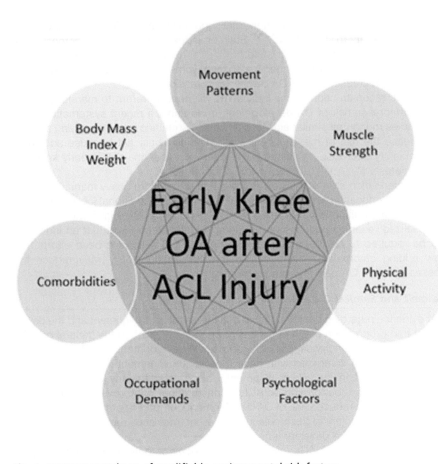

Fig. 1. Interconnectedness of modifiable environmental risk factors.

self-management strategies will be required to minimize the risk and burden of OA development and progression over time.

CLINICS CARE POINTS

- Osteoarthritis causes high costs to global society.
- Individuals with anterior cruciate ligament injury have a high risk of developing early onset knee osteoarthritis.
- There are non-modifiable risk factors for knee osteoarthritis, including previous joint injury, sociodemographic characteristics, and genetics.
- There are modifiable risk factors for knee osteoarthritis, including body mass, physical activity, muscle strength, movement patterns, psychological factors, comorbidities, occupational demands, and anatomic alignment.
- An interdisciplinary team is required to properly address all modifiable risk factors in patients at risk of developing or progression of osteoarthritis.

DISCLOSURE

There are no commercial or financial conflicts of interest to report for any of the author team.

REFERENCES

1. Safiri S, Kolahi AA, Smith E, et al. Global, regional and national burden of osteoarthritis 1990-2017: a systematic analysis of the Global Burden of Disease Study 2017. Ann Rheum Dis 2020;79(6):819–28.
2. USBaJ Inititative. The burden of musculoskeletal diseases in the United States (BMUS). 4th edition 2018.
3. Kellgren JH, Lawrence JS. Radiological assessment of osteo-arthrosis. Ann Rheum Dis 1957;16(4):494–502.
4. Wright EA, Katz JN, Cisternas MG, et al. Impact of knee osteoarthritis on health care resource utilization in a US population-based national sample. Med Care 2010;48(9):785–91.
5. Murphy LB, Cisternas MG, Pasta DJ, et al. Medical expenditures and earnings losses among US adults with arthritis in 2013. Arthritis Care Res (Hoboken) 2018;70(6):869–76.
6. Kotlarz H, Gunnarsson CL, Fang H, et al. Insurer and out-of-pocket costs of osteoarthritis in the US: evidence from national survey data. Arthritis Rheum 2009;60(12):3546–53. https://doi.org/10.1002/art.24984.
7. Kotlarz H, Gunnarsson CL, Fang H, et al. Osteoarthritis and absenteeism costs: evidence from US National Survey Data. J Occup Environ Med 2010;52(3): 263–8.
8. Osteoarthritis and you: patient information from the CDC. J Pain Palliat Care Pharmacother 2010;24(4):430–1.
9. Zhang W, Gignac MA, Beaton D, et al. Productivity loss due to presenteeism among patients with arthritis: estimates from 4 instruments. J Rheumatol 2010; 37(9):1805–14.
10. Oliveria SA, Felson DT, Reed JI, et al. Incidence of symptomatic hand, hip, and knee osteoarthritis among patients in a health maintenance organization. Arthritis Rheum 1995;38(8):1134–41.
11. Deshpande BR, Katz JN, Solomon DH, et al. Number of persons with symptomatic knee osteoarthritis in the us: impact of race and ethnicity, age, sex, and obesity. Arthritis Care Res (Hoboken) 2016;68(12):1743–50.
12. Katz JN, Arant KR, Loeser RF. Diagnosis and treatment of hip and knee osteoarthritis: a review. Jama 2021;325(6):568–78.
13. Allen KD, Thoma LM, Golightly YM. Epidemiology of osteoarthritis. Osteoarthritis Cartilage 2022;30(2):184–95.
14. Xie F, Kovic B, Jin X, et al. Economic and humanistic burden of osteoarthritis: a systematic review of large sample studies. Pharmacoeconomics 2016;34(11): 1087–100.
15. Prior JA, Jordan KP, Kadam UT. Variations in patient-reported physical health between cardiac and musculoskeletal diseases: systematic review and meta-analysis of population-based studies. Health Qual Life Outcomes 2015;13:71.
16. Park JI, Jung HH. Estimation of years lived with disability due to noncommunicable diseases and injuries using a population-representative survey. PLoS One 2017;12(2):e0172001.

17. Kurtz S, Ong K, Lau E, et al. Projections of primary and revision hip and knee arthroplasty in the United States from 2005 to 2030. J Bone Joint Surg Am 2007;89(4):780–5.

18. Whittaker JL, Runhaar J, Bierma-Zeinstra S, et al. A lifespan approach to osteoarthritis prevention. Osteoarthritis Cartilage 2021;29(12):1638–53.

19. Ravi B, Croxford R, Reichmann WM, et al. The changing demographics of total joint arthroplasty recipients in the United States and Ontario from 2001 to 2007. Best Pract Res Clin Rheumatol 2012;26(5):637–47.

20. Bayliss LE, Culliford D, Monk AP, et al. The effect of patient age at intervention on risk of implant revision after total replacement of the hip or knee: a population-based cohort study. Lancet 2017;389(10077):1424–30.

21. Brown TD, Johnston RC, Saltzman CL, et al. Posttraumatic osteoarthritis: a first estimate of incidence, prevalence, and burden of disease. J Orthop Trauma 2006;20(10):739–44.

22. Bodkin SG, Werner BC, Slater LV, et al. Post-traumatic osteoarthritis diagnosed within 5 years following ACL reconstruction. Knee Surg Sports Traumatol Arthrosc 2020;28(3):790–6.

23. Lohmander LS, Ostenberg A, Englund M, et al. High prevalence of knee osteoarthritis, pain, and functional limitations in female soccer players twelve years after anterior cruciate ligament injury. Arthritis Rheum 2004;50(10):3145–52.

24. Griffin LY, Albohm MJ, Arendt EA, et al. Understanding and preventing noncontact anterior cruciate ligament injuries: a review of the Hunt Valley II meeting, January 2005. Am J Sports Med 2006;34(9):1512–32.

25. Spector TD, MacGregor AJ. Risk factors for osteoarthritis: genetics. Osteoarthritis Cartilage 2004;12(Suppl A):S39–44.

26. Metcalfe D, Perry DC, Claireaux HA, et al. Does This Patient Have Hip Osteoarthritis?: The Rational Clinical Examination Systematic Review. Jama 2019;322(23):2323–33.

27. Pollard TCB, Batra RN, Judge A, et al. Genetic predisposition to the presence and 5-year clinical progression of hip osteoarthritis. Osteoarthritis Cartilage 2012;20(5):368–75.

28. Altman R, Alarcón G, Appelrouth D, et al. The American College of Rheumatology criteria for the classification and reporting of osteoarthritis of the hip. Arthritis Rheum 1991;34(5):505–14.

29. Valdes AM, Doherty SA, Muir KR, et al. The genetic contribution to severe posttraumatic osteoarthritis. Ann Rheum Dis 2013;72(10):1687–90.

30. Arundale AJH, Bizzini M, Giordano A, et al. Exercise-Based Knee and Anterior Cruciate Ligament Injury Prevention. J Orthop Sports Phys Ther 2018;48(9):A1–42.

31. Gourlay M, Richy F, Reginster JY. Strategies for the prevention of hip fracture. Am J Med 2003;115(4):309–17.

32. Rivera MJ, Winkelmann ZK, Powden CJ, et al. Proprioceptive Training for the Prevention of Ankle Sprains: An Evidence-Based Review. J Athl Train 2017;52(11):1065–7.

33. Lameijer CM, Ten Duis HJ, Dusseldorp IV, et al. Prevalence of posttraumatic arthritis and the association with outcome measures following distal radius fractures in non-osteoporotic patients: a systematic review. Arch Orthop Trauma Surg 2017;137(11):1499–513.

34. Cahueque M, Martínez M, Cobar A, et al. Early reduction of acetabular fractures decreases the risk of post-traumatic hip osteoarthritis? J Clin Orthop Trauma 2017;8(4):320–6.

35. Briffa N, Pearce R, Hill AM, et al. Outcomes of acetabular fracture fixation with ten years' follow-up. J Bone Joint Surg Br 2011;93(2):229–36.
36. Valderrabano V, Horisberger M, Russell I, et al. Etiology of ankle osteoarthritis. Clin Orthop Relat Res 2009;467(7):1800–6.
37. Muthuri SG, McWilliams DF, Doherty M, et al. History of knee injuries and knee osteoarthritis: a meta-analysis of observational studies. Osteoarthritis Cartilage 2011;19(11):1286–93.
38. Pernin J, Verdonk P, Si Selmi TA, et al. Long-term follow-up of 24.5 years after intra-articular anterior cruciate ligament reconstruction with lateral extra-articular augmentation. Am J Sports Med 2010;38(6):1094–102.
39. Curado J, Hulet C, Hardy P, et al. Very long-term osteoarthritis rate after anterior cruciate ligament reconstruction: 182 cases with 22-year' follow-up. Orthop Traumatol Surg Res 2020;106(3):459–63.
40. Patterson BE, Culvenor AG, Barton CJ, et al. Worsening Knee Osteoarthritis Features on Magnetic Resonance Imaging 1 to 5 Years After Anterior Cruciate Ligament Reconstruction. Am J Sports Med 2018;46(12):2873–83.
41. Svantesson E, Hamrin Senorski E, Kristiansson F, et al. Comparison of concomitant injuries and patient-reported outcome in patients that have undergone both primary and revision ACL reconstruction-a national registry study. J Orthop Surg Res 2020;15(1):9.
42. Grindem H, Snyder-Mackler L, Moksnes H, et al. Simple decision rules can reduce reinjury risk by 84% after ACL reconstruction: the Delaware-Oslo ACL cohort study. Br J Sports Med 2016;50(13):804–8.
43. Kyritsis P, Bahr R, Landreau P, et al. Likelihood of ACL graft rupture: not meeting six clinical discharge criteria before return to sport is associated with a four times greater risk of rupture. Br J Sports Med 2016;50(15):946–51.
44. Srikanth VK, Fryer JL, Zhai G, et al. A meta-analysis of sex differences prevalence, incidence and severity of osteoarthritis. Osteoarthritis Cartilage 2005; 13(9):769–81.
45. Jeong Y, Lee SW, Kim Y, et al. Relationship of sociodemographic and anthropometric characteristics, and nutrient and food intakes with osteoarthritis prevalence in elderly subjects with controlled dyslipidaemia: a cross-sectional study. Asia Pac J Clin Nutr 2019;28(4):837–44.
46. Dunlop DD, Manheim LM, Song J, et al. Arthritis prevalence and activity limitations in older adults. Arthritis Rheum 2001;44(1):212–21.
47. Callahan LF, Cleveland RJ, Shreffler J, et al. Associations of educational attainment, occupation and community poverty with knee osteoarthritis in the Johnston County (North Carolina) osteoarthritis project. Arthritis Res Ther 2011; 13(5):R169.
48. Duarte N, Rodrigues AM, Branco JDC, et al. Health and Lifestyles Factors Associated With Osteoarthritis among Older Adults in Portugal. Front Med (Lausanne) 2017;4:192.
49. Ziedas A, Abed V, Swantek A, et al. Social Determinants of Health Influence Access to Care and Outcomes in Patients Undergoing Anterior Cruciate Ligament Reconstruction: A Systematic Review. Arthroscopy 2021. https://doi.org/10.1016/j.arthro.2021.06.031.
50. Li LT, Bokshan SL, McGlone PJ, et al. Decline in Racial Disparities for United States Hospital Admissions After Anterior Cruciate Ligament Reconstruction From 2007 to 2015. Orthop J Sports Med 2020;8(11). 2325967120964473.
51. Bokshan SL, DeFroda SF, Owens BD. Risk Factors for Hospital Admission After Anterior Cruciate Ligament Reconstruction. Arthroscopy 2017;33(7):1405–11.

52. Bram JT, Talathi NS, Patel NM, et al. How Do Race and Insurance Status Affect the Care of Pediatric Anterior Cruciate Ligament Injuries? Clin J Sport Med 2020; 30(6):e201–6.
53. Perrone GS, Webster KE, Imbriaco C, et al. Risk of Secondary ACL Injury in Adolescents Prescribed Functional Bracing After ACL Reconstruction. Orthop J Sports Med 2019;7(11). 2325967119879880.
54. Webster KE, Feller JA, Leigh WB, et al. Younger patients are at increased risk for graft rupture and contralateral injury after anterior cruciate ligament reconstruction. Am J Sports Med 2014;42(3):641–7.
55. Pierce TP, Kurowicki J, Kelly JJ, et al. Risk Factors for Requiring a Revision Anterior Cruciate Ligament Reconstruction: A Case-Control Study. J Knee Surg 2021;34(8):859–63.
56. Sadigursky D, Braid JA, De Lira DNL, et al. The FIFA 11+ injury prevention program for soccer players: a systematic review. BMC Sports Sci Med Rehabil 2017;9:18.
57. Alliance OA. 2022. Available at: https://oaaction.unc.edu/resource-library/modules/.
58. Harding GT, Hubley-Kozey CL, Dunbar MJ, et al. Body mass index affects knee joint mechanics during gait differently with and without moderate knee osteoarthritis. Osteoarthritis Cartilage 2012;20(11):1234–42.
59. Eckstein F, Maschek S, Wirth W, et al. One year change of knee cartilage morphology in the first release of participants from the Osteoarthritis Initiative progression subcohort: association with sex, body mass index, symptoms and radiographic osteoarthritis status. Ann Rheum Dis 2009;68(5):674–9.
60. Bucknor MD, Nardo L, Joseph GB, et al. Association of cartilage degeneration with four year weight gain–3T MRI data from the Osteoarthritis Initiative. Osteoarthritis Cartilage 2015;23(4):525–31.
61. Culvenor AG, Felson DT, Wirth W, et al. Is local or central adiposity more strongly associated with incident knee osteoarthritis than the body mass index in men or women? Osteoarthritis Cartilage 2018;26(8):1033–7.
62. Batsis JA, Zbehlik AJ, Barre LK, et al. Impact of obesity on disability, function, and physical activity: data from the Osteoarthritis Initiative. Scand J Rheumatol 2015;44(6):495–502.
63. Messier SP, Resnik AE, Beavers DP, et al. Intentional Weight Loss in Overweight and Obese Patients With Knee Osteoarthritis: Is More Better? Arthritis Care Res (Hoboken) 2018;70(11):1569–75.
64. Messier SP, Mihalko SL, Legault C, et al. Effects of intensive diet and exercise on knee joint loads, inflammation, and clinical outcomes among overweight and obese adults with knee osteoarthritis: the IDEA randomized clinical trial. Jama 2013;310(12):1263–73.
65. Hunter DJ, Beavers DP, Eckstein F, et al. The Intensive Diet and Exercise for Arthritis (IDEA) trial: 18-month radiographic and MRI outcomes. Osteoarthritis Cartilage 2015;23(7):1090–8.
66. Salis Z, Sainsbury A, IK H, et al. Weight loss is associated with reduced risk of knee and hip replacement: a survival analysis using Osteoarthritis Initiative data. Int J Obes (Lond) 2022. https://doi.org/10.1038/s41366-021-01046-3.
67. Veronese N, Koyanagi A, Stubbs B, et al. Mediterranean diet and knee osteoarthritis outcomes: A longitudinal cohort study. Clin Nutr 2019;38(6):2735–9.
68. Chopp-Hurley JN, Wiebenga EG, Keller HH, et al. Diet and Nutrition Risk Affect Mobility and General Health in Osteoarthritis: Data from the Canadian Longitudinal Study on Aging. J Gerontol A Biol Sci Med Sci 2020;75(11):2147–55.

69. Chen SX, Bomfim FA, Youn HA, et al. Predictors of the effect of bariatric surgery on knee osteoarthritis pain. Semin Arthritis Rheum 2018;48(2):162–7.

70. Springer BD, Carter JT, McLawhorn AS, et al. Obesity and the role of bariatric surgery in the surgical management of osteoarthritis of the hip and knee: a review of the literature. Surg Obes Relat Dis 2017;13(1):111–8.

71. Üstün I, Solmaz A, Gülçiçek OB, et al. Effects of bariatric surgery on knee osteoarthritis, knee pain and quality of life in female patients. J Musculoskelet Neuronal Interact 2019;19(4):465–71.

72. Whittaker JL, Woodhouse LJ, Nettel-Aguirre A, et al. Outcomes associated with early post-traumatic osteoarthritis and other negative health consequences 3-10 years following knee joint injury in youth sport. Osteoarthritis Cartilage 2015; 23(7):1122–9.

73. Myer GD, Faigenbaum AD, Foss KB, et al. Injury initiates unfavourable weight gain and obesity markers in youth. Br J Sports Med 2014;48(20):1477–81.

74. MacAlpine EM, Talwar D, Storey EP, et al. Weight Gain After ACL Reconstruction in Pediatric and Adolescent Patients. Sports Health 2020;12(1):29–35.

75. Jones MH, Spindler KP. Risk factors for radiographic joint space narrowing and patient reported outcomes of post-traumatic osteoarthritis after ACL reconstruction: Data from the MOON cohort. J Orthop Res 2017;35(7):1366–74.

76. Kluczynski MA, Bisson LJ, Marzo JM. Does body mass index affect outcomes of ambulatory knee and shoulder surgery? Arthroscopy 2014;30(7):856–65.

77. Spindler KP, Warren TA, Callison JC Jr, et al. Clinical outcome at a minimum of five years after reconstruction of the anterior cruciate ligament. J Bone Joint Surg Am 2005;87(8):1673–9.

78. Barenius B, Ponzer S, Shalabi A, et al. Increased risk of osteoarthritis after anterior cruciate ligament reconstruction: a 14-year follow-up study of a randomized controlled trial. Am J Sports Med 2014;42(5):1049–57.

79. Fernandes L, Hagen KB, Bijlsma JW, et al. EULAR recommendations for the non-pharmacological core management of hip and knee osteoarthritis. Ann Rheum Dis 2013;72(7):1125–35.

80. Kolasinski SL, Neogi T, Hochberg MC, et al. 2019 American College of Rheumatology/Arthritis Foundation Guideline for the Management of Osteoarthritis of the Hand, Hip, and Knee. Arthritis Care Res (Hoboken) 2020;72(2):149–62.

81. Shih M, Hootman JM, Kruger J, et al. Physical activity in men and women with arthritis National Health Interview Survey, 2002. Am J Prev Med 2006;30(5): 385–93.

82. Hootman JM, Macera CA, Ham SA, et al. Physical activity levels among the general US adult population and in adults with and without arthritis. Arthritis Rheum 2003;49(1):129–35.

83. Rosemann T, Kuehlein T, Laux G, et al. Osteoarthritis of the knee and hip: a comparison of factors associated with physical activity. Clin Rheumatol 2007;26(11): 1811–7.

84. Rosemann T, Kuehlein T, Laux G, et al. Factors associated with physical activity of patients with osteoarthritis of the lower limb. J Eval Clin Pract 2008;14(2): 288–93.

85. Qin J, Barbour KE, Nevitt MC, et al. Objectively Measured Physical Activity and Risk of Knee Osteoarthritis. Med Sci Sports Exerc 2018;50(2):277–83.

86. Øiestad BE, Juhl CB, Eitzen I, et al. Knee extensor muscle weakness is a risk factor for development of knee osteoarthritis. A systematic review and meta-analysis. Osteoarthritis Cartilage 2015;23(2):171–7.

87. Master H, Thoma LM, Dunlop DD, et al. Joint Association of Moderate-to-vigorous Intensity Physical Activity and Sedentary Behavior With Incident Functional Limitation: Data From the Osteoarthritis Initiative. J Rheumatol 2021;48(9):1458–64.

88. White DK, Niu J, Zhang Y. Is symptomatic knee osteoarthritis a risk factor for a trajectory of fast decline in gait speed? Results from a longitudinal cohort study. Arthritis Care Res (Hoboken) 2013;65(2):187–94.

89. Master H, Thoma LM, Neogi T, et al. Daily Walking and the Risk of Knee Replacement Over 5 Years Among Adults With Advanced Knee Osteoarthritis in the United States. Arch Phys Med Rehabil 2021;102(10):1888–94.

90. White DK, Tudor-Locke C, Zhang Y, et al. Daily walking and the risk of incident functional limitation in knee osteoarthritis: an observational study. Arthritis Care Res (Hoboken) 2014;66(9):1328–36.

91. Fenton SAM, Neogi T, Dunlop D, et al. Does the intensity of daily walking matter for protecting against the development of a slow gait speed in people with or at high risk of knee osteoarthritis? An observational study. Osteoarthritis Cartilage 2018;26(9):1181–9.

92. White DK, Lee J, Song J, et al. Potential Functional Benefit From Light Intensity Physical Activity in Knee Osteoarthritis. Am J Prev Med 2017;53(5):689–96.

93. Kraus VB, Sprow K, Powell KE, et al. Effects of Physical Activity in Knee and Hip Osteoarthritis: A Systematic Umbrella Review. Med Sci Sports Exerc 2019;51(6):1324–39.

94. Bannuru RR, Osani MC, Vaysbrot EE, et al. OARSI guidelines for the non-surgical management of knee, hip, and polyarticular osteoarthritis. Osteoarthritis Cartilage 2019;27(11):1578–89.

95. Alentorn-Geli E, Samuelsson K, Musahl V, et al. The Association of Recreational and Competitive Running With Hip and Knee Osteoarthritis: A Systematic Review and Meta-analysis. J Orthop Sports Phys Ther 2017;47(6):373–90.

96. Timmins KA, Leech RD, Batt ME, et al. Running and Knee Osteoarthritis: A Systematic Review and Meta-analysis. Am J Sports Med 2017;45(6):1447–57.

97. Bartels EM, Juhl CB, Christensen R, et al. Aquatic exercise for the treatment of knee and hip osteoarthritis. Cochrane Database Syst Rev 2016;3:Cd005523.

98. Bell DR, Pfeiffer KA, Cadmus-Bertram LA, et al. Objectively Measured Physical Activity in Patients After Anterior Cruciate Ligament Reconstruction. Am J Sports Med 2017;45(8):1893–900.

99. Triplett AN, Kuenze CM. Characterizing body composition, cardiorespiratory fitness, and physical activity in women with anterior cruciate ligament reconstruction. Phys Ther Sport 2021;48:54–9.

100. Kuenze C, Lisee C, Pfeiffer KA, et al. Sex differences in physical activity engagement after ACL reconstruction. Phys Ther Sport 2019;35:12–7.

101. Wellsandt E, Kallman T, Golightly Y, et al. Knee joint unloading and daily physical activity associate with cartilage T2 relaxation times 1 month after ACL injury. J Orthop Res 2021. https://doi.org/10.1002/jor.25034.

102. Feucht MJ, Cotic M, Saier T, et al. Patient expectations of primary and revision anterior cruciate ligament reconstruction. Knee Surg Sports Traumatol Arthrosc 2016;24(1):201–7.

103. Ardern CL, Webster KE, Taylor NF, et al. Return to sport following anterior cruciate ligament reconstruction surgery: a systematic review and meta-analysis of the state of play. Br J Sports Med 2011;45(7):596–606.

104. Lai CCH, Feller JA, Webster KE. Fifteen-Year Audit of Anterior Cruciate Ligament Reconstructions in the Australian Football League From 1999 to 2013: Return to Play and Subsequent ACL Injury. Am J Sports Med 2018;46(14):3353–60.

105. Haberfield MJ, Patterson BE, Crossley KM, et al. Should return to pivoting sport be avoided for the secondary prevention of osteoarthritis after anterior cruciate ligament reconstruction? A prospective cohort study with MRI, radiographic and symptomatic outcomes. Osteoarthritis Cartilage 2021;29(12):1673–81.

106. Øiestad BE, Holm I, Risberg MA. Return to pivoting sport after ACL reconstruction: association with osteoarthritis and knee function at the 15-year follow-up. Br J Sports Med 2018;52(18):1199–204.

107. Kuenze C, Collins K, Pfeiffer KA, et al. Assessing Physical Activity After ACL Injury: Moving Beyond Return to Sport. Sports Health 2021. https://doi.org/10.1177/19417381211025307.

108. Kuenze C, Cadmus-Bertram L, Pfieffer K, et al. Relationship Between Physical Activity and Clinical Outcomes After ACL Reconstruction. J Sport Rehabil 2019;28(2):180–7.

109. Gay C, Chabaud A, Guilley E, et al. Educating patients about the benefits of physical activity and exercise for their hip and knee osteoarthritis. Systematic literature review. Ann Phys Rehabil Med 2016;59(3):174–83.

110. Physical activity guidelines for Americans. 2nd edition. US Department of Health and Human Services; 2021. Available at: http://www.health.gov/PAGuidelines. Accessed January 15, 2022.

111. Filbay SR, Grindem H. Evidence-based recommendations for the management of anterior cruciate ligament (ACL) rupture. Best Pract Res Clin Rheumatol 2019; 33(1):33–47.

112. Kemnitz J, Wirth W, Eckstein F, et al. Longitudinal change in thigh muscle strength prior to and concurrent with symptomatic and radiographic knee osteoarthritis progression: data from the Osteoarthritis Initiative. Osteoarthritis Cartilage 2017;25(10):1633 40.

113. Ruhdorfer A, Wirth W, Eckstein F. Longitudinal Change in Thigh Muscle Strength Prior to and Concurrent With Minimum Clinically Important Worsening or Improvement in Knee Function: Data From the Osteoarthritis Initiative. Arthritis Rheumatol 2016;68(4):826–36.

114. Glass NA, Torner JC, Frey Law LA, et al. The relationship between quadriceps muscle weakness and worsening of knee pain in the MOST cohort: a 5-year longitudinal study. Osteoarthritis Cartilage 2013;21(9):1154–9.

115. Takagi S, Omori G, Koga H, et al. Quadriceps muscle weakness is related to increased risk of radiographic knee OA but not its progression in both women and men: the Matsudai Knee Osteoarthritis Survey. Knee Surg Sports Traumatol Arthrosc 2018;26(9):2607–14.

116. Good Life with osteoArthritis in Denmark. 2022. Available at: https://gladinternational.org/.

117. Roos EM, Grønne DT, Skou ST, et al. Immediate outcomes following the GLA:D® program in Denmark, Canada and Australia. A longitudinal analysis including 28,370 patients with symptomatic knee or hip osteoarthritis. Osteoarthritis Cartilage 2021;29(4):502–6.

118. Messier SP, Mihalko SL, Beavers DP, et al. Effect of High-Intensity Strength Training on Knee Pain and Knee Joint Compressive Forces Among Adults With Knee Osteoarthritis: The START Randomized Clinical Trial. Jama Feb 16 2021;325(7):646–57. https://doi.org/10.1001/jama.2021.0411.

119. Brinlee AW, Dickenson SB, Hunter-Giordano A, et al. ACL Reconstruction Rehabilitation: Clinical Data, Biologic Healing, and Criterion-Based Milestones to Inform a Return-to-Sport Guideline. Sports Health 2021. 19417381211056873.

120. Pietrosimone B, Lepley AS, Harkey MS, et al. Quadriceps Strength Predicts Self-reported Function Post-ACL Reconstruction. Med Sci Sports Exerc 2016;48(9): 1671–7.

121. Ithurburn MP, Paterno MV, Ford KR, et al. Young Athletes With Quadriceps Femoris Strength Asymmetry at Return to Sport After Anterior Cruciate Ligament Reconstruction Demonstrate Asymmetric Single-Leg Drop-Landing Mechanics. Am J Sports Med 2015;43(11):2727–37.

122. Toole AR, Ithurburn MP, Rauh MJ, et al. Young Athletes Cleared for Sports Participation After Anterior Cruciate Ligament Reconstruction: How Many Actually Meet Recommended Return-to-Sport Criterion Cutoffs? J Orthop Sports Phys Ther 2017;47(11):825–33.

123. Arhos EK, Thoma LM, Grindem H, et al. Association of Quadriceps Strength Symmetry and Surgical Status with Clinical Osteoarthritis 5 Years after Anterior Cruciate Ligament Rupture. Arthritis Care Res (Hoboken) 2020. https://doi.org/10.1002/acr.24479.

124. Van Wyngaarden JJ, Jacobs C, Thompson K, et al. Quadriceps Strength and Kinesiophobia Predict Long-Term Function After ACL Reconstruction: A Cross-Sectional Pilot Study. Sports Health 2021;13(3):251–7.

125. Brunst C, Ithurburn MP, Zbojniewicz AM, et al. Return-to-sport quadriceps strength symmetry impacts 5-year cartilage integrity after anterior cruciate ligament reconstruction: A preliminary analysis. J Orthop Res 2022;40(1):285–94.

126. Hipsley A, Hall M, Saxby DJ, et al. Quadriceps muscle strength at 2 years following anterior cruciate ligament reconstruction is associated with tibiofemoral joint cartilage volume. Knee Surg Sports Traumatol Arthrosc 2022. https://doi.org/10.1007/s00167-021-06853-9.

127. Andrade R, Pereira R, van Cingel R, et al. How should clinicians rehabilitate patients after ACL reconstruction? A systematic review of clinical practice guidelines (CPGs) with a focus on quality appraisal (AGREE II). Br J Sports Med 2020;54(9):512–9. https://doi.org/10.1136/bjsports-2018-100310.

128. Wright RW, Haas AK, Anderson J, et al. Anterior Cruciate Ligament Reconstruction Rehabilitation: MOON Guidelines. Sports Health 2015;7(3):239–43.

129. Logerstedt DS, Scalzitti D, Risberg MA, et al. Knee Stability and Movement Coordination Impairments: Knee Ligament Sprain Revision 2017. J Orthop Sports Phys Ther 2017;47(11):A1–47.

130. Meuffels DE, Poldervaart MT, Diercks RL, et al. Guideline on anterior cruciate ligament injury. Acta Orthop 2012;83(4):379–836.

131. van Melick N, van Cingel RE, Brooijmans F, et al. Evidence-based clinical practice update: practice guidelines for anterior cruciate ligament rehabilitation based on a systematic review and multidisciplinary consensus. Br J Sports Med 2016;50(24):1506–15.

132. van Tunen JAC, Dell'Isola A, Juhl C, et al. Association of malalignment, muscular dysfunction, proprioception, laxity and abnormal joint loading with tibiofemoral knee osteoarthritis - a systematic review and meta-analysis. BMC Musculoskelet Disord 2018;19(1):273.

133. Foroughi N, Smith R, Vanwanseele B. The association of external knee adduction moment with biomechanical variables in osteoarthritis: a systematic review. Knee 2009;16(5):303–9.

134. Bennell KL, Bowles KA, Wang Y, et al. Higher dynamic medial knee load predicts greater cartilage loss over 12 months in medial knee osteoarthritis. Ann Rheum Dis 2011;70(10):1770–4.

135. Iijima H, Shimoura K, Ono T, et al. Proximal gait adaptations in individuals with knee osteoarthritis: A systematic review and meta-analysis. J Biomech 2019;87: 127–41.

136. Ismailidis P, Hegglin L, Egloff C, et al. Side to side kinematic gait differences within patients and spatiotemporal and kinematic gait differences between patients with severe knee osteoarthritis and controls measured with inertial sensors. Gait Posture 2021;84:24–30.

137. Master H, Neogi T, Callahan LF, et al. The association between walking speed from short- and standard-distance tests with the risk of all-cause mortality among adults with radiographic knee osteoarthritis: data from three large United States cohort studies. Osteoarthritis Cartilage 2020;28(12):1551–8.

138. Hart HF, Culvenor AG, Collins NJ, et al. Knee kinematics and joint moments during gait following anterior cruciate ligament reconstruction: a systematic review and meta-analysis. Br J Sports Med 2016;50(10):597–612.

139. Ismail SA, Button K, Simic M, et al. Three-dimensional kinematic and kinetic gait deviations in individuals with chronic anterior cruciate ligament deficient knee: A systematic review and meta-analysis. Clin Biomech (Bristol, Avon) 2016;35: 68–80.

140. Robbins SM, Pelletier JP, Abram F, et al. Gait risk factors for disease progression differ between non-traumatic and post-traumatic knee osteoarthritis. Osteoarthritis Cartilage 2021;29(11):1487–97.

141. Wellsandt E, Gardinier ES, Manal K, et al. Decreased Knee Joint Loading Associated With Early Knee Osteoarthritis After Anterior Cruciate Ligament Injury. Am J Sports Med 2016;44(1):143–51.

142. Titchenal MR, Williams AA, Chehab EF, et al. Cartilage Subsurface Changes to Magnetic Resonance Imaging UTE-T2* 2 Years After Anterior Cruciate Ligament Reconstruction Correlate With Walking Mechanics Associated With Knee Osteoarthritis. Am J Sports Med 2018;46(3):565–72.

143. Kumar D, Su F, Wu D, et al. Frontal Plane Knee Mechanics and Early Cartilage Degeneration in People With Anterior Cruciate Ligament Reconstruction: A Longitudinal Study. Am J Sports Med 2018;46(2):378–87.

144. Slater LV, Hart JM, Kelly AR, et al. Progressive Changes in Walking Kinematics and Kinetics After Anterior Cruciate Ligament Injury and Reconstruction: A Review and Meta-Analysis. J Athl Train 2017;52(9):847–60.

145. Sharma L, Chang AH, Jackson RD, et al. Varus Thrust and Incident and Progressive Knee Osteoarthritis. Arthritis Rheumatol 2017;69(11):2136–43.

146. Capin JJ, Zarzycki R, Ito N, et al. Gait mechanics in women of the ACL-SPORTS randomized control trial: interlimb symmetry improves over time regardless of treatment group. J Orthop Res 2019;37(8):1743–53.

147. Pfeiffer S, Harkey MS, Stanley LE, et al. Associations Between Slower Walking Speed and T1ρ Magnetic Resonance Imaging of Femoral Cartilage Following Anterior Cruciate Ligament Reconstruction. Arthritis Care Res (Hoboken) 2018;70(8):1132–40.

148. Capin JJ, Zarzycki R, Arundale A, et al. Report of the primary outcomes for gait mechanics in men of the ACL-SPORTS trial: secondary prevention with and without perturbation training does not restore gait symmetry in men 1 or 2 years after ACL reconstruction. Clin Orthop Relat Res 2017;475(10):2513–22.

149. Hartigan E, Axe MJ, Snyder-Mackler L. Perturbation training prior to ACL reconstruction improves gait asymmetries in non-copers. J Orthop Res 2009;27(6): 724–9.

150. Decker MJ, Torry MR, Noonan TJ, et al. Gait retraining after anterior cruciate ligament reconstruction. Arch Phys Med Rehabil 2004;85(5):848–56.

151. Ghaderi M, Letafatkar A, Thomas AC, et al. Effects of a neuromuscular training program using external focus attention cues in male athletes with anterior cruciate ligament reconstruction: a randomized clinical trial. BMC Sports Sci Med Rehabil 2021;13(1):49.

152. Buckthorpe M. Recommendations for Movement Re-training After ACL Reconstruction. Sports Med 2021;51(8):1601–18.

153. Stubbs B, Aluko Y, Myint PK, et al. Prevalence of depressive symptoms and anxiety in osteoarthritis: a systematic review and meta-analysis. Age Ageing 2016; 45(2):228–35.

154. Sjöberg L, Karlsson B, Atti AR, et al. Prevalence of depression: Comparisons of different depression definitions in population-based samples of older adults. J Affect Disord 2017;221:123–31.

155. Rosemann T, Gensichen J, Sauer N, et al. The impact of concomitant depression on quality of life and health service utilisation in patients with osteoarthritis. Rheumatol Int 2007;27(9):859–63.

156. Sharma A, Kudesia P, Shi Q, et al. Anxiety and depression in patients with osteoarthritis: impact and management challenges. Open Access Rheumatol 2016; 8:103–13.

157. Rathbun AM, Shardell MD, Ryan AS, et al. Association between disease progression and depression onset in persons with radiographic knee osteoarthritis. Rheumatology (Oxford) 2020;59(11):3390–9.

158. Giesinger JM, Kuster MS, Behrend H, et al. Association of psychological status and patient-reported physical outcome measures in joint arthroplasty: a lack of divergent validity. Health Qual Life Outcomes 2013;11:64.

159. Wang L, Zhang L, Yang L, et al. Effectiveness of pain coping skills training on pain, physical function, and psychological outcomes in patients with osteoarthritis: A systemic review and meta-analysis. Clin Rehabil 2021;35(3):342–55.

160. Briani RV, Ferreira AS, Pazzinatto MF, et al. What interventions can improve quality of life or psychosocial factors of individuals with knee osteoarthritis? A systematic review with meta-analysis of primary outcomes from randomised controlled trials. Br J Sports Med 2018;52(16):1031–8.

161. Hall M, Dobson F, Van Ginckel A, et al. Comparative effectiveness of exercise programs for psychological well-being in knee osteoarthritis: A systematic review and network meta-analysis. Semin Arthritis Rheum 2021;51(5):1023–32.

162. Truong LK, Mosewich AD, Holt CJ, et al. Psychological, social and contextual factors across recovery stages following a sport-related knee injury: a scoping review. Br J Sports Med 2020;54(19):1149–56.

163. Nwachukwu BU, Adjei J, Rauck RC, et al. How Much Do Psychological Factors Affect Lack of Return to Play After Anterior Cruciate Ligament Reconstruction? A Systematic Review. Orthop J Sports Med 2019;7(5). 2325967119845313.

164. Filbay SR, Ackerman IN, Dhupelia S, et al. Quality of Life in Symptomatic Individuals After Anterior Cruciate Ligament Reconstruction, With and Without Radiographic Knee Osteoarthritis. J Orthop Sports Phys Ther 2018;48(5): 398–408.

165. Davis-Wilson HC, Thoma LM, Longobardi L, et al. Quality of Life Associates With Moderate to Vigorous Physical Activity Following Anterior Cruciate Ligament Reconstruction. J Athl Train 2021. https://doi.org/10.4085/1062-6050-0670.20.
166. Miller RP, Kori S, Todd D. The Tampa Scale: A measure of kinesiophobia. Clin J Pain 1991;7(1):51–2.
167. Zigmond AS, Snaith RP. The hospital anxiety and depression scale. Acta Psychiatr Scand 1983;67(6):361–70.
168. Webster KE, Feller JA. Development and Validation of a Short Version of the Anterior Cruciate Ligament Return to Sport After Injury (ACL-RSI) Scale. Orthop J Sports Med 2018;6(4). 2325967118763763.
169. Thomeé P, Währborg P, Börjesson M, et al. A new instrument for measuring self-efficacy in patients with an anterior cruciate ligament injury. Scand J Med Sci Sports 2006;16(3):181–7.
170. Meierbachtol A, Obermeier M, Yungtum W, et al. Advanced training enhances readiness to return to sport after anterior cruciate ligament reconstruction. J Orthop Res 2022;40(1):191–9.
171. Coronado RA, Sterling EK, Fenster DE, et al. Cognitive-behavioral-based physical therapy to enhance return to sport after anterior cruciate ligament reconstruction: An open pilot study. Phys Ther Sport 2020;42:82–90.
172. Calders P, Van Ginckel A. Presence of comorbidities and prognosis of clinical symptoms in knee and/or hip osteoarthritis: A systematic review and meta-analysis. Semin Arthritis Rheum 2018;47(6):805–13.
173. Khor A, Ma CA, Hong C, et al. Diabetes mellitus is not a risk factor for osteoarthritis. RMD Open 2020;6(1). https://doi.org/10.1136/rmdopen-2019-001030.
174. Hall AJ, Stubbs B, Mamas MA, et al. Association between osteoarthritis and cardiovascular disease: Systematic review and meta-analysis. Eur J Prev Cardiol 2016;23(9):938–46.
175. Golightly YM, Alvarez C, Arbeeva LS, et al. Associations of Comorbid Conditions and Transitions Across States of Knee Osteoarthritis in a Community-Based Cohort. ACR Open Rheumatol 2021;3(8):512–21.
176. Best MJ, Harris AB, Marrache M, et al. Risk Factors for Readmission following Anterior Cruciate Ligament Reconstruction. J Knee Surg 2021. https://doi.org/10.1055/s-0041-1736200.
177. Brophy RH, Wright RW, Huston LJ, et al. Factors associated with infection following anterior cruciate ligament reconstruction. J Bone Joint Surg Am 2015;97(6):450–4.
178. Meehan WP, Weisskopf MG, Krishnan S, et al. Relation of Anterior Cruciate Ligament Tears to Potential Chronic Cardiovascular diseases. Am J Cardiol 2018;122(11):1879–84.
179. van der Molen HF, Hulshof CT, Kuijer PPF. How to improve the assessment of the impact of occupational diseases at a national level? The Netherlands as an example. Occup Environ Med 2019;76(1):30–2.
180. Jensen LK. Knee osteoarthritis: influence of work involving heavy lifting, kneeling, climbing stairs or ladders, or kneeling/squatting combined with heavy lifting. Occup Environ Med 2008;65(2):72–89.
181. Palmer KT. Occupational activities and osteoarthritis of the knee. Br Med Bull 2012;102:147–70.
182. McWilliams DF, Leeb BF, Muthuri SG, et al. Occupational risk factors for osteoarthritis of the knee: a meta-analysis. Osteoarthritis Cartilage 2011;19(7):829–39.

183. Perry TA, Wang X, Gates L, et al. Occupation and risk of knee osteoarthritis and knee replacement: A longitudinal, multiple-cohort study. Semin Arthritis Rheum 2020;50(5):1006–14.

184. Verbeek J, Mischke C, Robinson R, et al. Occupational Exposure to Knee Loading and the Risk of Osteoarthritis of the Knee: A Systematic Review and a Dose-Response Meta-Analysis. Saf Health Work 2017;8(2):130–42.

185. Bahns C, Bolm-Audorff U, Seidler A, et al. Occupational risk factors for meniscal lesions: a systematic review and meta-analysis. BMC Musculoskelet Disord 2021;22(1):1042.

186. Visser S, van der Molen HF, Kuijer PP, et al. Stand up: comparison of two electrical screed levelling machines to reduce the work demands for the knees and low back among floor layers. Ergonomics 2016;59(9):1224–31.

187. Xu H, Jampala S, Bloswick D, et al. Evaluation of knee joint forces during kneeling work with different kneepads. Appl Ergon 2017;58:308–13.

188. Bastick AN, Belo JN, Runhaar J, et al. What Are the Prognostic Factors for Radiographic Progression of Knee Osteoarthritis? A Meta-analysis. Clin Orthop Relat Res 2015;473(9):2969–89.

189. Robbins SM, Raymond N, Abram F, et al. The effect of alignment on knee osteoarthritis initiation and progression differs based on anterior cruciate ligament status: data from the Osteoarthritis Initiative. Clin Rheumatol 2019;38(12):3557–66.

190. Smith TO, Postle K, Penny F, et al. Is reconstruction the best management strategy for anterior cruciate ligament rupture? A systematic review and meta-analysis comparing anterior cruciate ligament reconstruction versus non-operative treatment. Knee 2014;21(2):462–70.

191. Petersen W, Karpinski K, Bierke S, et al. A systematic review about long-term results after meniscus repair. Arch Orthop Trauma Surg 2021. https://doi.org/10.1007/s00402-021-03906-z.

192. Wang L, Zhang K, Liu X, et al. The efficacy of meniscus posterior root tears repair: A systematic review and meta-analysis. J Orthop Surg (Hong Kong) 2021;29(1). 23094990211003350.

193. Santoso MB, Wu L. Unicompartmental knee arthroplasty, is it superior to high tibial osteotomy in treating unicompartmental osteoarthritis? A meta-analysis and systemic review. J Orthop Surg Res 2017;12(1):50.

194. Belsey J, Yasen SK, Jobson S, et al. Return to Physical Activity After High Tibial Osteotomy or Unicompartmental Knee Arthroplasty: A Systematic Review and Pooling Data Analysis. Am J Sports Med 2021;49(5):1372–80.

195. Stride D, Wang J, Horner NS, et al. Indications and outcomes of simultaneous high tibial osteotomy and ACL reconstruction. Knee Surg Sports Traumatol Arthrosc 2019;27(4):1320–31.

196. Gupta A, Tejpal T, Shanmugaraj A, et al. Surgical Techniques, Outcomes, Indications, and Complications of Simultaneous High Tibial Osteotomy and Anterior Cruciate Ligament Revision Surgery: A Systematic Review. HSS J 2019;15(2):176–84.

Targeting Environmental Risks to Prevent Rheumatic Disease

Kevin D. Deane, MD, PhD

KEYWORDS

- Rheumatic disease • Environmental risk factors • Prevention • Public health
- Preclinical rheumatic disease • Personalized prevention

KEY POINTS

- Targeting environmental factors may result in decreased incidence of the clinical onset of rheumatic diseases (RDs).
- Broad public health measures may reduce the incidence of RDs.
- An ability to identify an individual who is at high-risk for a future RD may allow for personalization of environmental modification to prevent disease.
- Environmental risk factor modification may be an important addition to pharmacologic interventions in RD prevention.

BACKGROUND

Prevention is an important goal for a variety of health conditions. Although typically thought about in diseases such as infections, cardiovascular diseases, and cancer, there are also efforts for prevention in rheumatic diseases (RDs). In particular, clinicians have long sought to prevent the worsening of a primary RD or to prevent the development and impact of comorbidities in individuals with an established clinical diagnosis of an RD. For example, in individuals with rheumatoid arthritis (RA), therapies are initiated to control disease and prevent future joint destruction. Individuals with gout can be counseled to reduce or eliminate risk factors such as alcohol consumption to prevent future flares of acute arthritis. Furthermore, across a wide range of RDs, lifestyle changes and pharmacologic treatments are recommended to prevent future osteoporotic fractures or reduce risk for cardiovascular disease events, and vaccines are given to prevent adverse outcomes from infections.

However, there is also an emerging understanding that for many RDs there is a "predisease" state that is highly predictive of future development of clinically-apparent disease. This has culminated in a general model of RD development presented in **Fig. 1**.

Division of Rheumatology, University of Colorado Denver Anschutz Medical Campus, Barbara Davis Center (M20), 1775 Aurora Court, Mail Stop B-115, Aurora, CO 80045, USA
E-mail address: kevin.deane@cuanschutz.edu

Rheum Dis Clin N Am 48 (2022) 931–943
https://doi.org/10.1016/j.rdc.2022.06.011
0889-857X/22/© 2022 Elsevier Inc. All rights reserved.

In this model, genetic and environmental factors trigger processes that over time can propagate and lead to clinically-apparent symptoms and findings, and a diagnosis of a particular RD.

Depending on the type of RD, the initiating and propagating processes can be auto-immune such as the development of breaks in tolerance (eg, autoantibodies in RA or lupus). In particular, for RA, multiple studies have demonstrated that disease-related autoantibodies such as rheumatoid factor (RF) and antibodies to citrullinated protein antigens (ACPA) can be abnormal on-average 3 to 5 years before the onset of clinically-apparent inflammatory arthritis.[1] In addition, in lupus, disease-related auto-antibodies such as antinuclear antibodies (ANAs) have been identified years before the first clinically-apparent manifestations of disease,[2] and similar findings have been demonstrated in scleroderma[3] and some forms of vasculitis.[4] For other RDs such as gout, "preclinical" processes can involve rising uric acid, and in osteoarthritis (OA), preclinical processes may be subtle cartilage damage.

Importantly, predisease states can be identified through biomarker testing as well as or other approaches that include genetic testing, family history, and even early nonspecific symptoms, and in some cases imaging. Although additional studies are needed, in many situations, this allows for fairly accurate identification of individuals who are at high risk for personally progressing to a clinically-apparent RD.

Of further importance, the ability to identify individuals who are at high-risk for a future RD makes the identification of modifiable factors—either environmental or phar-macologic—highly relevant for personal preventive interventions that can be designed to prevent the first clinically-apparent manifestations of an RD. For example, interven-tions to prevent the first swollen joint in RA or prevent the development of psoriatic arthritis in an individual with existing psoriatic skin disease.

Indeed, there are research efforts underway to identify individuals who exhibit some degree of immune dysregulation/abnormality and are therefore at high-risk for pro-gression to a clinically-apparent RD, and then identify effective approaches to prevent progression to additional manifestations of disease. These include multiple completed or ongoing clinical trials of pharmacologic interventions for the prevention of the first onset of clinically-apparent inflammatory arthritis in individuals at high-risk for RA development because they have serum elevations of RA-related autoantibodies (e.g. ACPA)[5–10] (and reviewed in ref[11]). In addition, there are clinical trials studies un-derway or in development to use pharmacologic agents to prevent progression to pre-vent new clinically-apparent manifestations in lupus,[12] as well as transition from psoriatic skin disease to clinically-apparent arthritis,[13] and in prevention of OA.[14]

These approaches to prevention of the first clinically-apparent onset of RDs are thus far largely based on pharmacologic interventions. However, there is also a great po-tential to develop environmental factor-targeted approaches for prevention. In partic-ular, addressing environmental risk factors for disease progression may be critically important adjuvant approaches to pharmacologic interventions for prevention, as well as stand-alone interventions.

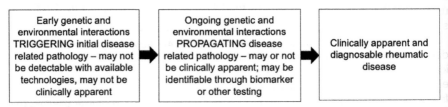

Fig. 1. Natural history of development of rheumatic diseases.

With these issues in mind, the following discussion will review the importance of understanding disease stage-specific environmental risk factors, discussion of public health-level interventions and targeting high-risk individuals with "personalized" modification of environmental factors, and additional challenges and opportunities to use modifications of environmental factors to implement RD prevention (**Boxes 1** and **2**).

Understanding Mechanisms and Stage-specific Environmental Risk Factors in the Development of Rheumatic Diseases

There are numerous published studies identifying environmental risk factors that are associated with a wide range of RDs. Some examples are associations of exposure to tobacco smoke and occupational dust within increased risk for RA as well as other RDs,[15] obesity and lack of exercise associated within increased risk for RDs,[16–18] dietary factors such as increased intake of saturated fats and salt with increased risk for several RDs,[19] protection from the development of RDs associated with diets such as the Mediterranean diet,[20] and exposures to pesticides with increased risk for several RDs including RA and lupus.[21] Furthermore, certain dietary patterns have been shown to be associated with reduced risk for incident gout (eg, dietary approaches to stop hypertension diet[22]). In addition, some factors likely related to some extent to environmental exposures are associated with decreased risk for RDs; some examples include studies that suggest lower vitamin D levels are associated with increased risk for several RDs,[23] and multiple studies have found that modest alcohol intake is protective against the future development of RA.[24,25]

There are also more specific environmental exposures that are associated with the subsequent development of an RD; these include medication-induced RDs such as drug-induced lupus and vasculitis,[26,27] as well as exposures to toxic oils resulting in eosinophilic fasciitis.[28] Furthermore, if one considers microbial factors as "environmental," rheumatic fever that results from infection with certain Streptococcal strains can be considered an environmentally caused RD.[29] There is also a large body of literature supporting certain infections as "triggers" of reactive arthritis, and there is growing data that organisms such as *Prevotella* may play a role in the development of RA,[30,31] and that viral infections such as Epstein Barr virus (EBV) may play a role in the pathogenesis of several RDs,[32,33] as well as other autoimmune diseases such as multiple sclerosis.[34] Indeed, the area of microbial influences with or without mucosal inflammation as triggering and propagating factors in RD development is advancing rapidly[35,36]; however, there remain challenges and controversies in determining if microbiomes truly trigger and propagate RDs, or are secondarily altered as part of the primary RD processes.

Broad Public Health Environmental Interventions to Prevent Rheumatic Diseases

In aggregate, the understanding that certain environmental factors may trigger and/or propagate RDs has led to hope that these factors could be manipulated to reduce the first onset of clinical RDs **Boxes 1 2**. This could be applied in a large population-based approach to reduce incident RDs. For example, based on observational data, tobacco use cessation programs and promotion of exercise, healthy weights, and potentially specific diets (eg, Mediterranean) may reduce the incidence of many RDs.

A caveat is that most data associating environmental factors with the risk for RDs is derived from observational studies. Ideally, one would have data from controlled clinical trials of environmental interventions to "prove" that a particular intervention was effective at reducing risk for a future RA as well as support robust recommendations from public health agencies that make policy and guidelines for populations (eg, World Health Organization, the USA-based Department of Health and Human Services, and the Department of Agriculture). However, such trials are costly and could take years to complete. As such, although there is limited data from interventional studies that these approaches are effective to reduce risk for RDs, these approaches could be goals for public health entities especially given modification of risk factors for RDs also have broad health benefits for society. These could include policies to reduce exposures to factors such as tobacco, toxic oils, and occupational dust, as well as diet and exercise recommendations—and indeed many of these interventions/recommendations are already in place, although not specifically for the prevention of RDs. Ultimately, such broad public health approaches to RD prevention may also include interventions directed toward specific infections; for example, if EBV is proven to be an etiologic factor in RDs, then vaccines may lead to RD prevention (as well as improvements incidence of other EBV-related diseases such as nasopharyngeal and others cancers[37]). Importantly, a further challenge is uptake of such recommendations by the general public, especially because it is already difficult to implement these general health strategies for the prevention of high prevalence diseases such as diabetes, heart disease, and cancer.[38,39]

Personalized Risk Assessment and Environmental Interventions to Prevent Rheumatic diseases

Beyond broad public health measures, the growing ability to identify specific individuals as being at increased risk for a future RD although approaches such as identifying a family history of an RD, and/or testing for circulating biomarkers or other factors has also led to excitement about personalizing preventive approaches in such high-risk individuals (see **Boxes 1 and 2**)

Box 1
Levels of targeting environmental factors for rheumatic disease prevention

Large-scale public health
- Examples: tobacco cessation, population-wide recommendations on diet and exercise, regulation of toxins and protection from occupational exposures, vaccines (?)

Personalized risk assessment and environment modification
- May include assessment of family history, and genetic and biomarker testing for a specific rheumatic disease, as well as personalized assessment of environmental risk factors
- Includes a tailored approach to prevention based on personal factor

---

Box 2
Steps to implementing targeting environmental factors for rheumatic disease prevention

- Demonstrate that an environmental factor is related to the development of rheumatic disease
  Includes understanding mechanisms, gene-environment interactions, andrisk estimations (population level and individual level)

- Demonstrate that altering that factor improves outcomes
  Outcomes may be clinical disease or surrogate biomarkers

- Demonstrate that interventions have public health benefit

- Identify barriers and facilitators to implementation of preventive strategies (ie, implementation science)

Importantly though, many of the studies that have identified certain environmental risk factors for RDs have been performed in a case-control manner where groups of individuals with well-established RDs are compared in a cross-sectional fashion to individuals without RDs. These may lead to important and "true" findings of relationships between an exposure and an RD and may help support public health measures targeting environmental factors to reduce RDs. However, if RDs have a preclinical stage (see **Fig. 1**), it may also be that the environmental factors that affect the disease development are acting years before the symptomatic onset and diagnosis of a disease; furthermore, the factors that were identified as related to disease by studying individuals with clinical diagnoses may not truly be relevant in earlier triggering and propagating stages.

Although data are limited in "preclinical" RDs, some studies do support that environmental factors truly precede the development of RDs; for example, use of hydralazine before the development of drug-induced lupus (and resolution of lupus with drug cessation).[26] There are also robust data suggesting that exposure to tobacco smoke precedes in the development of clinically-apparent RA,[40–42] although in both of these situations, the exact pathologic mechanisms by-which the environmental factor drives disease is unknown.

It may also be that there are some factors that drive early initiation of pathologic processes of an RD, and similar or different factors that drive a later propagation from a preclinical state to full-blown disease with clinical manifestations that are diagnosable as an RD. This can be critically important if an individual is identified in the "preclinical" stage of disease by methods such as a circulating autoantibody, and one may wish to alter an environmental factor in this specific high-risk individual to prevent them from progressing further to clinically-apparent disease. In such a scenario, one would need to know if a certain factor either was meaningful in preventing further progression or had already acted to trigger initial autoimmunity and therefore would not be productive to address because it is no longer driving the disease progression. An example is exposure to tobacco and the risk for future RA. Some data support that exposure to tobacco may trigger early RA-related autoimmunity and early symptoms but that other factors are needed for the transition to clinically-apparent inflammatory arthritis.[40] A caveat to this example is that the full story of RA development related to smoking is not yet understood; however, the concept here is that an intervention for smoking cessation may be useful in reducing early RA-related immunity but not as useful in reducing an individual's risk from progressing from a preclinical state to clinical disease once some degree of immune dysfunction has already developed. Another (and somewhat hypothetical) example is that if indeed microbes are part of triggering initial autoimmunity in an RD; it may be that once circulating autoimmunity has developed, a certain microbe no longer plays a role in disease progression; as such, intervening on that microbe may not have any effect on the development of clinical disease.

Importantly, it may well be that for each RD there are differing environmental factors that act to trigger and propagate disease within specific individuals. For example, in lupus, in some individuals, an exposure to ultraviolet light may be associated with their initial flare of clinically-apparent disease, whereas in others, it may be other factors. There are also likely factors specific to individuals (ie, "host" factors) that affect whether or not certain environmental factors impact an individual's risk for an RD. As an example, the average age of onset of incident RA is ~10 years earlier in women than men, and for RA, lupus as well as other RDs the rate in women far exceeds that in men. This suggests that even if the environmental risks are the same, there are sex-related differences in response and timing of disease development that would need to be considered in any approaches to tailor environmental interventions for prevention. Furthermore, there may be different impacts of risk factors for disease between men and women; for example, smoking seems to be a stronger risk factor for RA in men compared with women, although the reasons for this are not yet clear.[43]

As to other "host" factors that affect environmental risks, there are gene–environment interactions that influence the development of RDs.[21,44] As an example, in RA, the presence of certain human leukocyte antigen (HLA) alleles known to be associated with RA and tobacco use are much more strongly associated with the presence of RA-related autoantibodies.[41] In reactive arthritis, uveitis, and perhaps other forms of spondyloarthritis, the presence of HLA B27 alleles is thought to enhance risk for disease after exposure to certain environmental factors, such as bacteria.[45,46] Furthermore, in rheumatic fever, it is thought that a certain type of Streptococcal organisms in addition to certain host genetic factors are needed for disease to develop.[47]

Importantly, these host factors as well as gene–environment interactions may influence risk for disease, as well as the efficacy of a modification of a risk factor in prevention. There are some suggestions of this in RA where a potentially modifiable risk factor of omega 3 fatty acid levels seemed to be more strongly associated with positivity for RA-related autoantibodies in individuals without arthritis who had one or more HLA risk alleles for RA.[48] Although not specifically related to prevention of incident RD, a clinical correlate here is the association of the *HLA-B*58:01* allele with increased risk for adverse allopurinol reactions, and emerging data that using testing for this allele in determining treatment with allopurinol can help prevent the development of adverse allopurinol reactions.[49]

With these issues in mind, one can envision that in a certain individual, their RD is triggered and propagated by interactions between genetic factor "X" and environmental factor "Y," whereas another individual may have different risk factors. Importantly, if indeed there are "personal" environmental as well as genetic and gene–environmental risk factors for RDs, and these would need to be assessed and addressed with actionable prevention interventions that are appropriate for their stage of RD development (**Fig. 2**).

Such assessments would need to be through instruments that could evaluate an individual's "personal" risk factors for RDs, with these factors including genetic, environmental, and perhaps other factors such as an individual's level of a certain disease-related autoantibody or other biomarker. In addition, as discussed above, the disease stage-specific status of an individual may need to be determined so that a stage-specific intervention could be considered. Furthermore, this assessment would need to account for the type of RD considered because there is likely variable "baseline" risk, and therefore, not all individuals may need personalized assessments

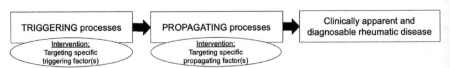

Fig. 2. Targeting stage-specific processes to prevent future rheumatic disease. In this model, there are stage-specific environmental processes that affect the development of a rheumatic disease. As such, there may be stage-specific approaches to prevention. Understanding and individual's stage and relevant environmental processes is critical to developing effective preventive interventions.

or interventions to prevent certain RDs such as lupus or vasculitis, whereas others may be at very high risk of other diseases such as gout or RA.

These types of approaches have been evaluated in preventive approaches in non-RDs (eg, type 2 diabetes) with varying success.[39,50,51] There have also been studies in RA in this area in arthritis-free first-degree relatives (FDRs) of patients with diagnosed RA where an online "personalized risk estimator for RA" was used to educate FDRs about their risk as well as identify potential modifiable risk factors.[52-54]

Related to this is the "implementation science" aspect of addressing environmental risk factor modification to prevent RDs. In brief, implementation science addresses the barriers and facilitators to the uptake of a clinical innovation.[55] For RDs, this would be uptake of personal risk assessment and then uptake of interventions to reduce risk. There is also a growing body of studies evaluating the role of individuals' preferences for preventive interventions in RDs. Most studies have been done in RA and have centered on pharmacologic interventions although some have included assessment of individuals willingness to adopt lifestyle and other changes.[56-60] Such studies are an excellent start but will need to be further studied across a range of RDs.

Clinical Trials in Personalized Prevention

Although observational studies can provide important data relating an environmental risk factor to an incident RD, well-constructed clinical trials are a key component of proving that an environmental intervention results in improved outcomes such as reduced risk for incident RDs. This is because such trials can give direct evidence of the efficacy of a specific intervention in a specific studied population. For example, one can study if a particular diet is effective rather a more general recommendation of "eating healthy" and understand the exact phenotype of the individuals who would benefit from the intervention.

As mentioned above, there are ongoing or developing clinical trials of prevention for several RDs. These trials are largely evaluating the role of specific pharmacologic agents; however, one study that is currently underway may be thought of as an "environmental" risk reduction trial because a whole food plant-based diet along with exercise and stress reduction are being applied in a population at-risk for future RA.[61]

However, for a variety of reasons, it is difficult to perform clinical trials that assess an environmental intervention (reviewed in ref[62]). This is because the magnitude of the effect of the environmental factor may be small therefore requiring an expensive study with difficult-to-attain sample sizes to demonstrate efficacy. Furthermore, there may a long duration between an intervention and a measurable outcome. For example, a long-term observational study identified that tobacco cessation was associated with a decreased risk of a future clinical diagnosis of RA after approximately 10 years of follow-up.[42] That duration would be difficult to attain due to funding and attrition in a controlled clinical interventional trial although this duration could be shortened if there are surrogate markers of "improvement" in RD risk; for example, lowering of autoantibody levels.

Another consideration is that there can be a blurring of the lines between altering an environmental factor, and a medical/pharmaceutical intervention. For example, if tobacco cessation is the "intervention," the effects of that on the outcome of an RD could be confounded if agents (eg, serotonin inhibitors) are used to enhance cessation. Furthermore, dietary alterations may be considered altering "environmental" or "lifestyle" factors but they could potentially have pharmacologic effects (eg, culinary medicine[63]) — especially if supplements are part of the dietary intervention. If the microbiome is ultimately targeted for prevention in RDs, that may further blur the lines between addressing an environmental factor and pharmacologic therapy, and indeed, we may need new definitions of what we consider "environmental" and "pharmacologic" in the future.

In clinical trials of environmental factors, there is also the possibility of "control" subjects adopting the intervention, thereby diminishing the ability of a study to determine how effective the primary intervention is. Notably, the VITAL (vitamin D and omega 3 trial) study that was originally performed to study the effects of these agents on cardiovascular disease and cancer found that the supplementation of vitamin D or omega 3 fatty acids reduced the incidence of an aggregate of autoimmune RDs including RA, polymyalgia rheumatica, and psoriasis.[64] The results from this trial may spur further beneficial approaches to RD prevention; however, the results may also lead to individuals who are at risk for RDs to take these agents in an uncontrolled fashion, which could confound future studies.

Because of the difficulties in performing clinical trials of a primary environmental intervention, it may be that there will need to be alterations of environmental factors integrated into pharmacologic trials. An example may be to recommend tobacco cessation to all subjects in an RA prevention trial, record ongoing use of tobacco after that, and integrate rates of cessation into the primary study analyses. This may still confound studies but yet be a reasonable approach that balances feasibility and ethical issues to learn more about the role of altering environmental factors in preventing RDs.

To the Future: Implementation of Targeting Environmental Factors for Rheumatic Disease Prevention

Clinical trials in RD prevention will hopefully soon provide information into specific pharmacologic agents and approaches (eg, duration of use) that can be used in actionable prevention of RDs. In addition, it is hoped that future observational studies and controlled clinical trials will provide additional information needed to identify meaningful risk factors for RDs—as well as to improve our understanding of stage-specific effects of environmental risks factors in order to develop "personalized" preventive approaches for individuals at risk for future RDs.

Importantly, completing ongoing studies as well as launching new ones will require significant effort by multiple stakeholders including researchers, funders, regulatory agencies, and perhaps most importantly populations and individuals who are at risk for RDs because these individuals will need to participate in research studies to identify effective preventions, as well as ultimately participate in the interventions once they are integrated into clinical care.

There will also need to be a consideration for how to integrate research findings into practical interventions that have been uptaken by society to lead to meaningful improvements in health outcome. For example, if it is found that a successful approach to prevention of knee OA is avoidance of contact sports in high school, will it be appropriate or even feasible to address that? It may also be that preventive interventions that reduce the risk for an RD may have other less beneficial effects and therefore should be avoided. An example of this is that modest alcohol use may decrease the risk for future RA; however, there are adverse effects from alcohol that have precluded it being recommended for the prevention of other conditions such as cardiovascular disease,[65] and indeed alcohol may worsen the risk for other RDs such as gout. These issues will need to be addressed on a case-by-case basis as potential effective preventive interventions are discovered.

Although the above issues are being addressed, individuals who are at high-risk for a future RD are presenting to clinical care on a regular basis. These may be individuals who have arthralgia and an elevated RA-related autoantibody but no detectable inflammatory arthritis. Individuals are also presenting with similar situations with lupus-related autoimmunity as well as other RDs. These individuals as well as their providers have a desire to know if there are effective preventive interventions—environmental, lifestyle, pharmacologic, or other—that can reduce their risk from developing a "full-blown" RD. These are challenging situations, and the field will need to await further studies to have evidence-based approaches. However, it may be reasonable to recommend environmental (and lifestyle) approaches that have broad general health benefits including tobacco cessation, regular exercise, healthy diet, and maintaining a healthy body weight (see "Clinics Care Points" section). An important caveat is that these recommendations have not been robustly studied in clinical trials for RD prevention, and details such as the type and duration of exercise, specific dietary changes for all RDs are not clearly known. Furthermore, such individuals should be followed closely clinically to ensure that evolving clinical disease can be identified and treated when it develops.

SUMMARY

Targeting environmental factors can be important way to reduce the incidence of RDs. Such approaches may be at population levels; furthermore, an emerging ability to identify an individual who is at very high risk for the development of a future RD can allow for personalized approaches to environmental modification for prevention. Some environmental and lifestyle interventions may reduce an individual's risk for future RDs (eg, tobacco cessation) although further studies are needed to identify actionable approaches to modification of environmental factors for prevention of RDs.

CLINICS CARE POINTS

- Environmental and lifestyle changes that may reduce the risk for the future development of an RD can include the following[a]:
  - Tobacco cessation
  - Regular aerobic exercise
  - Maintenance of a healthy body weight
  - Anti-inflammatory diet (eg, Mediterranean diet)
- Individuals at risk for future RD can be counseled to seek medical care if symptoms and signs of clinical disease develop.
- Future studies may identify specific "personalized" interventions that target environmental or lifestyle factors to reduce an individual's risk for developing a future clinically-apparent RD.

[a]A caveat is that the efficacies of these factors are largely identified in observational studies and have not been evaluated in prospective clinical trials.

DISCLOSURE

The author declares no competing interests. He is the Protocol Chair of an National Institutes of Health and National Institute of Allergy and Infectious Diseases (NIH/NIAID)-funded clinical trial for rheumatoid arthritis prevention (ClinicalTrials.gov identifier NCT02603146).

REFERENCES

1. Deane KD, Holers VM. Rheumatoid arthritis pathogenesis, prediction, and prevention: an emerging paradigm shift. Arthritis Rheum 2021;73:181–93.

2. Arbuckle MR, McClain MT, Rubertone MV, et al. Development of autoantibodies before the clinical onset of systemic lupus erythematosus. N Engl J Med 2003; 349(16):1526–33.

3. Burbelo PD, Gordon SM, Waldman M, et al. Autoantibodies are present before the clinical diagnosis of systemic sclerosis. PLoS One 2019;14(3):e0214202.

4. Berglin E, Mohammad AJ, Dahlqvist J, et al. Anti-neutrophil cytoplasmic anti-bodies predate symptom onset of ANCA-associated vasculitis. a case-control study. J Autoimmun 2021;117:102579.

5. Gerlag DM, Safy M, Maijer KI, et al. Effects of B-cell directed therapy on the pre-clinical stage of rheumatoid arthritis: the PRAIRI study. Ann Rheum Dis 2019; 78(2):179–85.

6. Bos WH, Dijkmans BA, Boers M, et al. Effect of dexamethasone on autoantibody levels and arthritis development in patients with arthralgia: a randomised trial. Ann Rheum Dis 2010;69(3):571–4.

7. van Boheemen L, Turk S, Beers-Tas MV, et al. Atorvastatin is unlikely to prevent rheumatoid arthritis in high risk individuals: results from the prematurely stopped STAtins to Prevent Rheumatoid Arthritis (STAPRA) trial. RMD Open 2021;7(1). https://doi.org/10.1136/rmdopen-2021-001591.

8. Al-Laith M, Jasenecova M, Abraham S, et al. Arthritis prevention in the pre-clinical phase of RA with abatacept (the APIPPRA study): a multi-centre, randomised, double-blind, parallel-group, placebo-controlled clinical trial protocol. Trials 2019;20(1):429.

9. Strategy for the prevention of onset of clinically-apparent rheumatoid arthritis (StopRA) ClinicalTrials.gov identifier NCT02603146. Available at: https://clinicaltrials.gov/ct2/show/NCT02603146.

10. Rech JO, Tascilar M, Hagen K, et al. Abatacept Reverses Subclinical Arthritis in Patients with High-risk to Develop Rheumatoid Arthritis -results from the Random-ized, Placebo-controlled ARIAA Study in RA-at Risk Patients [Abstract 0455]. Arthritis Rheumatol 2021;73(suppl 10).

11. Deane KD, Holers VM. Rheumatoid Arthritis Pathogenesis, Prediction, and Pre-vention: An Emerging Paradigm Shift. Arthritis Rheumatol 2021;73(2):181–93.

12. Olsen NJ, James JA, Arriens C, et al. Study of anti-malarials in incomplete lupus erythematosus (SMILE): study protocol for a randomized controlled trial. Trials 2018;19(1):694.

13. Scher JU, Ogdie A, Merola JF, et al. Preventing psoriatic arthritis: focusing on pa-tients with psoriasis at increased risk of transition. Nat Rev Rheumatol 2019;15(3): 153–66. https://doi.org/10.1038/s41584-019-0175-0.

14. Chu CR, Millis MB, Olson SA. Osteoarthritis: From Palliation to Prevention: AOA Critical Issues. J Bone Joint Surg Am 2014;96(15):e130.

15. Schmajuk G, Trupin L, Yelin EH, et al. Dusty trades and associated rheumatoid arthritis in a population-based study in the coal mining counties of Appalachia. Occup Environ Med 2022. https://doi.org/10.1136/oemed-2021-107899.

16. Fatima T, Nilsson PM, Turesson C, et al. The absolute risk of gout by clusters of gout-associated comorbidities and lifestyle factors-30 years follow-up of the Malmo Preventive Project. Arthritis Res Ther 2020;22(1):244.

17. Philippou E, Nikiphorou E. Are we really what we eat? Nutrition and its role in the onset of rheumatoid arthritis. Autoimmun Rev 2018;17(11):1074–7.

18. Lu B, Hiraki LT, Sparks JA, et al. Being overweight or obese and risk of devel-oping rheumatoid arthritis among women: a prospective cohort study. Ann Rheum Dis 2014;73(11):1914–22.

19. Sigaux J, Semerano L, Favre G, et al. Salt, inflammatory joint disease, and auto-immunity. Joint Bone Spine 2018;85(4):411–6.
20. Johansson K, Askling J, Alfredsson L, et al. Mediterranean diet and risk of rheu-matoid arthritis: a population-based case-control study. Arthritis Res Ther 2018; 20(1):175.
21. Woo JMP, Parks CG, Jacobsen S, et al. The role of environmental exposures and gene-environment interactions in the etiology of systemic lupus erythematous. J Intern Med 2022. https://doi.org/10.1111/joim.13448.
22. Rai SK, Fung TT, Lu N, et al. The Dietary Approaches to Stop Hypertension (DASH) diet, Western diet, and risk of gout in men: prospective cohort study. BMJ 2017;357:j1794.
23. Aranow C. Vitamin D and the immune system. J Investig Med 2011;59(6):881–6.
24. Sundstrom B, Johansson I, Rantapaa-Dahlqvist S. Diet and alcohol as risk factors for rheumatoid arthritis: a nested case-control study. Rheumatol Int 2015;35(3): 533–9.
25. van de Stadt LA, Witte BI, Bos WH, et al. A prediction rule for the development of arthritis in seropositive arthralgia patients. Ann Rheum Dis 2013;72(12):1920–6.
26. He Y, Sawalha AH. Drug-induced lupus erythematosus: an update on drugs and mechanisms. Curr Opin Rheumatol 2018;30(5):490–7.
27. Lenert P, Icardi M, Dahmoush L. ANA (+) ANCA (+) systemic vasculitis associ-ated with the use of minocycline: case-based review. Clin Rheumatol 2013;32(7): 1099–106.
28. Posada de la Paz M, Philen RM, Borda AI. Toxic oil syndrome: the perspective after 20 years. Epidemiol Rev 2001;23(2):231–47.
29. Shimanda PP, Shumba TW, Brunström M, et al. Preventive interventions to reduce the burden of rheumatic heart disease in populations at risk: a systematic review protocol. Syst Rev 2021;10(1):200.
30. Alpizar-Rodriguez D, Lesker TR, Gronow A, et al. Prevotella copri in individuals at risk for rheumatoid arthritis. Ann Rheum Dis 2019;78(5):590–3.
31. Scher JU, Sczesnak A, Longman RS, et al. Expansion of intestinal Prevotella copri correlates with enhanced susceptibility to arthritis. Elife 2013;2(0). https://doi.org/ 10.7554/eLife.01202.
32. Fechtner S, Berens H, Bemis E, et al. Antibody responses to epstein-barr virus in the preclinical period of rheumatoid arthritis suggest the presence of increased viral reactivation cycles. Arthritis Rheumatol 2021. https://doi.org/10.1002/art. 41994.
33. Houen G, Trier NH. Epstein-barr virus and systemic autoimmune diseases. Front Immunol 2020;11:587380.
34. Bjornevik K, Cortese M, Healy BC, et al. Longitudinal analysis reveals high prev-alence of Epstein-Barr virus associated with multiple sclerosis. Science 2022; 375(6578):296–301.
35. Holers VM, Demoruelle MK, Kuhn KA, et al. Rheumatoid arthritis and the mucosal origins hypothesis: protection turns to destruction. Nat Rev Rheumatol 2018; 14(9):542–57.
36. Konig MF. The microbiome in autoimmune rheumatic disease. Best Pract Res Clin Rheumatol 2020;34(1):101473.
37. Wong Y, Meehan MT, Burrows SR, et al. Estimating the global burden of Epstein-Barr virus-related cancers. J Cancer Res Clin Oncol 2022;148(1):31–46.
38. Wolfenden L, Goldman S, Stacey FG, et al. Strategies to improve the implemen-tation of workplace-based policies or practices targeting tobacco, alcohol, diet, physical activity and obesity. Cochrane Database Syst Rev 2018;11:CD012439.

39. Yates T, Davies M, Khunti K. Preventing type 2 diabetes: can we make the evidence work? Postgrad Med J 2009;85(1007):475–80.

40. Wouters F, Maurits MP, van Boheemen L, et al. Determining in which pre-arthritis stage HLA-shared epitope alleles and smoking exert their effect on the development of rheumatoid arthritis. Ann Rheum Dis 2021. https://doi.org/10.1136/annrheumdis-2021-220546.

41. Ishikawa Y, Terao C. The Impact of Cigarette Smoking on Risk of Rheumatoid Arthritis: A Narrative Review. Cells 2020;9(2). https://doi.org/10.3390/cells9020475.

42. Liu X, Tedeschi SK, Barbhaiya M, et al. Impact and timing of smoking cessation on reducing risk of rheumatoid arthritis among women in the nurses' health studies. Arthritis Care Res (Hoboken) 2019;71(7):914–24.

43. Deane KD, Demoruelle MK, Kelmenson LB, et al. Genetic and environmental risk factors for rheumatoid arthritis. Best Pract Res Clin Rheumatol 2017;31(1):3–18.

44. Karlson EW, Deane KD. Environmental and gene-environment interactions and risk of rheumatoid arthritis. Rheum Dis Clin North Am 2012;38:405–26. Not in File.

45. Rosenbaum JT, Asquith M. The microbiome and HLA-B27-associated acute anterior uveitis. Nat Rev Rheumatol 2018;14(12):704–13.

46. Kavadichanda CG, Geng J, Bulusu SN, et al. Spondyloarthritis and the Human Leukocyte Antigen (HLA)-B. Front Immunol 2021;12:601518.

47. Muhamed B, Parks T, Sliwa K. Genetics of rheumatic fever and rheumatic heart disease. Nat Rev Cardiol 2020;17(3):145–54.

48. Gan RW, Demoruelle MK, Deane KD, et al. Omega-3 fatty acids are associated with a lower prevalence of autoantibodies in shared epitope-positive subjects at risk for rheumatoid arthritis. Ann Rheum Dis 2017;76(1):147–52.

49. Yu KH, Yu CY, Fang YF. Diagnostic utility of HLA-B*5801 screening in severe allopurinol hypersensitivity syndrome: an updated systematic review and meta-analysis. Int J Rheum Dis 2017;20(9):1057–71.

50. Shubrook JH, Chen W, Lim A. Evidence for the Prevention of Type 2 Diabetes Mellitus. J Am Osteopath Assoc 2018;118(11):730–7.

51. Yates T, Davies M, Gorely T, et al. Effectiveness of a pragmatic education program designed to promote walking activity in individuals with impaired glucose tolerance: a randomized controlled trial. Diabetes Care 2009;32(8):1404–10.

52. Marshall AA, Zaccardelli A, Yu Z, et al. Effect of communicating personalized rheumatoid arthritis risk on concern for developing RA: A randomized controlled trial. Patient Educ Couns 2019;102(5):976–83.

53. Prado MG, Iversen MD, Yu Z, et al. Effectiveness of a web-based personalized rheumatoid arthritis risk tool with or without a health educator for knowledge of rheumatoid arthritis risk factors. Arthritis Care Res (Hoboken) 2018;70(10):1421–30.

54. Sparks JA, Iversen MD, Yu Z, et al. Disclosure of Personalized Rheumatoid Arthritis Risk Using Genetics, Biomarkers, and Lifestyle Factors to Motivate Health Behavior Improvements: A Randomized Controlled Trial. Arthritis Care Res (Hoboken) 2018;70(6):823–33.

55. Bauer MS, Kirchner J. Implementation science: What is it and why should I care? Psychiatry Res 2020;283:112376.

56. Wells I, Zemedikun DT, Simons G, et al. Predictors of interest in predictive testing for rheumatoid arthritis amongst first degree relatives of rheumatoid arthritis patients. Rheumatology (Oxford) 2021. https://doi.org/10.1093/rheumatology/keab890.

57. Falahee M, Finckh A, Raza K, et al. Preferences of Patients and At-risk Individuals for Preventive Approaches to Rheumatoid Arthritis. Clin Ther 2019;41(7): 1346–54.
58. Harrison M, Spooner L, Bansback N, et al. Preventing rheumatoid arthritis: Preferences for and predicted uptake of preventive treatments among high risk individuals. PLoS One 2019;14(4):e0216075.
59. Munro S, Spooner L, Milbers K, et al. Perspectives of patients, first-degree relatives and rheumatologists on preventive treatments for rheumatoid arthritis: a qualitative analysis. BMC Rheumatol 2018;2:18.
60. Finckh A, Escher M, Liang MH, et al. Preventive Treatments for Rheumatoid Arthritis: Issues Regarding Patient Preferences. Curr Rheumatol Rep 2016; 18(8):51.
61. Walrabenstein W, van der Leeden M, Weijs P, et al. The effect of a multidisciplinary lifestyle program for patients with rheumatoid arthritis, an increased risk for rheumatoid arthritis or with metabolic syndrome-associated osteoarthritis: the "Plants for Joints" randomized controlled trial protocol. Trials 2021;22(1):715.
62. Colditz GA, Taylor PR. Prevention trials: their place in how we understand the value of prevention strategies. Annu Rev Public Health 2010;31:105–20. https:// doi.org/10.1146/annurev.publhealth.121208.131051.
63. Asher RC, Shrewsbury VA, Bucher T, et al. Culinary medicine and culinary nutrition education for individuals with the capacity to influence health related behaviour change: A scoping review. J Hum Nutr Diet 2021. https://doi.org/10.1111/jhn.12944.
64. Hahn J, Cook NR, Alexander EK, et al. Vitamin D and marine omega 3 fatty acid supplementation and incident autoimmune disease: VITAL randomized controlled trial. BMJ 2022;376:e066452.
65. Roerecke M. Alcohol's Impact on the Cardiovascular System. Nutrients 2021; 13(10). https://doi.org/10.3390/nu13103419.

UNITED STATES POSTAL SERVICE ®

Statement of Ownership, Management, and Circulation
(All Periodicals Publications Except Requester Publications)

1. Publication Title	2. Publication Number	3. Filing Date
RHEUMATIC DISEASE CLINICS OF NORTH AMERICA	006 – 272	9/18/2022

4. Issue Frequency	5. Number of Issues Published Annually	6. Annual Subscription Price
FEB, MAY, AUG, NOV	4	$366.00

7. Complete Mailing Address of Known Office of Publication (Not printer) (Street, city, county, state, and ZIP+4®)

ELSEVIER INC.
230 Park Avenue, Suite 800
New York, NY 10169

Contact Person
Malathi Samayan

Telephone (Include area code)
91-44-4299-4507

8. Complete Mailing Address of Headquarters or General Business Office of Publisher (Not printer)

ELSEVIER INC.
230 Park Avenue, Suite 800
New York, NY 10169

9. Full Names and Complete Mailing Addresses of Publisher, Editor, and Managing Editor (Do not leave blank)

Publisher (Name and complete mailing address)

Dolores Meloni, ELSEVIER INC.
1600 JOHN F KENNEDY BLVD. SUITE 1800
PHILADELPHIA, PA 19103-2899

Editor (Name and complete mailing address)

JOANNA COLLETT, ELSEVIER INC.
1600 JOHN F KENNEDY BLVD. SUITE 1800
PHILADELPHIA, PA 19103-2899

Managing Editor (Name and complete mailing address)

PATRICK MANLEY, ELSEVIER INC.
1600 JOHN F KENNEDY BLVD. SUITE 1800
PHILADELPHIA, PA 19103-2899

10. Owner (Do not leave blank. If the publication is owned by a corporation, give the name and address of the corporation immediately followed by the names and addresses of all stockholders owning or holding 1 percent or more of the total amount of stock. If not owned by a corporation, give the names and addresses of the individual owners. If owned by a partnership or other unincorporated firm, give its name and address as well as those of each individual owner. If the publication is published by a nonprofit organization, give its name and address.)

Full Name	Complete Mailing Address
WHOLLY OWNED SUBSIDIARY OF REED/ELSEVIER, US HOLDINGS	1600 JOHN F KENNEDY BLVD. SUITE 1800 PHILADELPHIA, PA 19103-2899

11. Known Bondholders, Mortgagees, and Other Security Holders Owning or Holding 1 Percent or More of Total Amount of Bonds, Mortgages, or Other Securities. If none, check box. ► ☐ None

Full Name	Complete Mailing Address
N/A	

12. Tax Status (For completion by nonprofit organizations authorized to mail at nonprofit rates) (Check one)
The purpose, function, and nonprofit status of this organization and the exempt status for federal income tax purposes:
☒ Has Not Changed During Preceding 12 Months
☐ Has Changed During Preceding 12 Months (Publisher must submit explanation of change with this statement)

PS Form **3526**, July 2014 [Page 1 of 4 (see instructions page 4)] PSN: 7530-01-000-9931 PRIVACY NOTICE: See our privacy policy on www.usps.com.

---

13. Publication Title	14. Issue Date for Circulation Data Below
RHEUMATIC DISEASE CLINICS OF NORTH AMERICA	MAY 2022

15. Extent and Nature of Circulation			Average No. Copies Each Issue During Preceding 12 Months	No. Copies of Single Issue Published Nearest to Filing Date
a. Total Number of Copies (Net press run)			179	165
b. Paid Circulation (By Mail and Outside the Mail)	(1)	Mailed Outside-County Paid Subscriptions Stated on PS Form 3541 (Include paid distribution above nominal rate, advertiser's proof copies, and exchange copies)	85	79
	(2)	Mailed In-County Paid Subscriptions Stated on PS Form 3541 (Include paid distribution above nominal rate, advertiser's proof copies, and exchange copies)	0	0
	(3)	Paid Distribution Outside the Mails Including Sales Through Dealers and Carriers, Street Vendors, Counter Sales, and Other Paid Distribution Outside USPS®	56	51
	(4)	Paid Distribution by Other Classes of Mail Through the USPS (e.g., First-Class Mail®)	0	0
c. Total Paid Distribution (Sum of 15b (1), (2), (3), and (4))		►	141	130
d. Free or Nominal Rate Distribution (By Mail and Outside the Mail)	(1)	Free or Nominal Rate Outside-County Copies Included on PS Form 3541	24	21
	(2)	Free or Nominal Rate In-County Copies Included on PS Form 3541	0	0
	(3)	Free or Nominal Rate Copies Mailed at Other Classes Through the USPS (e.g., First-Class Mail)	0	0
	(4)	Free or Nominal Rate Distribution Outside the Mail (Carriers or other means)	0	0
e. Total Free or Nominal Rate Distribution (Sum of 15d (1), (2), (3) and (4))		►	24	21
f. Total Distribution (Sum of 15c and 15e)		►	165	151
g. Copies not Distributed (See Instructions to Publishers #4 (page #3))		►	14	14
h. Total (Sum of 15f and g)		►	179	165
i. Percent Paid (15c divided by 15f times 100)		►	85.45%	86.09%

* If you are claiming electronic copies, go to line 16 on page 3. If you are not claiming electronic copies, skip to line 17 on page 3.

16. Electronic Copy Circulation		Average No. Copies Each Issue During Preceding 12 Months	No. Copies of Single Issue Published Nearest to Filing Date
a. Paid Electronic Copies	►		
b. Total Paid Print Copies (Line 15c) + Paid Electronic Copies (Line 16a)	►		
c. Total Print Distribution (Line 15f) + Paid Electronic Copies (Line 16a)	►		
d. Percent Paid (Both Print & Electronic Copies) (16b divided by 16c × 100)	►		

☒ I certify that 50% of all my distributed copies (electronic and print) are paid above a nominal price.

17. Publication of Statement of Ownership
☒ If the publication is a general publication, publication of this statement is required. Will be printed
in the NOVEMBER 2022 issue of this publication. ☐ Publication not required.

18. Signature and Title of Editor, Publisher, Business Manager, or Owner

Malathi Samayan - Distribution Controller

Malathi Samayan Date 9/18/2022

I certify that all information furnished on this form is true and complete. I understand that anyone who furnishes false or misleading information on this form or who omits material or information requested on the form may be subject to criminal sanctions (including fines and imprisonment) and/or civil sanctions (including civil penalties).

PS Form **3526**, July 2014 (Page 3 of 4) PRIVACY NOTICE: See our privacy policy on www.usps.com